RADIOLOGY REVIEW

Radiologic Physics

Background of the Author

Dr. Edward L. Nickoloff was born in Harrisburg, Pennsylvania, and completed his public school education there. After high school, he attended Carnegie Mellon University and Lebanon Valley College, where he received his B.S. degree in physics. He received his M.S. degree in nuclear physics from the University of New Hampshire. Dr. Nickoloff obtained his doctor of science degree (D.Sc.) from the Johns Hopkins University in 1977; the title of his thesis dissertation was "The Physics of Left Ventricular Performance Measurement with Radioactive Tracers." After completion of his degree, Dr. Nickoloff was employed as an assistant professor and acting director of physics and engineering in the department of radiology at the Johns Hopkins Medical Institutions. In 1981, Dr. Nickoloff was recruited by Columbia University, where he is a professor of clinical radiology and chief hospital physicist. Dr. Nickoloff is board certified by the American College of Radiology, the American Board of Medical Physics, and the American Board of Health Physics. He was awarded the title of Fellow by the American College of Radiology, the American Association of Physicists in Medicine, and the American College of Medical Physics.

Dr. Nickoloff has taught radiologic physics to residents and graduate students for more than 25 years in Baltimore, New York, and Tampa, Florida. He has received several awards for the quality of his teaching. Dr. Nickoloff has also been an examiner for the American Board of Medical Physics and the American Board of Radiology. He has authored more than 45 peer-reviewed publications, 25 published book chapters or books, 57 published abstracts, and more than 100 presentations at professional meetings.

RADIOLOGY
REVIEW
Radiologic Physics

Edward L. Nickoloff, DSc, FACR, FACMP, FAAPM
Professor of Clinical Radiology
Chief Hospital Physicist
Department of Radiology
Columbia University College of Physicians and Surgeons
New York, New York

Consulting Editor
Naveed Ahmad, MD
Department of Radiology
Medical College of Wisconsin
Froedtert Hospital
Milwaukee, Wisconsin

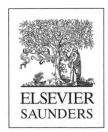

ELSEVIER
SAUNDERS

ELSEVIER
SAUNDERS

The Curtis Center
170 S Independence Mall W 300E
Philadelphia, Pennsylvania 19106

RADIOLOGY REVIEW: RADIOLOGIC PHYSICS ISBN 1-4160-2260-0
Copyright © 2005, Elsevier Inc.

Library of Congress Cataloging-in-Publication Data

Nickoloff, Edward L.
   Radiology review : radiologic physics / Edward L. Nickoloff, Naveed Ahmad.— 1st ed.
      p. cm.
   ISBN 1–4160–2260–0
   1. Medical physics—Outlines, syllabi, etc. 2. Physicians—Licenses—United
States—Examinations—Study guides. I. Ahmad, Naveed, M.D. II. Title.

R896.5.N53 2005
616.07′57′076–dc22   2004051481

Acquisitions Editor: *Allan Ross*
Developmental Editor: *Edward Pontee*
Publishing Services Manager: *Tina Rebane*
Project Manager: *Linda Van Pelt*

Printed in the United States of America.

Last digit is the print number: 9 8 7 6 5 4 3 2 1

This book would not have been possible without the many individuals who have encouraged me and contributed to my education and professional development over a period of many years. First, I want to thank my parents and grandparents, who instilled in me the value of education and high moral standards and financially supported me through my undergraduate training. They taught me to be proud of my Macedonian origins (which include Alexander the Great) and to work to make the world a better place.

I am grateful to my professors in college, such as Dr. Jacob Rhodes, who was my advisor and physics professor at Lebanon Valley College; he was dedicated to his students and was instrumental in securing the financial support that allowed me to go to graduate school. I appreciate the support and direction of my advisor and professor at the University of New Hampshire, Dr. John Lockwood. His encouragement and guidance were crucial to the completion of my masters degree in nuclear physics. I am particularly indebted to my first wife, Dr. Eileen L. Nickoloff, who both motivated me to complete my doctoral degree and financially supported me during the process. My mentor for my doctoral degree was Dr. Henry N. Wagner, Jr. Dr. Wagner inspired many careers in nuclear medicine and medical physics with his logic, humor, and innovative scientific approaches. He was instrumental in many ways to the completion of my doctoral degree. Dr. Wagner and a number of other professors at Johns Hopkins Medical Institutions taught me to be creative and at the same time meticulous, and they helped me understand some of the complexities of medical imaging and diagnoses.

I want to thank the current Chairman of Radiology at Columbia University and the Columbia University Medical Center, Dr. Philip O. Alderson, for his support of more than 20 years.

I also want to express my appreciation to many of my colleagues in medical physics who have helped me grow professionally during my career. The many radiology residents whom I taught over several decades at the Johns Hopkins Medical Institutions, the Columbia University Medical Center, Harlem Hospital, and the University of South Florida have also inadvertently made contributions to my career and to the formulation of this book. Finally, I want to express appreciation to my wife, Diane, and children, Eddie and Andrea, who allowed me to devote a significant portion of my free time during the past two years to this project.

Similar to the great pyramids in Egypt, which required the efforts of many individuals to build, most accomplishments owe their success to a host of direct and indirect contributions from many individuals. It is to this group of individuals that I dedicate this book.

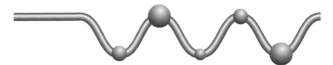

Preface

This book is intended for the review of the basic principles of the physics involved in diagnostic radiology. It was developed from many years of teaching radiology residents and graduate students about the science behind radiology imaging. This book covers many different topics, such as x-ray production, x-ray interactions with matter, x-ray equipment, image quality, quality control, safety/dosimetry, and regulatory requirements. It also covers different areas of imaging, such as radiography, fluoroscopy, computed tomography, magnetic resonance imaging, ultrasonography, and nuclear medicine. It also includes information on new technology, such as computed radiography, digital radiography, computers, PACS (picture archiving, communications, and storage), flat-panel detectors, and positron emission tomography, that is missing from some older textbooks.

In this book, key factors are listed in an outline format. Terminology and important concepts are in bold italics. Following the presentation of important facts, each chapter contains a series of multiple-choice review questions. The answers to these study questions are provided in each chapter as well, with a full explanation of both the correct and incorrect choices. Hints are provided for easy selection of the appropriate answers.

A CD is included, which contains about 1500 Microsoft PowerPoint slides that can be used to supplement the written material and to clarify concepts that are difficult to understand. The CD is organized in sections that correspond to the chapters of the book. It can be used as a teaching tool for those reviewing the physics of radiology imaging. Authorization is not provided, however, for reproduction or copying of this disk; this constitutes a violation of copyright laws. The CD can also be used with a personal computer to study the physics of radiology imaging on an individual basis.

This book is highly recommended for radiology residents and graduate students who are preparing for examinations containing questions about radiologic physics, image quality, quality control, and safety. This book could also be useful to instructors teaching these topics to professionals and various members of the medical facility staff. Because studying can be done individually by using the book and CD, this publication provides a method of covering the material without the need for a formal radiology physics course (if deemed appropriate). The book could also be used to train new users of fluoroscopy who do not have any training in radiology physics and x-ray equipment. In addition, it can be used to supplement radiation safety training and preparation for various accreditation programs and regulatory inspections.

The author hopes that his many years of teaching physics, and the simplified fashion in which major concepts and principles are explained, will be beneficial to the readers of this review book.

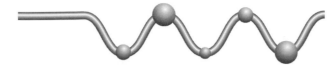

Acknowledgments

The author wishes to acknowledge the following individuals, who reviewed this book: Dr. Terry M. Button of the State University of New York, Stony Brook, Health Science Center in Long Island; Dr. Mahadevappa Mahesh of the Johns Hopkins Medical Institutions in Baltimore; Philip L. Rauch of the Henry Ford Health Systems in Detroit; and Dr. Zheng Feng Lu of the Columbia University Medical Center in New York. The suggestions and corrections from these individuals resulted in modifications that enhanced the content of the book. For any blatant errors or lack of clarity, the author assumes sole responsibility.

The author also acknowledges Dr. Naveed Ahmad for providing the motivation to begin the project and for his efforts to facilitate its publication. Dr. Ahmad persuaded me to write a review book on radiologic physics based on my teaching notes and slides; I probably would never have embarked on the project without his instigation. Dr. Ahmad and his colleagues are in the process of planning companion books reviewing clinical aspects of diagnostic radiology.

The author is also grateful for the efforts of the design, editorial, production, and advertising departments of Elsevier, which brought this book to fruition. In particular, the author wishes to acknowledge Allan Ross and Edward Pontee for their communications and coordination efforts over a period of many months.

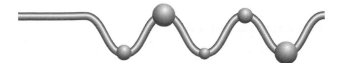

Contents

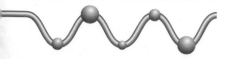

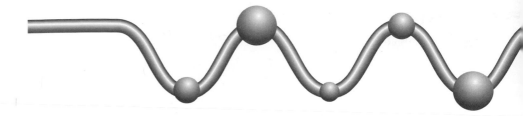

CHAPTER ONE

Properties of X-rays

A. Important Concepts

The following are the main characteristics of x-rays that are important.

1. X-rays are electromagnetic waves that travel at the speed of light in a vacuum.

2. The speed of light in a vacuum (c) is 186,400 miles per second or $3.0 \times 10^{+8}$ meters per second.

3. X-rays are packets of energy in the form of electric and magnetic fields that are rapidly changing in intensity with time. The rate of change determines their wavelength and frequency. One measure of energy is an *eV*. One eV is the kinetic energy of motion gained by an electron accelerated by one volt of electrical potential (voltage).

4. X-rays are known as **transverse waves**. The electric and magnetic fields are perpendicular (transverse) to the direction of motion.

5. By contrast, ultrasound waves have compressions and rarefactions in the same direction as the direction of travel. They are called **longitudinal waves**. Moreover, ultrasound waves are mechanical waves. They do *not* travel at the speed of light and do *not* have their energy stored as electromagnetic fields.

6. The distance between peaks in the intensity of the electromagnetic waves is called the **wavelength** (λ). The intensity varies according to a sine wave.

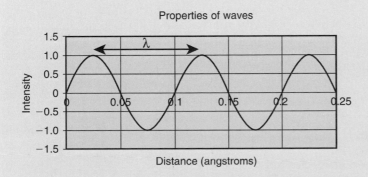

Properties of waves

7. The **frequency** (ν) is the number of wavelengths that pass a point in space in 1 second. A wavelength (or cycle) crossing a point per second is called a **hertz (Hz)**.

8. For electromagnetic waves, the product of wavelength and frequency equals the speed of light:

$$\lambda \times \nu = c$$

Hence, if one knows either the wavelength or the frequency, the other descriptor of the x-ray wave can be determined:

$$\lambda = c/\nu \quad \text{and} \quad \nu = c/\lambda.$$

9. Frequency and wavelength are inversely related. Short-wavelength x-rays have high frequencies. X-rays with long wavelengths have lower frequencies.

10. X-rays used in clinical radiology typically have wavelengths between 0.08 and 1.24 angstroms, where **1 angstrom = 0.00000001 cm or 1×10^{-8} cm** in length.

11. X-rays used in clinical radiology have frequencies between $2.4 \times 10^{+18}$ and $3.7 \times 10^{+19}$ Hz.

12. A single x-ray is the smallest packet of electromagnetic energy; this is called a **photon** or **quantum**.

13. **Planck's law** states that the energy (E) of an x-ray is directly proportional to its frequency (ν):

$$E = h \times \nu$$

where h = Planck's constant. That is, high-frequency x-rays have more energy than lower frequency x-rays.

14. Because frequency and wavelength are inversely related, x-rays with the shortest wavelengths (highest frequency) have the highest energy.

15. The energy of x-rays can be easily calculated if either the wavelength or frequency is known:

$$E \text{ (in keV)} = 12.4/\lambda \text{ (in angstroms)} \quad \text{or} \quad E \text{ (in keV)} = (4.13 \times 10^{-18}) \times \nu \text{ (in Hz)}$$

16. X-rays used in clinical radiology typically have energies between 10 and 150 keV.

17. *One keV is the energy gained by accelerating a single electron by a electrical potential difference of 1000 volts.*

18. **The most penetrating x-rays have high energy, short wavelengths, and high frequency**.

19. If x-rays penetrate better, fewer x-rays incident upon the patient are required in order to have a sufficient number passing through the patient into the image receptor to create a usable radiograph. This feature means that **more penetrating x-rays result in lower radiation doses to the patient** because fewer incident x-rays are absorbed and, thus, fewer x-rays can be used.

20. There are a number of different types of electromagnetic waves differentiated by their wavelengths.

21. Electromagnetic waves listed from the shortest wavelengths to the longest wavelengths are gamma rays, x-rays, ultraviolet (UV) waves, visible light, infrared (IR) waves, microwaves, and radio waves. If the list were ordered according to increasing frequency, the items would appear in reverse.

B. Questions

1-1. All of the following are electromagnetic waves, *except* _____.

    (a) Heat   (b) Radiation used in magnetic resonance imaging (MRI)
    (c) Sunlight   (d) Sound   (e) FM radio signals

1-2. If the wavelength of an x-ray is reduced to half, its energy is _____.

    (a) Increased by 4   (b) Increased by 2   (c) Unchanged
    (d) Decreased to 0.5   (e) Decreased by 0.25

1-3. If the wavelength of an x-ray is reduced to half, its speed is _____.

(a) Increased by 4   (b) Increased by 2   (c) Unchanged
(d) Decreased to 0.5   (e) Decreased by 0.25

1-4. If the wavelength of an x-ray is reduced by half, its frequency is _____.

(a) Increased by 4   (b) Increased by 2   (c) Unchanged
(d) Decreased to 0.5   (e) Decreased by 0.25

1-5. The x-rays that penetrate best through patient tissue have the smallest

_____.

(a) Frequency   (b) Energy   (c) Speed   (d) Wavelength   (e) Quanta

1-6. The wavelength of a 60-keV x-ray is about _____.

(a) 4.5 microns   (b) 0.2 angstroms   (c) 0.001 mm
(d) 1.25×10^{-8} cm   (e) 6.3 MB

1-7. As the energy of the x-rays is increased, the x-rays have _____.

(a) Faster speed   (b) Lower frequency   (c) Shorter wavelength
(d) Longer wavelength   (e) The same speed, wavelength, and frequency

1-8. For equal image quality, radiographs have lower radiation doses if the x-rays have _____.

(a) Higher frequency   (b) Longer wavelengths   (c) Faster speeds
(d) More quanta   (e) Longer period

1-9. All of the following are transverse waves, *except* _____.

(a) Gamma rays   (b) Ultraviolet waves   (c) Microwaves   (d) X-rays
(e) Diathermy waves

1-10. To make certain that the x-rays have dissipated after clinical radiography, one should wait at least _____ before entering the room.

(a) 50 nanoseconds   (b) 50 microseconds   (c) 50 femtoseconds
(d) 50 milliseconds   (e) 50 deciseconds

C.   **Answers to Sample Questions**

1-1. Answer = (d). As listed in the Important Concepts section, gamma rays, x-rays, ultraviolet waves, infrared waves, light (of all types), microwaves, and radio waves are all electromagnetic waves. All forms of heat are IR radiation.

MRI uses radio waves at frequencies 43 to 87 MHz (dependent upon the strength of the magnet) to excite and receive the signals of the hydrogen atoms. Sunlight is a form of visible light composed of various colors (from the longest wavelength to the shortest wavelength, the colors of visible light are red, orange, yellow, green, blue, and violet). FM radio is a form of radio electromagnetic waves with frequencies of 60 to 110 MHz. These MRI and FM radio waves have wavelengths about 3 to 7 meters (each meter is about 3 feet) in length. The MRI and FM radio wavelengths can be compared with x-rays, which are around 1×10^{-10} meter (1 angstrom) in length. X-ray wavelengths are extremely short. Sound is a longitudinal pressure wave that travels at about 330 meters per second; it is not an electromagnetic wave.

1-2. Answer = (b). The relationship between energy and wavelength is E (in keV) = $12.4/\lambda$ (in angstroms). Hence, if the wavelength becomes smaller and the wavelength is in the denominator, the energy increases. Energy is inversely related to wavelength. If the wavelength is decreased by half, $(E_2/E_1) = (\lambda_1/\lambda_2) = (\lambda/0.5\,\lambda) = 2.0$. Decreasing the wavelength by half makes the energy two times greater.

1-3. Answer = (c). All electromagnetic waves travel at the speed of light in a vacuum, regardless of their wavelength or corresponding frequency. That is, the speed does not change for electromagnetic waves; only the wavelength and frequency change.

1-4. Answer = (b). Wavelength and frequency are inversely proportional. If the wavelength becomes smaller, the frequency will increase. Conversely, if the wavelength becomes larger, the frequency will decrease. Frequency is given by the equation $\nu = c/\lambda$. Hence the following ratio is true: $(\nu_2/\nu_1) = (\lambda_1/\lambda_2) = \lambda/0.5\lambda = 2.0$. For a wavelength that is half of a specified value, the frequency is twice as large and the energy is double.

1-5. Answer = (d). The most penetrating x-rays have small wavelength. Short wavelengths correspond to high frequency and thus high energy. The speed of all electromagnetic waves is the same; it is the speed of light. Quanta refer to the number of x-rays. Increasing or decreasing the number of x-rays does not change the fraction that penetrates through tissue.

1-6. Answer = (b). Even before attempting to do the problem precisely, one should recall that the notes indicated that diagnostic x-rays with energies between 10 and 150 keV have wavelengths between 0.08 and 1.2 angstroms. Hence, one can guess the correct answer without doing any math. The equation given in the notes can be rearranged as follows: λ (in angstroms) = $12.4/E$ (in keV) = $12.4/60$ keV = 0.2.

Another learning point from this problem is that the answer could be in different units. 1 angstrom = 10^{-8} cm. 1 micron = $1\ \mu = 10^{-6}$ meter = 10^{-4} cm. 1 millimeter = 1 mm = 10^{-3} meter = 10^{-1} cm. MB refers to computer memory, not distance measurement. 1 MB = 1 megabyte = 1,000,000 bytes.

1-7. Answer = (c). The energy of x-rays is directly related to the frequency and inversely related to the wavelength. In other words, high-energy x-rays have higher frequencies and shorter wavelengths.

1-8. Answer = (a). To get the same image quality, one must have the same number of x-rays absorbed in the imaging device, whether it be film or a detector such as computed radiography (CR) or digital radiography (DR). If the x-rays penetrate through tissue better, a larger percentage of the x-rays that are incident upon a patient pass through the patient and reach the image receptor. Hence, with more penetrating x-rays, fewer incident x-rays can be used to obtain the same number reaching the image receptor. Reducing the number of x-rays that impinge upon the patient reduces the patient's radiation dose. In summary, fewer high-energy x-rays can be used to produce a given quality image than lower energy x-rays. This reduces the patient's radiation dose. As stated several times previously, high-energy x-rays mean both short wavelengths and correspondingly high frequencies.

1-9. Answer = (e). Transverse waves have their forces perpendicular to the direction of travel. All electromagnetic waves are transverse waves. Gamma rays, x-rays, ultraviolet light, visible light, infrared waves, and radio waves are electromagnetic waves that are transverse. Diathermy treatments use high-power ultrasound waves, which are longitudinal waves. For longitudinal waves, the force (mechanical pressure) is in the same direction as the motion of the waves.

1-10. Answer = (a). There are three teaching points to this question. X-rays either can be absorbed by the lead in the walls or the rooms or can scatter several times before they are absorbed. Even if the walls are 4 meters apart and the x-rays scatter four times at most, the total distance traveled by the x-rays would be 16 meters. The speed of the x-rays is $3 \times 10^{+8}$ meters/second. The time to travel four times across the room before the x-rays are absorbed is equal to the distance divided by the speed: 16 meters/$3 \times 10^{+8}$ meters/second = 5×10^{-8} seconds. This time is nearly instantaneous. *First point*, there is no need to wait to enter an x-ray room after an exposure; the radiation dissipates nearly instantaneously. *Second point*, because x-rays travel at the speed of light, they

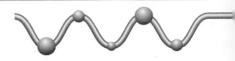

cover large distances quickly. *Third point*, one needs to know the various prefixes to units. Some of these prefixes are as follows:

femto- = 10^{-12}	tera- = 10^{+12}
nano- = 10^{-9}	giga- = 10^{+9}
micro- = 10^{-6}	mega- = 10^{+6}
milli- = 10^{-3}	kilo- = 10^{+3}
centi- = 10^{-2}	hecto- = 10^{+2}
deci- = 10^{-1}	deka- = 10^{+1}

The symbol for each of these prefixes is the first letter of the prefix. For prefixes less than one, use lowercase letters, and for prefixes greater than one, use uppercase (capital) letters. To avoid confusion for the two prefixes that use the same lowercase letter, "milli-" uses a lowercase "m" and "micro-" uses the Greek symbol "μ."

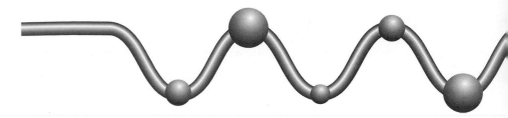

CHAPTER TWO

The X-ray Tube

A. Important Concepts

The accompanying drawing shows the important parts of an x-ray tube and the associated collimator assembly.

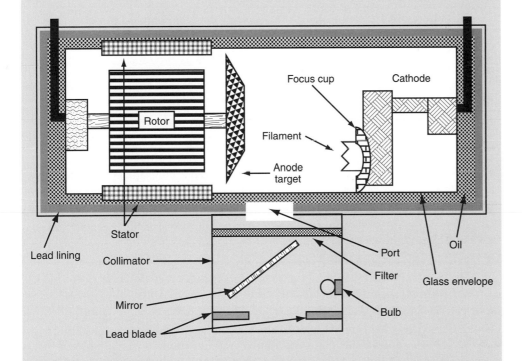

1. The x-ray tube has two basic parts. The **cathode** is the negatively charged portion of the x-ray tube. The cathode contains the filament wire (which generates the electrons used to produce x-rays), the focusing cup, and the structural support assembly. The positively charged portion of the x-ray tube is called the **anode**. The anode contains the target into which the bombarding electrons collide, the rotor stem, the bearing assembly (which is a ball bearing that facilitates rotation), the rotor (which is a portion of the motor that rotates the target), and the stator (stationary electrical coils that provide varying magnetic fields for rotation).

2. The job of the x-ray tube is to produce x-rays.

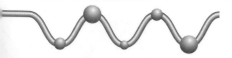

3. The mechanism of x-ray production has several steps.

   - First, as electricity is sent through the filament wire, it becomes hot.

   - Like a teakettle, as the wire gets hot, it "boils off" electrons from the surface of the filament wire. This is called ***thermionic emissions***.

   - As the electrical current through the filament wire increases, the number of electrons boiled off the surface of the filament increases.

   - The thermionically ejected electrons are then bombarded into the target of the x-ray tube.

   - High electrical voltages are used to accelerate these electrons.

   - The cathode is placed at a negative voltage, which repels the electrons, and the anode is placed at a high positive voltage, which attracts the electrons.

   - As larger electrical voltages are applied to the x-ray tube, the speed of the electrons increases, resulting in greater kinetic energy of motion. (These electrons approach speeds around one third the speed of light and become relativistic, gaining mass.)

   - The electrons then collide into a small area on the target of the x-rays tube called the ***focal spot***.

   - Approximately 99% of the energy of the electrons that bombard the target of the x-ray tube is converted into heat.

   - Only about 1% of the energy of the electrons that bombard the target of the x-ray tube is converted into x-rays, by processes described in the next chapter.

4. As the temperature of the filament wire is raised, more electrons are boiled off and a larger number of electrons hit the target of the x-ray tube. This flow of electrons is called the ***tube current*** and is measured in milliamperes ***(mA)***.

5. $1 \text{ mA} = 6.2 \times 10^{+15}$ electrons per second flowing from the cathode to the anode. (This is a very large number of electrons hitting the target of the x-ray tube.)

6. Typical clinically used x-ray tube currents in radiology range from 1 to 50 mA in fluoroscopy, 50 to 400 mA in computed tomography (CT), and 400 to 1000 mA in cardiac catheterization or angiography imaging.

7. The product of the tube current and the duration of current flow in seconds determines the total number of electrons that hit the target of the x-ray tube. The number is measured in units of ***mAs***.

8. The number of x-rays produced is directly proportional to the number of electrons hitting the target of the x-ray tube (the mAs). ***If the mAs is doubled, the number of x-rays produced is doubled***.

9. The energy of the x-rays is controlled by the amount of voltage applied between the anode and cathode of the x-ray tube. This voltage is measured in units of kilovolt peak potential (kVp). One kVp is equal to 1000 volts of electrical potential. For comparison, a D-cell flashlight battery has an electrical potential of 1.5 volts.

10. As the kVp is increased, the energy of the x-rays produced increases. The highest energy x-rays can have an energy only equal to the kinetic energy of the bombarding electrons. This energy is gained from the acceleration provided by the applied voltage between the anode and the cathode.

11. The kinetic energy gained by the bombarding electrons is measured in units of keV. One keV is the energy gained by one electron accelerated by an electrical potential of 1 kVp (1000 volts). X-ray photon energies are also measured in units of keV.

12. In review, an electron accelerated in an x-ray tube by a voltage of 100 kVp gains a kinetic energy of motion of 100 keV, and the highest energy x-ray that

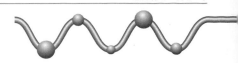

can be produced by this electron when it hits the target of the x-ray tube is 100 keV. (However, it could produce x-rays with less than all its kinetic energy; this phenomenon is discussed in the next chapter.)

13. Once again, mA controls only the number of x-rays produced. kVp affects the energy of the x-rays; therefore, it influences how well the x-rays penetrate through tissue.

14. In addition, kVp has an effect on the number of x-rays produced. In fact, the x-ray intensity increases as the kVp squared (kVp^2). If the applied voltage is increased from 60 to 120 kVp, the measured x-ray exposure increases by approximately four times. However, the measured x-ray exposure would only double for a change from 100 to 200 mA.

15. Typical clinical x-ray tube voltages range from 25 to 30 kVp for mammography, 60 kVp for bone radiographs, 70 to 80 kVp for angiography and cardiac catheterization, and 110 to 130 kVp for chest radiographs to 120 to 140 kVp for CT scans.

16. One of the factors that controls **image quality** is the **size of the focal spot**, the region of the anode from which the x-rays are produced.

    - Small focal spots produce less image blur, which improves the ability to visualize small objects **(spatial resolution)**.

    - Thick and dense body tissue requires the use of a large number of x-rays, which means that large mA values are needed.

    - To produce large mA values, the filament wire must be long, which results in a wide electron beam and large focal spot sizes.

    - Hence, large mA values can *not* be used for small focal spot sizes.

    - Small focal spot sizes can be obtained only with smaller mA values, and they produce smaller numbers of x-rays.

    - Some x-ray tubes have several filaments of different lengths. Each filament length produces a different focal spot size and has a different range of mA values that it can use.

    - Most x-ray tubes have at least two or three filaments, resulting in two or three different focal spot sizes. Each focal spot is capable of producing a different number of x-rays. Larger focal spot sizes are used to produce a greater number of x-rays and result in more image blur.

17. The **line focus principle** is used to minimize the effective size of the focal spots. The line focus principle uses a beveled anode. The bombarding electrons from the cathode distribute their impact and heat over the hypotenuse of the triangle shown in the figure (see next page). Meanwhile, from the perspective of the image receptor, the region from which the x-rays seem to emerge (the base of the triangle) appears to be smaller. That is, a beveled anode distributes heat better while making the **effective focal spot size** appear smaller.

18. The **anode angle** is the angle between the surface of the anode target and a perpendicular line drawn from the anode to the image receptor. Small anode angles have very little bevel. A large anode angle means that the target of the anode has significant bevel.

    - The anode angle on most diagnostic x-ray tubes is 12.5 degrees.

    - For the same effective focal spot size, small anode angles dissipate heat better.

    - For the same effective focal spot size, small anode angles have more heel effect. (See explanation later.)

    - For the same actual focal spot size, the effective focal spot size depends on the location at the image receptor surface. The effective focal spot size appears larger and has more image blur on the cathode side, and it appears

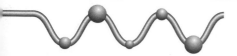

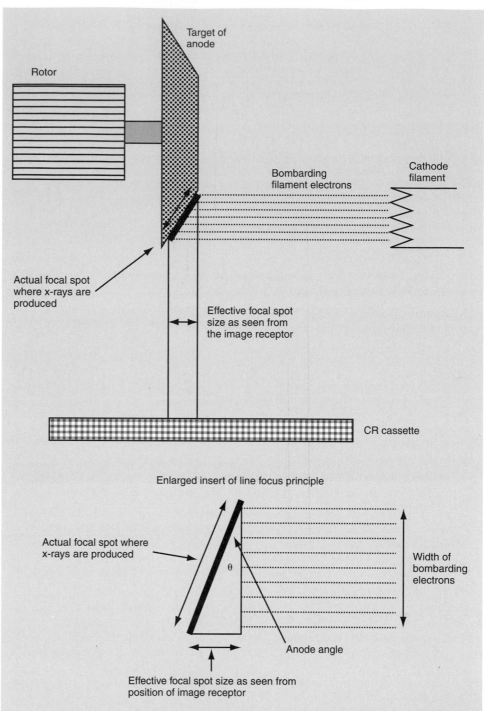

Enlarged insert of line focus principle

to be smaller and has less blur on the anode side of the image receptor—because of the line focus principle.

19. ***Heel effect*** is the reduction of the amount of x-ray radiation on the anode side in comparison with the cathode side.

- Heel effect is due to attenuation of the x-rays as they emerge through the target of the x-ray tube.

- The path lengths through the anode are greater if the x-rays emerge toward the anode in comparison with the cathode direction.

- There is complete "cutoff" of the x-rays at an angle of 1 degree less than the anode angle in the anode direction.

- There is no cutoff in the cathode direction.

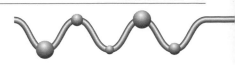

- Cutoff means that no image can be seen beyond a certain distance on the image receptor in the anode direction.

- Cutoff is more severe for small anode angles and short distances between the x-ray tube and the image receptor (*source-to-image receptor distance = SID*).

- For a 12.5-degree anode angle, there is no heel effect cutoff at 40 inches to the image receptor (SID) with a 14 inch × 17 inch (35 cm × 43 cm) cassette. However, the darkness (density) of the image decreases as one moves from the cathode side toward the anode side.

20. The *focusing cup* is used to keep the electron beam from spreading and increasing the focal spot size.

21. A high kVp produces a smaller effective focal spot size than a lower kVp. The explanation is that electrons repel each other and tend to spread the impact region on the target of the anode. With a high kVp, the electrons travel faster and have less time to spread out.

22. A high mA produces larger effective focal spot sizes. The explanation is that there are more electrons at a high mA and more electrostatic repulsion, which spreads the beam and impact area.

23. *Off-focus radiation* means that the electrons sometimes strike the anode and bounce and hit the anode again outside the normal focal spot. Hence, it is a region of low x-ray production outside the normal focal spot. This creates a low-intensity shadow image outside the collimated region.

24. The *rotor* causes the target area of the x-ray tube to spin and to distribute the heat created by the electron impact over the entire circular area of the target.

25. The *stator* consists of the electrical windings wrapped around the outside of the x-ray tube, which create time-varying electromagnetic fields that force the rotor to spin.

26. The x-ray tube is surrounded with a glass envelope that is evacuated. The vacuum removes the air, which would collide with electrons traveling from the anode to the cathode.

27. The glass envelope is surrounded by oil. The oil acts as an electrical insulator, a mechanical "shock absorber" to prevent damage to the glass, and a transfer mechanism for heat.

28. The entire structure resides inside a steel case.

29. Lead lines the inside of the steel case, except at the port of the x-ray tube. X-rays traveling in any direction (except where the port and collimator assembly are located) are severely attenuated by the lead lining.

30. *Leakage radiation* is the small amount of radiation that passes through the lead lining of the x-ray tube.

- These x-rays are a radiation hazard.

- Leakage radiation is *limited to less than 100 milliroentgens per hour* (100 mR/hr) at maximum kVp and maximum continuous mA at a distance of 1 meter from the tube.

- Leakage radiation must be considered when shielding an x-ray room, but leakage radiation does not produce any useful image quality.

- Leakage radiation (just like scattered x-rays) travels in all directions.

- *Secondary radiation* is the scattered radiation plus the leakage radiation.

31. The purpose of the *collimator assembly* is to restrict the x-ray beam to a limited size.

- The collimator assembly contains a light and mirror to show the location of the main x-ray beam that travels through the port of the x-ray tube.

- *Primary radiation* refers to the main x-ray beam that has been neither attenuated nor deflected in any way.

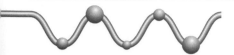

- The agreement between the light location and the real x-ray beam must be within 2% of the SID distance in each orthogonal direction.

- Some units have automated collimators that sense the cassette size and restrict the x-ray field size to the cassette size. This automated collimation system is called **positive beam limitation (PBL)**. The alignment between the light location and the x-ray edge on PBL systems must be less than 3% of the SID in any one orthogonal direction, and a sum of errors for two orthogonal directions must be less than 4%.

- The purpose of the collimator is to prevent tissue that is not being imaged from being exposed to radiation. Moreover, wide x-ray fields of view (FoV) have more scattered radiation, which degrades image contrast.

- The collimator assembly may also contain extra x-ray beam filtration.

B. Questions

2-1. The x-rays that penetrate through the housing of the x-ray tube are called _____ radiation.

(a) Off focus   (b) Primary   (c) Heel effect   (d) Leakage   (e) Secondary

2-2. Having fewer x-rays on the anode side of the image receptor in comparison with the cathode side is called _____.

(a) Off focus   (b) Heel effect   (c) Line focus principle
(d) Effective focal spot   (e) Positive beam limitation

2-3. _____ produces images of reduced intensity outside the edges of the collimated field of view.

(a) Off focus   (b) Heel effect   (c) Line focus principle
(d) Effective focal spot   (e) Positive beam limitation

2-4. That the effective focal spot size is smaller than the area where the x-rays are actually produced because of the beveled angle of the x-ray tube target is called _____.

(a) Off focus   (b) Heel effect   (c) Line focus principle   (d) Collimation
(e) Positive beam limitation

2-5. _____ is attributed to attenuation within the target of the x-ray tube.

(a) Off focus   (b) Heel effect   (c) Line focus principle
(d) Effective focal spot   (e) Positive beam limitation

2-6. Federal regulations limit leakage radiation at a distance of 1 meter to an amount less than _____ mR/hr at highest kVp and maximum continuous mA.

(a) 1   (b) 2   (c) 10   (d) 25   (e) 100

2-7. If the mA used during measurement of the effective focal spot of an x-ray tube is increased, the measured dimension of the focal spot size _____.

(a) Is increased   (b) Remains the same   (c) Decreases   (d) Oscillates
(e) Cannot be determined

2-8. If the kVp used during measurement of the effective focal spot of an x-ray tube is increased, the measured dimension of the focal spot size _____.

(a) Is increased   (b) Remains the same   (c) Decreases   (d) Oscillates
(e) Cannot be determined

2-9. For the same effective focal spot size, the _____ as the anode angle is decreased from 12 to 8 degrees.

(a) Filament size decreases   (b) Heat distribution improves
(c) Focal blur increases   (d) Heel effect is less
(e) Secondary radiation decreases

2-10. X-ray radiation levels at the image receptor increase with an increase in all of the following parameters, *except* _____.

(a) SID   (b) KVp   (c) mA   (d) Exposure duration (seconds)
(e) Anode angle

2-11. The cutoff on the anode side of the image receptor is more severe when _____.

(a) Anode angle increases   (b) Image receptor is smaller in dimension
(c) SID is smaller   (d) Effective focal spot is smaller
(e) Added filtration is decreased

2-12. One of the two key purposes of x-ray beam collimation is to _____.

(a) Limit heel effect   (b) Reduce the scattered radiation
(c) Control off-focus radiation   (d) Reduce anode heating
(e) Reduce leakage radiation

2-13. _____ percent of the bombarding electrons' energy is converted in x-ray production.

(a) 1   (b) 10   (c) 25   (d) 50   (e) 99

2-14. The part of the x-ray tube responsible for the heat distribution in the anode is the _____.

(a) Focusing cup   (b) Filter   (c) Cathode
(d) Filament   (e) Rotor

2-15. Secondary radiation consists of scattered x-rays plus _____.

(a) Off-focus radiation   (b) Thermionic emissions   (c) Primary radiation
(d) Leakage radiation   (e) Cutoff radiation

2-16. The main x-ray tube factor that affects the spatial resolution in the image is the _____.

(a) Anode angle   (b) KVp   (c) Filament size
(d) Effective focal spot size   (e) Stator

2-17. The spatial resolution in the image is always better _____.

(a) On the anode side   (b) For greater geometric magnification
(c) With small anode angles   (d) With the larger focal spot size
(e) With more collimation

2-18. The factor that results in the largest increase in the x-ray output is to ____.

(a) Triple the exposure time   (b) Double the kVp
(c) Double the mAs   (d) Half the anode angle
(e) One third the SID

2-19. For a constant filament size, all of the following cause more image blur, *except* _____.

(a) Smaller anode angle   (b) Lower kVp   (c) Higher mA
(d) Greater geometric magnification
(e) Longer exposure times

2-20. To prevent anode cutoff at 100 cm with the largest cassette (35 cm × 43 cm), the anode angle must be no less than _____ degrees.

(a) 7   (b) 10   (c) 13   (d) 15   (e) 20

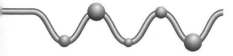

C. Answers

2-1. Answer = (d). When x-rays are produced inside the x-ray tube, they travel in all directions. By definition, leakage radiation is the amount of x-rays that penetrate through the lead internal lining of the x-ray tube. The primary x-rays are those that travel through the port of the x-ray tube with no lead, are collimated to a useful beam, and penetrate through the patient into the image receptor. Primary x-rays are the useful portion of the x-ray beam. X-rays that travel through the port of the x-ray tube and interact in the patient, causing them to be deflected, are called scattered x-rays. Leakage plus scattered x-rays is called secondary radiation. Secondary radiation degrades the image because it contains no useful information; secondary radiation is also a safety concern because the x-rays travel in areas outside the useful collimated x-ray beam. Off-focus radiation consists of the x-rays produced outside the true focal spots by electrons bouncing off the anode and hitting the target in some remote location. Heel effect is the reduction in the number of x-rays on the anode side of the image receptor related to self-attenuation in the target.

2-2. Answer = (b). Heel effect and some of the other terms were explained in answer 2-1. The line focus principle explains how the bevel angle (anode angle) of the anode target makes the actual focal spot size look small from the location of the image receptor. Positive beam limitation refers to the automatic collimation system that senses the size of the image receptor cassette and adjusts the collimator to restrict the x-ray beam to be no larger than the cassette.

2-3. Answer = (a). X-rays produced outside the actual focal spot (off-focus radiation) are not properly collimated and produce radiation outside the collimated x-ray beam. They are smaller in number than the useful primary x-ray beam. Thus, they image anatomy outside the collimated area, but the images appear with reduced density. Effective focal spot refers to the size the focal spot appears to be at the location of the image receptor. This size is smaller than the actual focal spot size because of the line focus principle—the beveled anode target area.

2-4. Answer = (c). The line focus principle is similar to the situation in which an individual turns sideways. In the anteroposterior projection, the person looks larger than in the lateral projection. Similarly, the angle on the target of the x-ray tube reduces the effective size as seen from the image receptor. As the anode angle becomes smaller, the effective focal spot becomes smaller. Collimation has no impact on the effective focal spot size.

2-5. Answer = (b). X-rays are produced below the surface of the x-ray tube target. The path length traveled by the x-rays as they emerge from the anode determines the degree of reduction of the x-ray beam. To travel to the anode side of the image receptor, the path lengths through the anode are longer, and the number of emerging x-rays is reduced more by interactions with the atoms in the anode.

2-6. Answer = (e). The regulatory value for leakage radiation is a number that must be memorized.

2-7. Answer = (a). As the mA is increased, there are more electrons bombarding the anode target. Because like charges repel each other, more electrons result in the bombarding electrons spreading out as they travel from the cathode to the anode. Because the bombarding electrons are spread, the area on the target where they strike is larger with more electrons. This larger impact area means a larger actual focal spot size. Thus, as mA increases, the focal spot increases slightly in size and the resulting image blurs slightly more, which decreases the spatial resolution.

2-8. Answer = (c). As the kVp is increased, the bombarding electrons achieve greater speed and travel from the cathode to the anode in less time. Thus, there is less time for the bombarding electrons to spread. Hence, higher kVp means the actual focal spot size decreases slightly, and the image blur is slightly less. None of these effects is very large; the changes are on the order of 10% to 20%.

2-9. Answer = (b). For the same effective focal spot size, a smaller anode angle requires a larger filament. The smaller anode angle increases the actual focal spot size (area where bombarding electrons strike) without changing the effective focal spot size—provided the filament is redesigned by increasing its length. If the effective focal spot size does not change, the image blur neither decreases nor increases. Image quality depends on the effective focal spot size as seen at the image receptor; it does not depend on the size of the impact area of the bombarding electrons (actual focal spot size). Heel effect becomes more pronounced as the anode angle is decreased. The cutoff on the anode side extends only to 1 degree less than the anode angle. Thus, as the angle decreases, the coverage area where the image is recorded also decreases. The anode angle has no effect at all on the secondary radiation. Secondary radiation increases as the kVp increases and as the collimated FoV increases.

2-10. Answer = (a). The x-ray production increases as the kVp is squared. The x-ray production is directly related to the mA and time duration. The radiation produced increases with the product of these two terms (mAs). If the mAs is doubled, the x-ray radiation level doubles. The x-ray production increases only very slightly with anode angle because of slightly less attenuation of the x-rays with the anode target material. However, the x-ray radiation levels at the image receptor decrease significantly as the distance between the focal spot and the image receptor (SID) becomes larger. In fact, the radiation levels decrease as $(1/SID)^2$, the "inverse square law."

2-11. Answer = (c). The *heel effect* becomes less as the anode angle is increased. The cutoff distance is determined by drawing a line at an angle 1 degree less than the anode angle (on the anode side of the central ray) from the focal spot to the image receptor. If the cassette size is larger, there is a greater region of cutoff. The cassette is centered under the focal spot, and larger cassettes extend farther in the anode direction beyond the cutoff line. Smaller cassettes have the opposite effect. The focal spot size affects image blur and spatial resolution, but it has no impact on the heel effect cutoff. Similarly, the filtration affects the number of x-rays emerging from the collimator and how well the x-rays penetrate through tissue. However, filtration has no impact on the heel effect cutoff. As the image receptor moves closer to the anode, the same angle cuts off more of the cassette surface. For example, consider your side vision—close and far away. Although the angle is the same, far away from your face you can see greater distances to each side of the center.

2-12. Answer = (b). The collimation has no effect whatsoever on heel effect, off-focus radiation, anode heating, or leakage radiation. The two goals of collimation are to prevent radiation exposure of tissue outside the region of interest and to reduce the scattered radiation. A smaller FoV is associated with less scattered radiation than are larger areas.

2-13. Answer = (a). Approximately 99% of the energy of the bombarding electrons is converted to heat, and only 1% results in x-ray production.

2-14. Answer = (e). The rotor and the stator cause the target to rotate. Thus, the bombarding electrons strike a different section of anode, distributing the heat. The job of the focusing cup is to push the bombarding electrons together as they travel from the cathode to the anode. The purpose of the filter is to remove preferentially low-energy x-rays, which are highly attenuated in the patient's tissue. Most of these low-energy x-rays contribute to radiation dose but never reach the image receptor. The filament is the part of the cathode that produces the electrons, and the cathode is negative to repel the electrons. Neither the filament nor the cathode has anything to do with heat distribution.

2-15. Answer = (d). Leakage radiation is the radiation that penetrates through the lead lining inside the x-ray tube housing. Because it is not part of the primary x-ray beam used to do the imaging, it is called secondary radiation. Off-focus radiation refers to the small amount of x-rays produced outside the main region of the actual focal spot. Thermionic emissions are the electrons that are boiled off the filament. Cutoff radiation is not related to either primary or secondary radiation. There is a cutoff angle beyond which there are no x-rays.

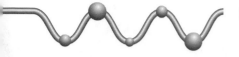

2-16. Answer = (d). The effective focal spot size and the geometric magnification influence the focal spot blur, which contributes to a degradation of spatial resolution.

kVp has only a minor influence on the focal spot size; the reduction at high kVp is typically less than 10%. The anode angle has no effect on the effective focal spot size. X-ray tubes can be manufactured with a variety of anode angles and still have the same effective focal spot size. For a given anode angle, the filament is adjusted in size to produce a specified effective focal spot size. X-ray tubes are designed for a given heat distribution by selecting the anode angle and for a specified effective focal spot size. Once these items are selected, the x-ray tube is designed. The filament size is then manufactured to provide the appropriate effective focal spot size. The rotor function is related to heat distribution.

2-17. Answer = (a). Because of the line focus principle, the effective focal spot is smaller on the anode side of the image receptor and larger on the cathode side. The spatial resolution depends directly on the effective focal spot size. Hence, the spatial resolution is better on the anode side of the image receptor.

2-18. Answer = (e). Triple the exposure time results in triple the radiation. Doubling the kVp results in four times the radiation because the radiation output increases with the square of the kVp. Doubling the mAs results in double the radiation.

The anode angle has only very minor effects on the radiation levels. Because the radiation changes as one divided by the square of the SID, using ⅓ for the SID (being closer to the x-ray tube) increases the radiation by a factor of 9.

2-19. Answer = (a). Anything that increases either the effective focal spot size or the geometric magnification increases image blur and degrades spatial resolution. Although x-ray tubes are not designed for a fixed filament size, changing to a smaller angle actually reduces the effective focal spot size and reduces blur. Lower kVp and higher mA slightly increases the effective focal spot size. Longer exposure times have no influence on the effective focal spot size, but longer x-ray durations affect motion blur.

2-20. Answer = (c). As stated in the notes, full coverage of a 35 × 43-cm cassette at 100 cm (40 inches) requires a 12.5-degree anode angle. The needed anode angle decreases for larger SIDs or a smaller image receptor. Most radiology x-ray tubes have 12.5-degree anode angles. The exceptions are some CT scanners and some angiography x-ray tubes, which have smaller anode angles in order to provide better heat distribution. Mammography x-ray tubes have assorted anode angles.

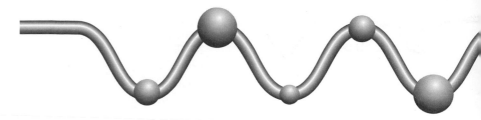

CHAPTER THREE

X-ray Tube Heat Loading Characteristics

A. Important Concepts

1. Because 99% of the energy of the electrons that hit the anode is converted into heat, it is important to limit the heat to levels that will not damage the anode.

2. The damage occurs when the heat increases the temperature of the anode to the melting point.

3. The melting point of tungsten (which is the most common anode) is 3370° C, and it is 2320° C for molybdenum (the anode of mammography x-ray tubes).

4. There are four major parameters that are used to assess and limit the heat to the anode:

- KW rating
- Single exposure rating
- Anode heat capacity
- Housing heat rating

5. The **kW rating** is the maximum instantaneous heat load that the anode can receive without damage, even if the exposure is as short as 0.10 second = 100 milliseconds in duration.

- $kW = (kVp \times mA)/1000$
- There is a maximum combination of kVp and mA that cannot be exceeded without damaging the anode.
- The kW rating is dependent on focal spot size. It increases with the focal spot size to the 1.5 power ($f^{1.5}$).
- The kW rating is higher for smaller anode bevel angles.
- The kW rating is greater for higher rotation rates of the anode.
- The kW rating is less for single-phase x-ray generators.
- The kW rating is dependent on the melting point temperature and specific heat constant of the anode material (metal).

6. ***Single exposure anode heat ratings*** restrict the maximum combination of kVp, mA, and exposure duration (time), which cannot be exceeded without damaging the anode.

   ● Heat is measured in heat units (HUs).

   ● HU = constant × kVp × mA × time (sec) where constant = 1.0 for single-phase, 1.35 for three-phase, and 1.41 for constant potential.

   ● Single exposure heat rating depends on focal spot size, ***kVP waveform***, anode angle, rotation speed of the anode, anode diameter, and anode material.

   ● The permissible kVp, mA, and time are determined from graphs provided by the manufacturers of the x-ray tubes. An example is shown in the figure.

   ● The kVp is located on the vertical axis, and a line is drawn horizontally until it intersects the mA to be used. At this point, a line is dropped vertically to determine the maximum exposure time allowed.

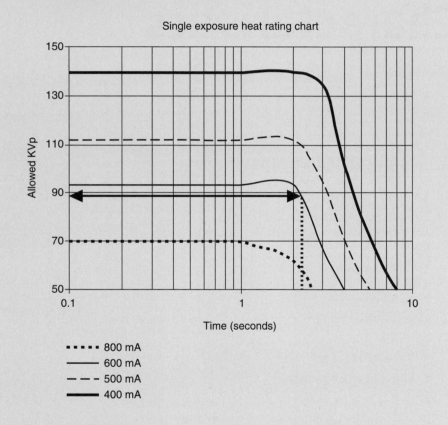

Single exposure heat rating chart

····· 800 mA
——— 600 mA
– – – 500 mA
▬▬▬ 400 mA

7. ***Anode heat capacity*** is the total heat from a series of x-ray exposures that is distributed over the entire anode without raising the temperature so high that damage occurs.

   ● The HU values from the individual x-ray exposures are added together.

   ● 1 kHU = 1000 HU

   ● 1 MHU = 1,000,000 HU

   ● Typical values are about 300 kHU for radiographic tubes, 1 to 3 MHU for angiography, and 5 MHU for CT scanner x-ray tubes.

   ● Typically, cooling times are in the order of 10 to 15 minutes.

   ● Anode heat capacity does not depend on focal spot size, rotation speed, or anode angle.

   ● Anode heat capacity does depend on anode diameter, material, mass (kg), and surface texture.

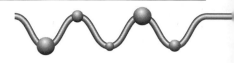

- An anode cooling graph is used to determine how long to wait between series of exposures. The typical curve in the figure indicates how long to wait after one 300,000-HU series before the same series can be repeated. The entry point at 300,000 HU is at 2 minutes. The heat must cool to 100,000 HU so that on adding 300,000 HU, it does not exceed the top of the graph, which is at 400,000 HU. The time to cool to 100,000 HU is 11 minutes. Hence, the cooling time is 11 minutes − 2 minutes = 9 minutes.

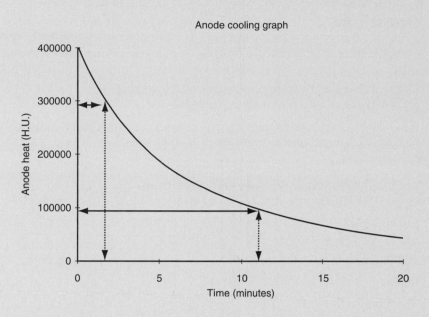

Anode cooling graph

8. **Housing heat capacity** represents the total heat that the entire x-ray tube assembly can tolerate before the tube is damaged.

   - It includes the x-ray tube, oil, and metal housing as heat storage devices.

   - Typical values for the housing are 1 to 4 MHU.

   - The housing takes a long time to cool—from 1 to 2 hours.

9. **There are three methods by which cooling** of heated items occurs.

   - **Conduction cooling** occurs by direct flow of heat by contact from one object or area to another.

     (dQ/dt) = heat flow = $(K \times A/L) \times [T_S - T_B]$.

     That is, the cooling increases with the difference in the temperature of a hot surface (T_S) and the cooler surrounding surface (T_B). Cooling increases for a large cross-sectional area (A) and decreases for a long path lengths (L).

   - **Radiative cooling** occurs by the emission of heat in the form of infrared electromagnetic waves. For very hot surfaces, this is the predominant form of cooling. This cooling is proportional to $[T_S^4 - T_B^4]$.

   - **Convection cooling** is the transfer of heat by means of a gas or liquid flowing past a hot surface. The heat transfer depends on whether the flow is smooth (laminar) or turbulent. Hence, the area of the surface and the speed of the flow are important. This heat transfer also depends on the first power of the temperature difference. Convection cooling does not occur inside an x-ray tube because the inside is a vacuum without a gas or fluid to transfer heat. Convection cooling does occur in the oil surrounding the glass insert and outside the tube housing.

10. During fluoroscopy, the heating is counterbalanced by cooling because fluoroscopy typically uses a lower mA or is not continuously activated in pulsed fluoroscopy. Usually, an x-ray tube never overheats during fluoroscopy.

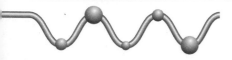

11. Some angiography and cardiac catheterization x-ray tubes use oil heat exchangers to circulate the hot oil in an x-ray tube to a cooling fin, which transfers heat to either air or a closed water system.

12. Most modern x-ray units automatically calculate x-ray tube heating and prevent exposures that would overheat the tubes and cause damage.

B. Questions

3-1. The kW rating of an x-ray tube depends on all the following factors, *except* _____.

(a) Focal spot size   (b) Exposure time   (c) Anode angle
(d) Rotation speed   (e) Anode material

3-2. According to the single exposure graph given in the Important Concepts section, the kW rating of the x-ray tube is about _____.

(a) 36   (b) 42   (c) 56   (d) 74   (e) 85

3-3. According to the single exposure graph given in the Important Concepts section, the longest exposure at 70 kVp and 400 mA is _____ seconds.

(a) 0.0   (b) 1.0   (c) 2.7   (d) 5.7   (e) 8.0

3-4. According to the single exposure graph given in the Important Concepts section, the longest exposure at 90 kVp and 800 mA is _____ seconds.

(a) 0.0   (b) 1.0   (c) 2.7   (d) 5.7   (e) 8.0

3-5. According to the single exposure graph given in the concepts section, the longest exposure at 70 kVp and 800 mA is _____ seconds.

(a) 0.0   (b) 1.0   (c) 2.7   (d) 5.7   (e) 8.0

3-6. The anode heat capacity depends on all of the following factors, *except* _____.

(a) Focal spot size   (b) Anode diameter   (c) Anode materials
(d) Anode mass   (e) Surface texture

3-7. Cooling of a very hot anode primarily occurs by _____.

(a) Conduction   (b) Convection   (c) Radiation
(d) Bremsstrahlung   (e) Cascade

3-8. *For a constant effective focal spot size*, the kW x-ray tube rating can be increased by using _____.

(a) Large anode angle   (b) High kVp values   (c) Low rotation speeds
(d) Small focal spot sizes   (e) Three-phase rather than single-phase generators

3-9. If a single-phase generator is used to take three x-rays at 100 kVp, 600 mA, and 100 milliseconds, the amount of heat units produced is about _____.

(a) 600   (b) 1800   (c) 6000   (d) 18,000   (e) 60,000

3-10. In general, x-ray tube overheating can be prevented by _____.

(a) Using high kVp   (b) Using high mA settings   (c) Using large anode angles
(d) Using small focal spots   (e) Allowing time between exposures

3-11. According to the anode cooling curve in the Important Concepts section, the maximum anode heat capacity is _____ kHU.

(a) 500   (b) 400   (c) 300   (d) 200   (e) 100

3-12. According to the anode cooling graph in the Important Concepts section, the shortest amount of time required to make three series of x-ray exposures that each deliver 200,000 HU to the anode is _____ minutes.

(a) 2   (b) 4   (c) 6   (d) 8   (e) 10

C. Answers

3-1. Answer = (b). The kW rating is the instantaneous heat rating for 0.10-second or shorter x-ray exposures. Hence, it does not depend on exposure duration. However, the kW rating increases with larger focal spot sizes, smaller anode angles, faster rotation speeds, and use of materials with higher specific heat constants and melting points.

3-2. Answer = (c). By selecting the flat portion of the kW graphs at the shortest times, one can determine that the kW rating is equal to the product of the kVp times mA for this portion of the curve divided by 1000. For example, 70 kVp × 800 mA/1000 = 56 kW.

3-3. Answer = (d). A horizontal line is drawn at 70 kVp until it intersects the curve for 400 mA. At the intersection, a vertical line is drawn down to the time axis and is read.

3-4. Answer = (a). A horizontal line drawn at 90 kVp never intersects the curve for 800 mA; the 800-mA curve lies below the value of 90 kVp. In fact, 90 kVp × 800 mA/1000 = 72 kW, which is greater than allowed for this x-ray tube. The maximum kW allowed is 56 kW, as shown in question 3-2.

3-5. Answer = (b). The horizontal curve at 70 kVp coincides with the 800-mA curve until the time exceeds 1 second. After 1 second, the 800-mA curve is below 70 kVp, and these exposures are not allowed.

3-6. Answer = (a). Once the heat is distributed over the entire anode as a result of a number of x-ray exposures over a short time interval, the size of the focal spot is not a factor in the anode heat capacity. The focal spot size is important for the kW rating and single exposure rating; it has no influence on the anode heat capacity and the housing heat capacity.

3-7. Answer = (c). When the anode is very hot, radiation cooling by the emission of infrared waves is the most important process because it is related to the fourth power of temperature. Conduction cooling is driven only by a difference of the temperature to the first power. Convection cooling does not occur because the inside of the x-ray tube is a vacuum. Bremsstrahlung refers to x-ray production, not cooling. Cascade refers to consecutive photon emission, such as those from ^{60}Co.

3-8. Answer = (e). For three-phase generators, the mA is relatively constant. For single-phase generators, the peak mA is about 1.41 times the average mA. To prevent damage during peak mA, the allowable kW rating must be reduced to prevent damage to the anode. Smaller anode angles give higher kW ratings than large anode angles. The kW rating is a product of kVp and mA, so at a high kVp, a lower mA is used. However, kVp does not alter the kW rating. The kW rating increases for higher rotation speeds (RPM, rotations per minute) of the anode. The kW rating is less for smaller focal spot sizes.

3-9. Answer = (d). The calculation is as follows: 3 exposures × 1 × 100 kVp × 600 mA × 0.1 seconds = 18,000 HU.

3-10. Answer = (e). Heat input to the anode increases with higher kVp and higher mA values. Small focal spots and larger anode angles concentrate the heat and cause greater damage. Spreading the x-ray exposures over time allows the anode to cool between x-ray exposures.

3-11. Answer = (b). The maximum anode heat capacity on an anode cooling curve is the value at time zero. On the graph shown, the value at time zero is 400,000 HU.

3-12. Answer = (b). Because the anode heat capacity (Problem 3-11) is 400 kHU, the first two 200-kHU can be done immediately one after the other. Once the anode reaches 400 kHU, it must cool from a start time of zero until the anode temperature decreases to 200 kHU. The time to 200 kHU is 4 minutes from the graph.

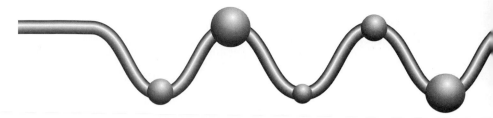

CHAPTER FOUR

X-ray Production

A. Important Concepts

This section lists the principal concepts related to the production of x-rays.

1. The **kinetic energy** (energy of motion) of the electrons hitting the target of the x-ray tube is gained by acceleration from the voltage (kVp).

2. The **kinetic energy** is converted into heat (99%) and x-rays (approximately 1%).

   - The percentage of x-ray production increases with the energy of the bombarding electrons.

   - The percentage of x-ray production increases with the atomic number (Z) of the target material.

   - The percentage of x-ray production = [E (keV) × Z]/8000.

3. Target materials for anodes are **tungsten** (symbol = W, Z = 74) for most x-ray tubes and **molybdenum** (symbol = Mo, Z = 42) and **rhodium** (symbol = Rh, Z = 43) for mammography x-ray tubes.

4. Electrons interact with the atoms in the target to **produce two types of x-rays**:

   - Bremsstrahlung x-rays (braking, or slowing down, radiation) = 85% to 100%

   - Characteristic x-rays = 0 to 15% (tungsten target at 50 to 150 kVp)

5. **Bremsstrahlung x-rays** occur when a bombarding electron approaches the nucleus of the tungsten atom of the x-ray tube target. The electron is negatively charged, and the nucleus of tungsten has 74 positively charged protons. The nucleus electrostatically attracts and slows the bombarding electrons. As the electrons are slowed, the lost energy is transferred to produce x-rays.

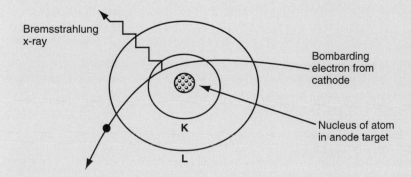

   - Electrons can make impact at different distances from the nucleus and thus are slowed by different amounts.

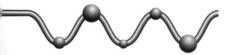

- Some electrons undergo numerous small interactions, producing many low-energy x-rays.

- Some x-rays undergo a single event in which all the energy is lost, producing a single high-energy x-ray.

- The highest energy x-rays can never exceed the kinetic energy of the bombarding electrons, which is numerically equal to the kVp (in units of keV).

- The lowest energy x-rays produced go down to zero keV; however, the lowest energy x-rays are never emitted.

- Low-energy x-rays are absorbed by the glass envelope of the x-ray tube and the filtration in the collimator assembly.

- More low-energy x-rays are produced than high-energy x-rays.

- ***Bremsstrahlung x-rays appear over a continuous distribution of energies***.

6. ***Characteristic x-rays*** are produced when a bombarding electron collides with the orbital electrons rotating around the nucleus of the atoms in the target material. If the bombarding electrons have sufficient energy to break the ***binding energy (BE),*** the orbital electrons are knocked out of the atom. The remaining electrons then rearrange themselves to fill the position of the missing orbital electron.

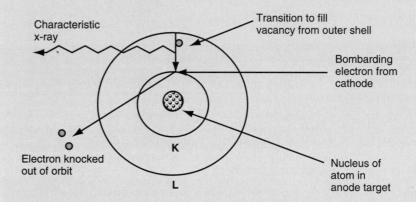

- Energy of characteristic x-rays = $[BE_{inner} - BE_{outer}]$.

- The transition is from an outer shell to fill a vacancy in an inner orbital shell.

- Binding energy is proportional to $[Z/n]^2$, where $n = 1$ for K-shell, $n = 2$ for L-shell, $n = 3$ for M-shell, and so on.

- The binding energy for the K-shell is much greater than for an outer shell.

- The binding energy of a low-Z target material is less than for a higher Z material.

- "Characteristic" refers to the fact that the binding energy is characteristic of the type of target material of the x-ray tube and therefore the energy of these x-rays.

- If the K-shell electron is knocked out of orbit, the x-rays are called "K-characteristic x-rays."

- If the L-shell electron is knocked out of orbit, the x-rays that are produced are called "L-characteristic x-rays."

- To produce K-characteristic x-rays, the bombarding electrons must have a kinetic energy exceeding the K-shell binding energy of the target material atoms. K-shell binding energies of various target materials are 69.5 keV for tungsten, 20 keV for molybdenum, and 23 keV for rhodium.

- When the voltage of a tungsten x-ray tube is less than 69.5 kVp, the bombarding electrons have less than 69.5 keV. The energy is insufficient to

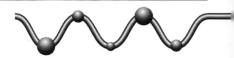

knock a K-shell orbital electron of a tungsten atom out of orbit, and no K-characteristic x-rays are produced.

- K-characteristic x-rays of tungsten appear at 57 to 59 keV (K-alpha) and 67 to 69.5 keV (K-beta).
- K-characteristic x-rays of molybdenum appear at 17 to 20 keV.
- K-characteristic x-rays of rhodium appear at 20–23 keV.
- L-characteristic x-rays are rarely seen because they have energies around 8 to 10 keV. These x-ray energies are so low that they are absorbed by the glass envelope of the x-ray tube and filtration in the collimator assembly.
- Unlike bremsstrahlung x-rays, *characteristic x-rays appear at only a few fixed (discrete) x-ray energies*.

7. An *x-ray spectrum* is a plot of the number of x-rays at each energy level versus the energy of the x-rays; see the accompanying plot.

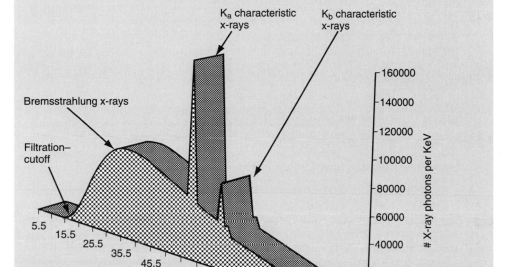

8. The mAs merely controls the number of x-rays. Doubling the mAs produces double the number of x-rays. However, the mAs does *not* affect the maximum x-ray energy, the average x-ray energy, or the characteristic x-ray energy.

9. The average energy of the x-rays is one third to one half of the kVp in units of keV.

10. As kVp is increased, the following happen:
- The maximum x-ray energy increases.
- The average x-ray energy increases.
- The number of bremsstrahlung x-rays increases.
- The number of characteristic x-rays increases, but their energy is the same.
- The minimum x-ray energy is not affected.
- The x-rays are more penetrating at higher kVp.
- If the kVp is below 69.5, no characteristic x-rays are produced.
- See examples of spectra shown in the figure on next page.

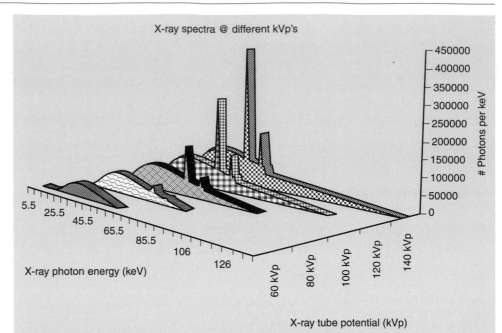

X-ray spectra @ different kVp's

11. Filters placed in the x-ray beams remove more lower energy x-rays than higher energy x-rays.

12. Filters increase the average energy (not the maximum energy) of an x-ray spectrum.

13. Filters reduce the total number of x-rays.

14. X-ray beams are described by two terms: quantity and quality.

15. *Quantity* measures the number of x-rays and the energy of the x-rays indirectly; the number of electrons knocked loose from air atoms (ion pairs) as x-rays pass through the air is measured. Quantity is the same as the radiation measurement called "exposure." One roentgen (R) is equal to $2.08 \times 10^{+9}$ ion pairs produced per cubic centimeter of air at standard temperature and pressure (STP). In new standard international (SI) units, exposure or quantity is measured in coulombs per kilogram of air.

16. $1 \text{ R} = 2.58 \times 10^{-4}$ coulombs per kg of air.

17. The quantity increases:
    - With the square of the kVp
    - Linearly with mAs
    - Linearly with atomic number of the anode material

18. The quantity decreases:
    - With the inverse square of the distance $[1/d^2]$
    - With added filtration of the x-ray beam

19. *Quality* is a measure of the penetration of the x-ray beam through matter. Quality is measured in units of *half-value layer (HVL)*. HVL is the thickness of the material needed to reduce the quantity of penetrating x-rays to 50%. HVL is measured in mm or cm of a particular material. HVL for diagnostic x-rays is usually measured in mm of aluminum.

20. The quality increases with:
    - Higher kVp
    - Added filtration of the x-ray beam

21. The HVL increases with higher kVp and greater filtration in the x-ray beam.

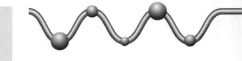

22. The typical HVL for 70- to 80-kVp x-rays from a tungsten target is about 2.1 to 3.5 mm of aluminum. However, the HVL is significantly greater for angiographic and cardiac catheterization x-ray beams that are filtered by 0.1 to 0.9 mm of copper.

23. As the quantity increases, the x-ray film image becomes darker.

24. For higher quality (HVL), the x-rays are more penetrating and fewer x-rays could be used. Thus, high-quality x-ray beams usually result in lower radiation doses to patients.

B. Questions

4-1. Bremsstrahlung x-ray production accounts for _____ % of all the x-rays.

(a) 85–100 (b) 70–85 (c) 55–70 (d) 30–45 (e) 15–30

4-2. The energy spectrum of bremsstrahlung x-rays is _____.

(a) Monoenergetic (b) Polychromatic
(c) Composed of multiple discrete peaks (d) Isotropic (e) Homogeneous

4-3. The shortest wavelength x-ray photons are dependent on _____.

(a) Characteristic x-rays (b) K-edge x-rays (c) kVp
(d) X-ray beam filtration (e) mAs settings

4-4. The longest wavelength x-ray photons are dependent on _____.

(a) Characteristic x-rays (b) K-edge x-rays (c) kVp
(d) X-ray beam filtration (e) mAs settings

4-5. The K-characteristic x-rays for a tungsten x-ray tube target have energies of about _____ keV.

(a) 17–20 (b) 20–23 (c) 30–50 (d) 50–70 (e) 70–88

4-6. The K-characteristic x-rays for a rhodium x-ray tube target have energies of about _____ keV.

(a) 17–20 (b) 20–23 (c) 30–50 (d) 50–70 (e) 70–88

4-7. The K-characteristic x-rays for a molybdenum x-ray tube target have an energy of about _____ keV.

(a) 17–20 (b) 20–23 (c) 30–50 (d) 50–70 (e) 70–88

4-8. The L-characteristic x-rays for a tungsten x-ray tube target are usually

_____.

(a) More penetrating than the K-characteristic x-rays
(b) More abundant with greater filtration
(c) A significant portion of the scattered x-rays
(d) An insignificant portion of the total x-ray production
(e) A significant contributor to the radiation dose to the patient's skin

4-9. A single bombarding electron that undergoes several bremsstrahlung interactions in the x-ray tube anode produces _____.

(a) A single high-energy x-ray (b) Several low-energy x-rays
(c) Only heat (d) Several high-energy x-rays
(e) Three characteristic x-rays

4-10. If the average energy of an x-ray spectrum is approximately 40 keV, the voltage across the x-ray tube must be around _____ kVp.

(a) 20–40 (b) 40–60 (c) 50–80 (d) 80–120 (e) 120–150

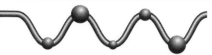

4-11. To be able to produce K-characteristic x-rays in a tungsten target x-ray tube, the x-ray tube voltage must be no lower than _____ kVp.

(a) 101.5   (b) 98.5   (c) 88.5   (d) 76.5   (e) 69.5

4-12. The x-ray quantity increases when the _____ is larger in magnitude.

(a) kVp   (b) mAs   (c) Filtration   (d) Both a and b
(e) Both a and c   (f) a, b, and c

4-13. The quality (ability of x-rays to penetrate through the patient's body) improves when the _____ is larger in magnitude.

(a) kVp   (b) mAs   (c) Filtration   (d) Both a and b   (e) Both a and c
(f) a, b, and c

4-14. The contrast in radiographic images degrades when the _____ is larger in magnitude.

(a) kVp   (b) mAs   (c) Filtration   (d) Both a and b   (e) Both a and c
(f) a, b, and c

4-15. The relative amount of scattered x-rays increases when the _____ is larger in magnitude.

(a) kVp   (b) mAs   (c) Filtration   (d) Both a and b   (e) Both a and c
(f) a, b, and c

4-16. The quantity of the bremsstrahlung x-rays depends on _____.

(a) kVp   (b) mAs   (c) Filtration   (d) Both a and b   (e) Both a and c
(f) a, b, and c

4-17. The quantity of the characteristic x-rays depends on all of the following, *except* _____.

(a) kVp   (b) Distance (SID)   (c) mAs   (d) Atomic number
(e) Mass number

4-18. If the x-ray tube voltage is increased from 60 to 120 kVp, the quantity is changed by _____ the previous value.

(a) 4.0 times   (b) 2.0 times   (c) 1 (same)   (d) 0.5 times
(e) 0.25 times

4-19. If the mAs is doubled, the quantity of the x-ray beam is changed by _____ the previous value.

(a) 4.0 times   (b) 2.0 times   (c) 1 (same)   (d) 0.5 times   (e) 0.25 times

4-20. Quantity is usually measured in units of _____.

(a) mm of aluminum   (b) keV   (c) kVp   (d) mR   (e) Calories

4-21. Quality is usually measured in units of _____.

(a) mm of aluminum   (b) keV   (c) kVp   (d) mR   (e) Calories

4-22. An increase in filtration with a corresponding increase in mAs in order to maintain radiographic film density constant results in _____ to the patient's skin entrance radiation dose.

(a) No effect   (b) An increase   (c) A decrease
(d) An effect that cannot be determined

4-23. The quality of the characteristic x-rays is affected by the _____.

(a) kVp   (b) mAs   (c) Added filtration   (d) Atomic number
(e) Distance (SID)

4-24. Higher amounts of _____ increase both the quantity and quality of an x-ray beam.

(a) kVp   (b) mAs   (c) Filtration   (d) Both a and b   (e) Both a and c
(f) a, b, and c

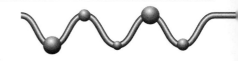

4-25. Higher amounts of _____ increase quantity without affecting quality.

(a) kVp   (b) mAs   (c) Filtration   (d) Both a and b   (e) Both a and c
(f) a, b, and c

C.   Answers

4-1. Answer = (a). In tungsten targets, no characteristic x-rays are produced at voltages of less than 69.5 kVp. In this event, the x-ray production is 100% bremsstrahlung production. At 150 kVP, the characteristic x-ray production is the largest fraction of the total at 15% of all the x-rays. Thus, bremsstrahlung x-ray production varies from 85% at 150 kVp to 100% at kVp values of less than 69.5 kVp.

4-2. Answer = (b). Monoenergetic means that the x-rays all have just a single energy. Bremsstrahlung x-rays have a distribution of x-ray energies that is called polyenergetic or polychromatic. Characteristic x-rays have multiple discrete energies because the energies are exactly the difference between the orbital electron binding energies of the atom in the anode. Isotropic means equal in all directions. Homogeneous means uniform. Water is homogeneous; however, the tissues in the lungs are nonhomogeneous.

4-3. Answer = (c). Characteristic x-ray energy is slightly less than the K-shell binding energy regardless of the kVp applied across the x-ray tube. K-edge refers to the K-shell binding energy; again, this value depends on the material of the anode and is fixed in energy. The shortest wavelength x-rays are the highest energy x-rays. These x-rays are numerically equal to the kVp. The x-ray beam filtration preferentially attenuates the lower energy x-rays. Filtration affects the longest wavelength x-rays. Typically, the filtration removes x-rays below 10 to 15 keV. mAs increases the total number of x-rays without affecting the distribution of x-ray energies or the spectrum.

4-4. Answer = (d). The longest wavelength x-rays are the lowest energy x-rays. As explained in answer 4-3, the amount of x-ray beam filtration determines the lowest energy x-rays that emerge from the x-ray tube. As the amount of filtration increases, the x-rays need higher energies to pass through the filter material. Hence, more filtration means that very low energy x-rays are attenuated, and the lowest energy emerging from the filter is higher than it would be without the filter.

4-5. Answer = (d). For a tungsten anode, the K-alpha x-rays are between 57 and 59 keV and the K-beta characteristic x-rays are between 67 and 69.5 keV. There are more K-alpha than K-beta x-rays. K-alphas represent transitions from the L-shell to a vacancy in the K-shell. K-beta characteristic x-rays represent transitions from the M- and N-shells to a vacancy in the K-shell.

4-6. Answer = (b). The K-shell binding energy for rhodium is only 23 keV, in comparison with the K-shell binding energy of tungsten, which is 69.5 keV.

4-7. Answer = (a). The K-shell binding energy of molybdenum is 20 keV. The average K-shell binding energy is about $13.6\ eV \times Z^2$. That is, the binding energy depends on the atomic number of the anode material.

4-8. Answer = (d). L-characteristic x-rays have much lower energies than K-characteristic x-rays. For a tungsten anode, the L-characteristic x-rays have energies 8 to 12 keV. These L-characteristic x-rays have such low energies that they are unable to penetrate through the glass envelope of the x-ray tube and the filtration in the collimator. Thus, they do not emerge from the x-ray tube and have no effect on the radiation dose or the x-ray produced.

4-9. Answer = (b). To produce very high energy x-rays, the bombarding electron must lose most of its energy in a single bremsstrahlung interaction. If it has several bremsstrahlung interactions, the total kinetic energy must be divided by the number of interactions, producing several low-energy x-rays. For the kinetic energy to be emitted as heat, ionization interactions must occur instead of bremsstrahlung. If there were more than one high energy x-ray produced, the

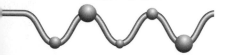

total energy of the x-rays would be greater than the energy of the bombarding electron, which is contrary to the principle of conservation of energy. A single electron must expend approximately 70 keV of energy to knock a K-shell electron out of orbit and produce a characteristic x-ray. For three characteristic x-rays, 210 keV would be necessary; however, diagnostic x-ray tubes produce a maximum of only 150 kVp, which imparts only 150 keV (at most) to a single bombarding electron.

4-10. Answer = (d). The average x-ray energy is about 0.33 to $0.5 \times$ kVp. In other words, the kVp must be two to three times the average x-ray beam energy. Two times 40 keV equals 80 kVp, and three times 40 keV would be 120 kVp.

4-11. Answer = (e). To knock a K-shell electron of tungsten from orbit, the bombarding electron must have an energy equal to or greater than the K-shell binding energy, which is 69.5 keV. Thus, the accelerating voltage across the x-ray tube must be greater than 69.5 kVp for the bombarding electrons to gain this kinetic energy.

4-12. Answer = (d). The kVp increases both the number and the energy of the x-rays. The mAs increases only the number of x-rays. Quantity is dependent on both the number and the energy of the x-rays. By contrast, filtration preferentially removes more of the lower energy x-rays, leaving a smaller total number of x-rays. However, the remaining x-rays have higher energy values. Thus, filtration decreases quantity; the higher energy x-rays remaining are more penetrating, resulting in higher quality.

4-13. Answer = (e). Raising the kVp increases the maximum x-ray energy and the average energy of the x-ray spectrum; thus, these x-rays would be more penetrating. Raising the mAs increases the total number of x-rays, but it does not affect the relative energy distribution. Additional x-ray beam filtration removes more of the lower energy x-rays, leaving the higher energy x-rays unchanged. Thus, the average x-ray energy of the x-ray spectrum increases, but the maximum x-ray energy is unchanged. The net effect is that the remaining x-rays are more penetrating. Hence, only kVp and filtration influence x-ray penetration.

4-14. Answer = (e). Higher energy x-rays produce less image contrast and more scattered x-rays, which further reduces the contrast. Again, higher kVp and more filtration result in higher energy x-rays.

4-15. Answer = (e). As explained in 4-14, higher energy x-rays reduce image contrast and produce more scattered x-rays. Raising the mAs increases the total number of x-rays, which would increase the absolute number of scattered x-rays. However, the ratio of the number of scattered x-rays to the total number of x-rays (the relative number of scattered x-rays) would not change because both would increase by the same amount. If the total number is doubled and the number scattered is doubled, the ratio (scattered to total) is the same.

4-16. Answer = (f). Raising the kVp and the mAs increases the total number of bremsstrahlung and characteristic x-rays. More filtration decreases the total number of x-rays because the low-energy x-rays are preferentially removed by the filtration. Because quantity depends on both the number and the energy of the x-rays, all the listed factors (kVp, mAs, and filtration) affect the quantity.

4-17. Answer = (e). Raising both kVp and mAs causes an increase in the number of characteristic x-rays. Larger distances reduce the number of both bremsstrahlung and characteristic x-rays according to the inverse square law [$1/d^2$]. If the anode target material has a higher atomic number, x-ray production increases [$Z \times E(\text{keV})/8000$]. Higher mass numbers have no effect on bremsstrahlung or characteristic x-ray production.

4-18. Answer = (a). The x-ray production is related to $(\text{kVp})^2$. Hence, if the kVp is doubled (from 60 to 120 kVp), the quantity is quadrupled (4 times).

4-19. Answer = (b). The quantity is directly proportional to the mAs. If the mAs is doubled, the x-ray quantity is also doubled.

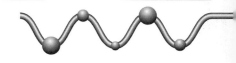

4-20. Answer = (d). Quantity is determined by the ionization created by the x-rays as they pass through air. The number of ion pairs created per cubic centimeter of air is termed exposure, and it can be measured in units of milliroentgens (mR). As the quantity increases, more ionization is created in the air through which the x-rays travel.

4-21. Answer = (a). Quality is a measure of the ability of the x-rays to penetrate through matter. The amount of material required to reduce the quantity to 50% is deemed the half-value layer (HVL). For diagnostic x-rays, the HVL is usually measured in millimeters of aluminum. As the energy of the x-rays increases and the x-rays penetrate better, more material is required to reduce the quantity to 50% of the initial quantity.

4-22. Answer = (c). The filtration removes the lower energy x-rays. Low-energy x-rays are not very penetrating and deposit their energy in the body, increasing the radiation dose to the patient. Eliminating these low-energy x-rays leaves higher energy x-rays, which can penetrate the body better. However, because the filter removes an appreciable number of low-energy x-rays, the mAs has to be increased somewhat to maintain film density. Usually, the net effect of more filtration with increased mAs is to reduce the patient's entrance radiation dose by 25% to 40%.

4-23. Answer = (d). Raising mAs increases the total number of all x-rays without changing their energy. Greater distances reduce the total number of all x-rays without changing their energy. Raising kVp increases the energy of the bremsstrahlung x-rays, but it increases only the number of the characteristic x-rays. The energy of characteristic x-rays depends on the binding energy of the K-shell electrons, which increases with atomic number. Added filtration removes the lower energy bremsstrahlung x-rays, but it does not change the energy of the characteristic x-rays, which is related to the Z of the target material.

4-24. Answer = (a). Raising kVp increases both the energy and the number of x-rays produced; both quantity and quality increase. Raising mAs increases quantity, but the quality is unchanged because the x-ray energy distribution is unchanged. More filtration reduces quantity, but it increases the quality.

4-25. Answer = (b). As explained in 4-24, raising mAs increases the quantity without any effect on the quality. Changes in kVp and filtration affect both quantity and quality.

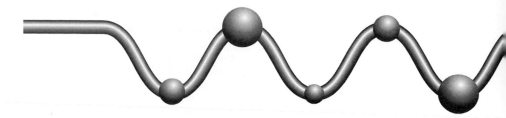

CHAPTER FIVE

X-ray Equipment Electronics

A. Basic Concepts

This chapter describes the electronic components of the x-ray equipment used to generate the x-ray tube voltage, the amount of x-rays produced, and the exposure time duration. It begins with a discussion of basic electronic components and continues on to different types of x-ray generator circuits.

1. There are two types of voltage: constant (direct current, DC) and sinusoidal time-varying voltage (alternating current, AC).

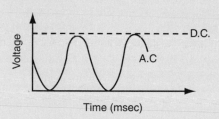

2. The **_resistor (R)_** is used to regulate the amount of electron flow (current $= I$).

- $I = (V/R)$, where V is voltage and R is resistance (ohms, Ω).

- As the resistance increases, the current decreases.

- As the voltage increases, the current increases.

- The schematic symbol for a resistor is shown in the figure.

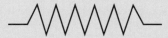

3. The **_capacitor (C)_** has several different functions. It can store electrical charge (electrons). The charge builds up exponentially at a speed related to $R \times C$.

Capacitors also block constant voltage (DC), but they allow time-varying voltage (AC) to be transmitted.

- Rate of Q accumulation:

    $Q = C \times V \times \{1 - \exp[-\text{time}/(R \times C)]\}$

- Capacitors are used in timer circuits.

- Capacitors are used to smooth the ripple in time-varying voltages.

- The schematic symbol for a capacitor is shown in the figure.

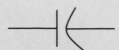

4. **Transformers** are used to increase or decrease the input voltage. The effect on the voltage depends on the number of windings on the secondary side compared with the primary side **(turns ratio, N_r)**.

   - Transformers with a turns ratio of greater than one ($N_r > 1$) increase the voltage and are called **step-up transformers**. Step-up transformers are used to increase the voltage across the x-ray tube.

   - Transformers with a turns ratio of less than one ($N_r < 1$) decrease the voltage and are called **step-down transformers**. Step-down transformers are used to decrease the voltage supplied to the filament of the x-ray tube.

   - The schematic symbol for a transformer is shown in the figure.

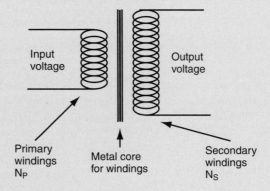

   - Turns ratio = $N_r = [N_S/N_P]$
   - Transformers work only with AC voltage. If DC input voltage is used, there is no output voltage.
   - The power on the primary and secondary windings of a transformer is constant:

     $$I_P \times V_P = I_S \times V_S$$

5. Rectifiers are used to let electrons flow in only one direction, like a one-way street sign. Rectifiers convert AC electron flow to DC electron flow.

   - Electron flow is opposite to the direction of the arrow in the drawn symbol.
   - Rectifiers typically consist of a stack of silicon or selenium diodes.
   - The schematic symbol for the rectifier is shown in the figure.

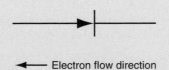

6. The **autotransformer** adjusts the input voltage to maintain a constant voltage into the electronics of the x-ray circuit. The **line voltage monitor** senses the input voltage and signals a motor to change the number of input windings so as to maintain a constant output voltage.

7. **Timer circuits** control the duration of the x-ray exposure. The timer turns on and off the kVp across the x-ray tube at the input to the step-up transformer. There are basically five different types of timer circuits.

   - Mechanical timers, which have increments in seconds

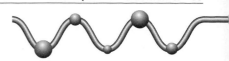

- Synchronous motor timers, which have increments in 1/60 second
- R-C timers, which use the duration of the charging of a capacitor through a variable resistor to adjust the time in increments of milliseconds
- mAs timers, which also use R-C circuits to control mAs instead of time
- **_Phototimers_** (also called **_automatic exposure control, AEC_**), which use a radiation detector to sense the amount of radiation passing through a patient into an image receptor. The detector terminates the x-rays when sufficient radiation has been incident upon the image receptor.
- Timer accuracy can be checked with radiation detectors attached to oscilloscopes.

8. **_kVp selectors_** are used to adjust the voltage applied to the x-ray tube.
- The selector is located between the autotransformer and the step-up transformer.
- The selection is performed by adjusting the number of windings on the output of the autotransformer.
- The major adjustments are in increments of 10 kVp.
- The minor adjustments are in increments of 1 kVp.

9. The **_filament adjustment_** circuit controls heating and thermionic emissions of filament.
- A step-down transformer decreases the voltage to the x-ray tube filament.
- A variable resistor controls the current through the filament.
- As the current passing through the filament of the x-ray tube increases, it becomes hotter, and more electrons are "boiled off" (thermionic emission).
- At low voltage across the x-ray tube, an electron cloud forms around the filament, which prevents additional electrons from traversing from the cathode to the anode. This repulsion is called the **_space charge effect_**.
- At a voltage of about 40 kVp, the electron cloud is removed, and most electrons emitted by the filament easily move to the anode without repulsion from the cloud. This voltage, at which the space charge effect is minimized, is called the **_saturation voltage_**.
- There is also a special circuit to maintain constant electron flow for a given mA setting regardless of the kVp. This compensating circuit is called the **_space charge circuit_**.
- Electron flow from cathode to anode is called **_tube current_**.
- For low tube currents (10 to 200 mA), a small filament is used that produces a small focal spot.
- For high tube currents (200 to 1000 mA), a larger filament size is used that produces a larger focal spot.

10. A block diagram of basic components of x-ray circuits is shown in the figure (see figure in the next page).

11. There are different types of high-voltage (step-up transformers and rectifiers) sections of x-ray equipment. These differences affect the ripple in the voltage to the x-ray tube and thus the radiation produced.

12. **_Ripple_** is the percent variation in the voltage across the x-ray tube during x-ray exposure. It can range from 0% (constant voltage) to 100% (voltage varies from peak to zero).

13. **_Pulses_** are the number of oscillations in the voltage each 1/60 second (or 16.7 milliseconds). Pulses can be listed as the number per second.

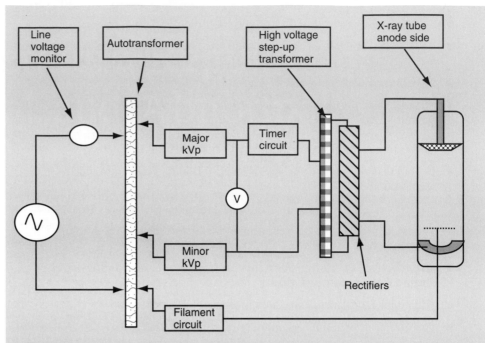

14. The amount of x-ray radiation produced per second is reduced as the amount of ripple increases.

15. The various types of x-ray generators and their characteristics are listed in the table.

GENERATOR TYPE	NO. OF DIODES	RIPPLE (%)	NO. OF PULSES PER 1/60 SECOND (PER 1 SEC)	RELATIVE RADIATION (mR/mAs) AT 1 METER (%)
Self-rectified	None	100	1 (60/sec)	25
Single-phase, half-wave rectified	2	100	1 (60/sec)	25
Single-phase, full-wave rectified	4	100	2 (120/sec)	50
3-phase, 6-pulse	6	12–15	6 (360/sec)	89
3-phase, 12-pulse	12	3–6	12 (720/sec)	95–98
High frequency	2–4	3–15	20–1500 (1K–100 K/sec)	89–98
Constant potential	12	0	None	100

16. Dental x-ray units are self-rectified units. Single-phase units are an older design for situations involving a low number of exposures. Most modern x-ray generators are high-frequency units.

17. High-frequency units are smaller in size than the other units—except dental ones.

18. mA waveforms can be either single phase or relatively constant. For single-phase mA, the peak mA is about 1.41 times greater than the average mA. For the other units, the average mA and peak mA values are almost the same.

19. The mA meter is located on the high-voltage side of the step-up transformer.

20. The **_amount of radiation_** measured depends on kVp, mAs, distance, filtration, and type of x-ray generator. The following formula provides an estimate of typical values. The constant C is 1.0 for constant potential generators and scales down for single-phase, half-wave rectified generators to 0.25 to 0.35.

$$\text{Radiation exposure} = C \times 10 \times (kVp/100)^2 \times mAs \times (100 \text{ cm/distance in cm})^2 \text{ (in units of mR)}$$

- For 100 kVp and 100 mAs at 100 cm with a constant potential generator, the expected radiation levels would be about 1000 mR or 1 roentgen. (1 roentgen = 2.58×10^{-4} coulombs per kg of air.)

B. Questions

5-1. The filament circuit uses _____.

(a) Step-up transformer   (b) Step-down transformer   (c) Rectifiers
(d) Autotransformer   (e) Inverter circuit

5-2. The line regulator uses _____.

(a) Step-up transformer   (b) Step-down transformer   (c) Rectifiers
(d) Autotransformer   (e) Inverter circuit

5-3. The high-voltage (kVp) circuit requires _____ and _____.

(a) Step-up transformer   (b) Step-down transformer   (c) Rectifiers
(d) Autotransformer   (e) Inverter circuit

5-4. A high-frequency generator requires _____.

(a) Step-up transformer   (b) Step-down transformer   (c) Rectifiers
(d) Autotransformer   (e) Inverter circuit

5-5. Changing AC current to DC current requires _____.

(a) Step-up transformer   (b) Step-down transformer   (c) Rectifiers
(d) Autotransformer   (e) Inverter circuit

5-6. The voltage required to remove most of the space charge around the filament and collect more of the thermionic emitted electrons is called the _____ voltage.

(a) Cascade   (b) Saturation   (c) Null   (d) Complex   (e) Focusing

5-7. The x-ray generator (high-voltage section) that produces the most x-rays per mAs at a given kVp and distance is _____.

(a) Single phase   (b) 3-phase, 6-pulse   (c) 3-phase, 12-pulse
(d) High frequency   (e) Constant potential

5-8. The generator that uses six diodes for the high-voltage rectification is _____.

(a) Single phase   (b) 3-phase, 6-pulse   (c) 3-phase, 12-pulse
(d) High frequency   (e) Constant potential

5-9. The x-ray generator that has the least penetrating x-rays and results in the highest radiation dose to the patient for the same kVp and same film density is the _____.

(a) Single phase   (b) 3-phase, 6-pulse   (c) 3-phase, 12-pulse
(d) High frequency   (e) Constant potential

5-10. The x-ray generator with the smallest transformer size is the _____.

(a) Single phase   (b) 3-phase, 6-pulse   (c) 3-phase, 12-pulse
(d) High frequency   (e) Constant potential

5-11. The x-ray generator that produces the smallest amount of x-rays for a given setting of kVp and mAs is _____.

(a) Single phase   (b) 3-phase, 6-pulse   (c) 3-phase, 12-pulse
(d) High frequency   (e) Constant potential

5-12. The x-ray generator that produces 180 pulses per 500-millisecond exposure is _____.

(a) Single phase   (b) 3-phase, 6-pulse   (c) 3-phase, 12-pulse
(d) High frequency   (e) Constant potential

5-13. The x-ray generator that has 100% ripple in the kVp waveform is the _____.

(a) Single phase   (b) 3-phase, 6-pulse   (c) 3-phase, 12-pulse
(d) High frequency   (e) Constant potential

5-14. The space charge effect dissipates at an x-ray tube potential of about _____ kVp.

(a) 25   (b) 40   (c) 50   (d) 69.5   (e) 88

5-15. The x-ray timer circuit that uses radiation measurements to terminate the exposure is called a(n) _____ timer.

(a) Mechanical   (b) mAs   (c) R-C   (d) Synchronous
(e) Automatic exposure control (AEC)

5-16. The most common x-ray exposure timer, which can adjust to exposure durations from several seconds to 1 millisecond, is the _____ timer.

(a) Mechanical   (b) Bridge   (c) R-C   (d) Synchronous   (e) Multiplexer

5-17. Timer circuits terminate x-ray exposures by interrupting the _____.

(a) Filament current   (b) Line compensation
(c) Primary current of the autotransformer
(d) Primary current of the step-up transformer
(e) Secondary current of the step-up transformer

5-18. The device that stores electrical charge and is used in timer circuits is called a _____.

(a) Resistor   (b) Capacitor   (c) Diode   (d) Transformer   (e) Inductor

5-19. The _____ allows electrons to flow in only one direction.

(a) Resistor   (b) Capacitor   (c) Diode   (d) Transformer   (e) Inductor

5-20. The equation for Ohm's law is _____.

(a) $P = IV$ (b) $R = V/I$ (c) $I = RV$ (d) $P = V^2/R$ (e) $V = I^2R$

5-21. The device that does not function with DC power is a _____.

(a) Resistor   (b) X-ray tube   (c) Transformer   (d) Filament
(e) Conductor

5-22. A transformer can regulate all the following electrical parameters, *except* _____.

(a) Voltage   (b) Current   (c) Phase   (d) Power   (e) Inductance

5-23. Ripple in the x-ray tube voltage is undesirable because it reduces _____.

(a) Contrast   (b) Resolution   (c) Exposure time   (d) X-ray production
(e) Patient's radiation dose

5-24. The x-ray tube current is monitored on the _____.

(a) Primary side of the autotransformer
(b) Primary side of the step-up transformer
(c) Secondary side of the autotransformer
(d) Secondary side of the step-up transformer
(e) Secondary side of the step-down transformer

5-25. Typical values for the filament current are around _____ mA, and typical values for the tube current are _____ mA.

(a) 100, 10   (b) 5000, 500   (c) 500, 500   (d) 50, 500   (e) 5, 10

C.   Answers

5-1.   Answer = (b). The filament circuit needs a large current but low voltage. Hence, a step-down transformer is used to reduce the voltage to the filament.

5-2.   Answer = (d). The line regulation circuit uses a single transformer to adjust the output voltage so that it is relatively constant for a variety of input voltages. The autotransformer is also used to adjust the voltage to the primary side of the step-up transformer.

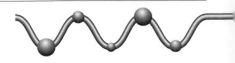

5-3. Answer = (a) and (c). It is necessary to increase the voltage to the x-ray tube and make certain the anode is always positive and the cathode is always negative.

The step-up transformer increases the voltage, and the rectifiers keep the current flowing in one direction from the cathode to the anode.

5-4. Answer = (e). Higher frequency generators first rectify the voltage to obtain a nearly constant DC voltage. Because transformers cannot function with DC voltage, the voltage must then be converted to a high-frequency pulsed DC voltage by using a rapid switch called a "chopper." The high-frequency pulsed DC voltage looks like AC voltage to a transformer. A step-up transformer then increases the voltage, and rectifiers are used to keep the direction constant from the x-ray tube cathode to the anode. This combination is called an ***inverter circuit***.

5-5. Answer = (c). Rectifiers keep the current (and voltage) applied in a single direction so that electrons flow from the cathode of the x-ray tube to the anode.

5-6. Answer = (b). Cascade refers to an isomer transition of a radioactive nucleus in which one photon emission is followed by a second photon emission. Null voltage refers to a Wheatstone bridge circuit in which the voltages are balanced, yielding no current flow. Complex voltage refers to a mathematical description in which there is a real and an imaginary component to the value. Focusing voltage refers to the voltage on the focusing cup surrounding the filament of the x-ray tube, which tends to keep those electrons bombarding the anode pushed closer together, resulting in a smaller focal spot size.

5-7. Answer = (e). A constant potential generator produces the most x-rays for a given kVp and mAs. A single-phase, half-wave rectified generator produces the smallest number of x-rays. The x-ray production increases with a more constant voltage (small ripple), when the voltage is applied constantly rather than pulsed.

5-8. Answer = (b). Reference to the table on page 36 indicates that single-phase generators use 2 diodes (half-wave) or 4 diodes (full-wave). Three-phase generators can use either 6 diodes (6-pulse) or 12 diodes (12-pulse). High-frequency generators are a special case; they are three-phase generators with many pulses and some capacitance smoothing of the waveform. Constant potential generators are three-phase, 12-pulse generators that chop off the ripple to make the voltage constant.

5-9. Answer = (a). In single-phase generators, there is a large variation in the voltage across the x-ray tube (100% ripple). A large ripple in the x-ray tube voltage results in both fewer x-rays being produced and a lower average energy of the x-rays. Low-energy x-rays do not penetrate the body very well. Hence, more of these x-rays are needed to obtain the number necessary to darken the film. The larger number of x-rays results in a higher radiation dose to the patient.

5-10. Answer = (d). As the number of pulses in the AC-voltage waveforms increases, the transformer becomes more efficient and can be made smaller in size.

Thus, high-frequency generators, which produce 10,000 to 100,000 pulses per second, are the smallest in size.

5-11. Answer = (a). As previously stated, the amount of x-ray production and the energy of the x-rays decrease as the ripple in the x-ray tube voltage increases.

Because single-phase generators have 100% ripple, they are associated with the least x-ray production, and the average energy of the x-rays is lower for any given kVp setting.

5-12. Answer = (b). If there are 180 pulses in 0.5 second, there are 360 pulses per second. The numbers of pulses per second are 60 for single-phase, half-wave; 120 for single-phase, full-wave; 360 for three-phase, 6-pulse; 720 for three-phase, 12-pulse; 10,000 or more for high frequency; and no pulses (no ripple) for constant potential.

5-13. Answer = (a). Single-phase generators have 100% ripple. See the data in the Basic Concepts section for the other generators.

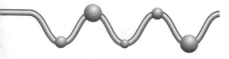

5-14. Answer = (b). The saturation voltage is around 40 kVp.

5-15. Answer = (e). A timer that uses a radiation detector to terminate the exposure is called either a phototimer or an AEC (automatic exposure control) circuit.

5-16. Answer = (c). A mechanical timer has exposure times of greater than 1 second. The shortest time for a synchronous timer is 1/60 second (or 16.7 milliseconds). An mAs timer does not adjust exposure time; it monitors the total amount of electron flow or mAs. AEC timers (with forced extinction circuits) can produce exposures down to 2 to 3 milliseconds, but the circuit does not allow the operator to select the exposure time. The most common timer circuit is the R-C circuit, which adjusts the time through a variable resistor, therefore affecting the time required to charge the capacitor in the circuit.

5-17. Answer = (d). The timer must operate at low voltages. It is a switch on the primary side of the step-up, high-voltage transformer.

5-18. Answer = (b). A capacitor stores charge. The rate of charge storage is an exponential function dependent on the product of resistance and capacitance.

5-19. Answer = (c). Resistors change the rate of electron flow. Capacitors and transformers function only with AC voltage. Capacitors store charge, and transformers either increase or decrease the voltage. Diodes allow the electrons to flow in only one direction. An inductor tries to maintain a steady current flow and causes a phase change in the AC waveform.

5-20. Answer = (b). Ohm's law can be written several ways: $I = V/R$, $V = IR$, and $R = V/I$.

5-21. Answer = (c). A transformer requires AC voltage, and it merely multiples the voltage. Resistors, filaments, and conductors (wires) can operate with either AC or DC voltage. An x-ray tube should only be operated with DC voltage, but dental (single-phase, self-rectified circuits) units operate with AC voltage directly applied to the x-ray tube.

5-22. Answer = (d). The power for the transformer is nearly 100% on both sides of the transformer; it does not change from the primary to the secondary side of the transformer.

5-23. Answer = (d). The most x-ray production is achieved with 0% ripple on the x-ray tube voltage. Ripple reduces x-ray production, and it has a lower average voltage on the x-ray tube. For these reasons, exposure time must increase for significant ripple; the patient radiation exposure increases for x-ray equipment that has considerable ripple, such as single-phase generators. The image contrast will increase owing to the lower energy x-rays produced.

5-24. Answer = (d). The tube current ammeter must be somewhere in the x-ray tube circuit at a low voltage. It is usually placed at the center tap on the secondary side of the step-up transformer. The center tap is usually grounded at near-zero voltage.

5-25. Answer = (b). A filament current of around 3 to 6 amps (3000 to 6000 mA) is usually required before the filament gets hot enough to release electrons by thermionic emissions. Regulating the filament current can release more or fewer electrons by heating the filament either more or less. The tube current can then be varied from 10 to 1000 mA, depending on the generator design.

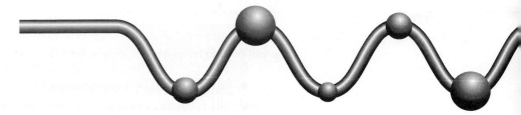

X-ray Interactions with Matter

A. Basic Concepts

1. X-ray transmission through matter is an exponential function.

- It depends on the **mass attenuation coefficient (μ/ρ),** expressed in cm^2/g.
- It depends on the density of the material, ρ, expressed in g/cm^3.
- It depends on the thickness of the material, t, expressed in cm.
- The incident x-ray intensity is I_0, and the intensity of the x-rays after they pass through the material is I_T.

  $I_T = I_0 \exp [-(\mu/\rho)\rho t]$

- The product of the mass attenuation coefficient and the density has a special name; it is called the **linear attenuation coefficient, μ.**

  $\mu = (\mu/\rho)\rho$

- The unit of the linear attenuation coefficient is cm^{-1}.

2. The thickness of any given material that reduces the x-ray intensity to 50% (half) is called the **half-value layer (HVL).**

3. The HVL depends on the atomic number of the material (Z), the density of the material, and the energy of the incident x-rays.

- HVL is related to the linear attenuation coefficient, μ.
- For a **monoenergetic** x-ray beam (which consists of x-rays with a single energy), each additional HVL reduces the intensity by another one half.

NO. OF HALF-VALUE LAYERS	% X-RAYS TRANSMITTED
1	50
2	25
3	12.5
4	6.25

  $HVL = [0.693/\mu]$ and $\mu = [0.693/HVL]$

- Thus, the HVL can be determined from the linear attenuation coefficient, and the linear attenuation can be determined from the HVL.
- For many calculations, the amount of x-rays penetrating through a material can be easily determined by using the number of HVLs. Using the HVL reduces the need to use the exponential equation for x-ray transmission.

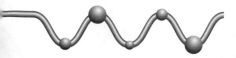

4. The mass attenuation coefficient is dependent on the material and the energy of the x-ray photons.

- It is not dependent on the density of the material.

- Various types of x-ray interactions occur in the material.

- These interactions are coherent scatter, photoelectric effect, Compton scatter, pair production, and photonuclear disintegration.

- Each type of interaction has its own mass attenuation coefficient.

- The total mass attenuation coefficient is the sum of the mass attenuation coefficients for the various types of interactions.

$$(\mu/\rho)_{TOTAL} = (\mu/\rho)_{COHERENT} + (\mu/\rho)_{PHOTOELECTRIC} + (\mu/\rho)_{COMPTON} + \cdots$$

- For diagnostic x-rays in the range of 10 to 150 keV, *coherent scatter, photoelectric effect, and Compton scatter are the predominant types of interactions*. The other types of interactions (pair production and photonuclear disintegration) occur only at much higher photon energies.

5. *Coherent scatter* contributes only 2% to 12% of all photon interactions in a material. In this interaction, the x-ray photon interacts with the orbital electrons of the atoms and the photon disappears. The orbital electrons are displaced by the input of energy and oscillate in an excited state for a very short period of time (10^{-24} second). The energy is released in the form of another photon of identical energy, but it travels in a different direction. The term coherent means no loss of energy. Other names for coherent scatter are elastic scatter, Raleigh scatter, and Thompson scatter.

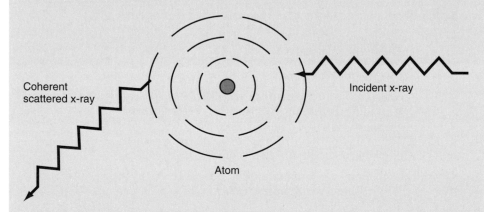

Coherent scattered x-ray

Incident x-ray

Atom

6. *Photoelectric effect* is strongly dependent on the x-ray energy and the atomic number of the material. In this interaction, the x-ray photon interacts with an inner shell electron of an atom. If the photon energy is greater than the binding energy, the x-ray photon disappears, and its energy is used to break the binding energy and impart the remaining energy to the dislodged electron as kinetic energy of motion (speed). After the removal of the inner shell electron, the other orbital electrons rearrange themselves to fill the vacancy; this rearrangement produces either a characteristic x-ray or an Auger electron. In body tissues, the characteristic x-rays are very low in energy, do not travel very far, and need not be considered.

- Energy of photoelectron = [energy of the incident x-rays] − [orbital binding energy of the material].

- For low-Z materials such as tissue and bone, the photoelectric effect is important only at low x-ray energies.

- For high-Z materials such as iodine contrast and barium, photoelectric interactions dominate at all diagnostic x-ray energies.

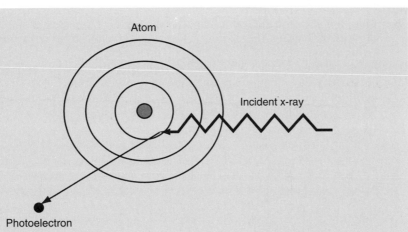

- The number of photoelectric interactions decreases rapidly at the higher x-ray energies.

$$(\mu/\rho)_{\text{PHOTOELECTRIC}} = \text{constant} \times [Z/E_x]^3$$

- For example, as the material is changed from tissue (Z ~ 7) to bone (Z ~ 14), the mass attenuation coefficient for the photoelectric effect increases $(14/7)^3 = 8$ times.

- For example, as the x-ray photon energy increases from 40 to 80 keV, the mass attenuation coefficient for the photoelectric effect decreases $(40/80)^3 = (1/8)$ times.

- There are no scattered photons from the photoelectric effect.

- All energy from the photoelectric effect is deposited locally and contributes significantly to the patient's radiation dose.

- The photoelectric effect produces the best tissue contrast of the various types of interactions, but low x-ray tube kVp values are necessary for this to be the dominant type of interaction.

7. **Compton scatter** interactions primarily depend on the electron density of the material. The electron density is related to the ratio Z/A, where A is the mass number of the material and Z is the effective atomic number. Except for hydrogen, where Z/A = 1.0, the electron density is nearly the same in all materials (Z/A ~ ½). Moreover, the mass attenuation coefficient for Compton scatter does not change much with energy in the diagnostic x-ray range. In this interaction, the x-ray photon usually collides with an outer shell electron of the material. The x-ray has a "billiard ball" type of collision with this electron. The x-ray imparts part of its energy to the outer shell electron (which has little binding energy), which is knocked loose from the atom. The x-ray is deflected at a angle (θ) and continues on its way in a different direction with reduced energy (longer wavelength).

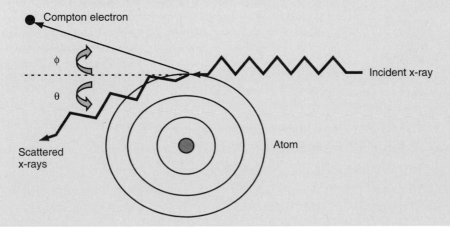

8. Compton scatter usually dominates at the higher x-ray energies because the photoelectric effect interactions are decreasing with higher x-ray energy. At some energy, the probabilities of photoelectric effect and Compton scatter are equal; this is called the ***crossover energy***. At x-ray energies above the crossover value, Compton scatter interactions dominate. Below this energy, the dominant interaction is the photoelectric effect. These crossover energies are listed in the table for various materials.

MATERIAL	CROSSOVER ENERGY
Fat	22 keV
Muscle	25 keV
Bone	44 keV
Iodine	240 keV
Barium	270 keV

9. The energy of Compton-scattered x-rays depends on the scatter angle.

   - The scattered x-rays have the most energy for zero angle scatter.

   - The x-rays have the least retained energy for 180-degree angle scatter.

   - In the diagnostic energy range, the 180-degree Compton-scattered x-rays still retain 65% to 80% of their initial (prior to scatter) energy.

   - At very high energies (5 MeV or higher), the 180-degree Compton-scattered x-rays retain only 0.25 MeV regardless of their initial energy.

   - The energy of a scattered photon (E') depends on the scatter angle (θ) and its initial energy (E_0):

     $$E' = E_0/[1 + \alpha(1 - \cos \theta)]$$

     where $\alpha = E_0/511$ keV.

10. ***Pair production*** can occur when a high-energy photon approaches the nucleus of an atom. If the incident photon has more than 1.02 MeV of energy, the photon can disappear and the energy is transformed to produce two particles: a negatively charged electron and a positively charged electron (positron). Each requires 0.511 MeV (511 keV) of energy to be created. Any additional energy provides kinetic energy (speed) to the particles.

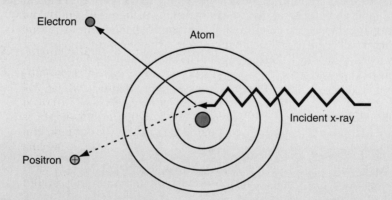

   - At 2.04 MeV, triplet production is possible: two electrons and a positron.

   - The photon disappears.

   - ***Pair production is not possible for energies of less than 1.02 MeV*** (or 1020 keV). Hence, it is not important for diagnostic radiology.

   - At the higher energies, pair production increases, whereas Compton and photoelectric interactions are of reduced probability.

11. In ***photonuclear disintegration***, a high-energy photon penetrates the nucleus and deposits its energy. The excess energy in the nucleus results in a particle being ejected from the nucleus. The ejected particle is often a neutron.

- The threshold energy for this interaction to occur is around 5 to 10 MeV.
- This interaction is therefore not important for diagnostic x-rays.

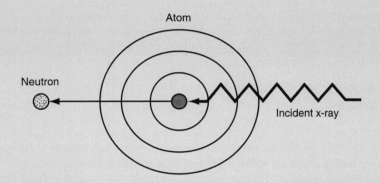

12. ***Summary:***

- For low x-ray energies and/or high atomic number (Z) materials, photoelectric interactions dominate. The photoelectric effect does not produce scattered x-rays.
- For higher diagnostic x-ray energies (more than 25 to 45 keV) with medium to low atomic number materials, Compton interactions dominate and produce scattered x-rays.
- For contrast materials such as iodine or barium, the high atomic number of the substance means that the photoelectric effect always dominates.
- When the photoelectric effect dominates, the tissue contrast differences are more pronounced.
- For air versus tissue, it is the large density difference that produces the difference in x-ray attenuation and affects the image contrast.

B. Questions

6-1. In _____ interactions between x-rays and matter, the scattered photon has a different direction and different energy.

(a) Photoelectric effect   (b) Compton scatter   (c) Coherent scatter
(d) Pair production   (e) Photonuclear disintegration   (f) All of the above

6-2. In _____ interactions between x-rays and matter, the scattered photon has a different direction and the same initial energy.

(a) Photoelectric effect   (b) Compton scatter   (c) Coherent scatter
(d) Pair production   (e) Photonuclear disintegration   (f) All of the above

6-3. The most prevalent x-ray interaction at diagnostic x-ray energies (60 to 150 kVp) in tissue is _____.

(a) Photoelectric effect   (b) Compton scatter   (c) Coherent scatter
(d) Pair production   (e) Photonuclear disintegration   (f) All of the above

6-4. The dominant interaction in iodine contrast media at diagnostic x-ray energies is _____.

(a) Photoelectric effect   (b) Compton scatter   (c) Coherent scatter
(d) Pair production   (e) Photonuclear disintegration   (f) All of the above

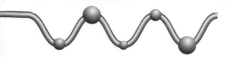

6-5. At diagnostic x-ray energies, the _____ interaction between x-rays and matter has the same mass attenuation coefficient in all elements of the atomic table (except for hydrogen).

(a) Photoelectric effect   (b) Compton scatter   (c) Coherent scatter
(d) Pair production   (e) Photonuclear disintegration   (f) All of the above

6-6. The _____ interaction between x-rays and matter depends strongly on the atomic number (Z) of the attenuation material.

(a) Photoelectric effect   (b) Compton scatter   (c) Coherent scatter
(d) Pair production   (e) Photonuclear disintegration   (f) All of the above

6-7. In the _____ interaction between x-rays and matter, the photon disappears, and an electron and a positron are created.

(a) Photoelectric effect   (b) Compton scatter   (c) Coherent scatter
(d) Pair production   (e) Photonuclear disintegration   (f) All of the above

6-8. The _____ interaction between x-rays and matter requires photon energies greater than 5 to 10 MeV.

(a) Photoelectric effect   (b) Compton scatter   (c) Coherent scatter
(d) Pair production   (e) Photonuclear disintegration   (f) All of the above

6-9. The _____ interaction between x-rays and matter requires photon energies greater than 1.02 MeV before it can occur.

(a) Photoelectric effect   (b) Compton scatter   (c) Coherent scatter
(d) Pair production   (e) Photonuclear disintegration   (f) All of the above

6-10. The probability of _____ interaction between x-rays and matter decreases in inverse proportion to the photon energy cubed.

(a) Photoelectric effect   (b) Compton scatter   (c) Coherent scatter
(d) Pair production   (e) Photonuclear disintegration   (f) All of the above

6-11. For incident photons with high energies, the _____ interaction between x-rays and matter results in photons that are scattered primarily in the forward direction.

(a) Photoelectric effect   (b) Compton scatter   (c) Coherent scatter
(d) Pair production   (e) Photonuclear disintegration   (f) All of the above

6-12. The probability of _____ interaction between x-rays and matter depends primarily on the electron density of the attenuation material.

(a) Photoelectric effect   (b) Compton scatter   (c) Coherent scatter
(d) Pair production   (e) Photonuclear disintegration   (f) All of the above

6-13. The _____ and _____ interactions do not occur at diagnostic x-ray energies.

(a) Photoelectric effect   (b) Compton scatter   (c) Coherent scatter
(d) Pair production   (e) Photonuclear disintegration   (f) All of the above

6-14. The probability of _____ interaction between x-rays and matter depends on the physical density of the attenuation material.

(a) Photoelectric effect   (b) Compton scatter   (c) Coherent scatter
(d) Pair production   (e) Photonuclear disintegration   (f) All of the above

6-15. The probability of _____ interaction between x-rays and matter depends on the thickness of the attenuation material.

(a) Photoelectric effect   (b) Compton scatter   (c) Coherent scatter
(d) Pair production   (e) Photonuclear disintegration
(f) All of the above

6-16. The primary shielding material for diagnostic x-rays is _____.

(a) Acrylic   (b) Concrete   (c) Steel   (d) Barium   (e) Lead

6-17. A 10-MeV x-ray that is Compton scattered through a 180-degree angle has an energy of about _____ MeV.

(a) 0.10   (b) 0.25   (c) 0.51   (d) 1.02   (e) 9.9

6-18. A 100-keV x-ray that is Compton scattered through a 180-degree angle has an energy of about _____ keV.

(a) 11   (b) 33   (c) 54   (d) 72   (e) 88

6-19. The x-ray energy at which Compton scatter and the photoelectric effect have an equal probability of occurring in tissue is _____ keV.

(a) 25   (b) 44   (c) 88   (d) 169   (e) 240

6-20. The x-ray energy at which Compton scatter and the photoelectric effect have an equal probability of occurring in bone is _____ keV.

(a) 25   (b) 44   (c) 88   (d) 169   (e) 240

6-21. The x-ray energy at which Compton scatter and the photoelectric effect have an equal probability of occurring in barium is _____ keV.

(a) 25   (b) 44   (c) 88   (d) 169   (e) 240

6-22. The photon interaction that is most responsible for contrast degradation in diagnostic radiographs is _____.

(a) Photoelectric effect   (b) Compton scatter   (c) Coherent scatter
(d) Pair production   (e) Photonuclear disintegration

6-23. The photon interaction that produces the greatest contrast differences in calcium clusters in mammography images is _____.

(a) Photoelectric effect   (b) Compton scatter   (c) Coherent scatter
(d) Pair production   (e) Photonuclear disintegration

6-24. The Compton-scattered x-rays lose the most energy at scatter angles of _____ degrees.

(a) 0   (b) 90   (c) 180   (d) 270   (e) 360

6-25. The approximate amount of x-ray scatter at a 90-degree angle is _____ % of the incident exposure at 1 meter from the scatter medium.

(a) 0.1   (b) 0.5   (c) 1.0   (d) 2.5   (e) 5.0   (f) 10.0

6-26. A 100-keV x-ray photon has a photoelectric interaction with the K-shell electron of a molybdenum atom. (Binding energy of the K-shell electron of molybdenum is about 20 keV.) The energy of the ejected electron is ____ keV.

(a) 20   (b) 50   (c) 70   (d) 80   (e) 100

6-27. Injected contrast medium influences the x-ray attenuation because of the property of _____.

(a) High density   (b) Lower density   (c) Higher atomic number (Z)
(d) None of the above   (e) All of the above

6-28. X-ray transmission through matter is mathematically modeled by a(n) _____ function.

(a) Logarithmic   (b) Exponential   (c) Power   (d) Inverse square
(e) Linear

6-29. After a photoelectric interaction, _____ can occur.

(a) Coherent scatter   (b) Compton scatter   (c) Photoelectric effect
(d) Characteristic x-ray emission   (e) Positron emission

6-30. The percent x-ray transmission increases when _____ is used.

(a) High kVp   (b) More kVp ripple   (c) Low x-ray beam filtration
(d) Increased mAs   (e) All of the above

C. Answers

6-1. Answer = (b). The answer requires a scattered photon. Photoelectric effect, pair production, and photonuclear disintegration do not produce scattered photons.

In coherent interactions, the x-rays do not lose any energy; they just change directions. In Compton scatter, the photons change direction and lose some energy to the ejected Compton (outer shell) electrons.

6-2. Answer = (c). See explanation in answer to Question 6-1.

6-3. Answer = (b). The average x-ray photon energy is about half the kVp in units of keV. So the average energy range of diagnostic x-rays (excluding mammography) is 30 to 75 keV. For tissue, Compton scatter dominates above 25 keV. Coherent scatter is not significant (<10% interactions) at these energies. Pair production and photonuclear disintegration do not occur until much higher photon energies.

6-4. Answer = (a). Because of the high atomic number of iodine, photoelectric interactions dominate throughout the diagnostic x-ray energies.

6-5. Answer = (b). Because Compton scatter interactions depend on electron density and the electron density is nearly the same for all elements except hydrogen, the mass attenuation coefficient is nearly the same for all elements at diagnostic x-ray energies.

6-6. Answer = (a). The mass attenuation coefficient for photoelectric interactions increases with $[Z/E_x]^3$.

6-7. Answer = (d). The incident photon disappears in the following interactions: photoelectric effect, pair production, and photonuclear disintegration. In the photoelectric effect, the photon disappears and an inner shell electron is knocked loose; later, a characteristic x-ray is emitted as the orbital electrons rearrange themselves. In pair production, an electron and a positron are produced. In photonuclear disintegration, a nuclear particle is knocked out of the nucleus.

6-8. Answer = (e). The incident photon needs considerable energy to penetrate into the nucleus and knock a nucleon out of the nucleus.

6-9. Answer = (d). The "$E = mc^2$" requires 0.511 MeV = 511 keV to create either an electron or a positron. To create both, double this energy is needed, or 1.02 MeV.

6-10. Answer = (a). The mass attenuation coefficient for photoelectric interactions depends on $[Z/E_x]^3$.

6-11. Answer = (b). Only two interactions result in scattered photons: Compton and coherent. In Compton scattering, the scattered photons are primarily aimed forward at high incident photon energies and are uniformly (isotropically) scattered at low energies.

6-12. Answer = (b). The mass attenuation coefficient for Compton scatter in the diagnostic x-ray range does not change much with energy or atomic number, except for hydrogen. The coefficient is dependent on the electron density of the attenuation material, which is nearly constant for all materials unless they contain considerable hydrogen.

6-13. Answer = (d) and (e). Pair production requires a minimum of at least 1.02 MeV before it can occur. Photonuclear disintegration requires very high energy photons in the 5 to 10 MeV region or higher.

6-14. Answer = (f). The transmission of x-rays is equal to $I = I_0 \exp[-(\mu/\rho) \times \rho \times t]$. Thus, all interactions depend on the density and thickness of the attenuation material.

6-15. Answer = (f). The transmission of x-rays is equal to $I = I_0 \exp[-(\mu/\rho) \times \rho \times t]$. Thus, all interactions depend on the density and thickness of the attenuation material.

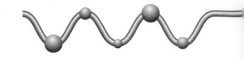

6-16. Answer = (e). Lead, because of its high atomic number (Z = 84) and density (ρ = 19.2), can attenuate diagnostic x-rays several orders of magnitude with a thickness of only 1.5 mm. It is relatively inexpensive and abundant, making it ideal for shielding x-ray radiation.

6-17. Answer = (b). All very high energy photons (above several MeV) result in 180-degree Compton scatter, producing 0.25-MeV photons. This is because the equation for Compton scatter reduces to $E_0/[1 + 2\alpha] \cong E_0/[2\alpha] = [E_0 \times 511 \text{ KeV}]/[2 \times E_0] = 511 \text{ keV}/2$.

6-18. Answer = (d). First, when low-energy x-rays are scattered—even through 180 degrees—they retain most of their energy. For x-rays below 100 keV, the 180-degree scattered x-rays retain 70% or more of their initial energy. So the answer must be either (d) or (e). The equation yields $100 \text{ keV}/[1 + 2\alpha] = 100 \text{ keV}/[1 + 0.4] = 71.4$.

6-19. Answer = (a). The equal probability of photoelectric effect and Compton scatter in tissue occurs at 25 keV. At higher energies, Compton scatter dominates. This is an important fact to remember.

6-20. Answer = (b). Because of the higher atomic number of bone (Z = 14), the energy at which Compton scatter dominates is higher. Because the Z of bone is about double that of tissue, the crossover energy should be about double that of tissue.

6-21. Answer = (e). The atomic number (Z) of barium is 56, which is about four times larger than the Z of bone. Thus, the crossover energy at which Compton scatter dominates over the photoelectric effect should be at least 4×44 keV. The actual value is even higher at 240 keV.

6-22. Answer = (b). For diagnostic x-rays, only three interactions with matter are dominant: coherent scatter, photoelectric effect, and Compton scatter. Coherent scatter accounts for only about 7% to 14% of all interactions at diagnostic energies; thus, it is not very significant. Compton scatter produces scattered x-rays, which degrade contrast in the images. The photoelectric effect does not produce scattered x-rays.

6-23. Answer = (a). As per the previous answer, only the photoelectric effect and Compton scatter are important for diagnostic x-rays. The relative amount of each type of interaction is independent of the density and thickness of the anatomy. In addition, the photoelectric effect depends on the cube of the atomic number of the material, whereas Compton scatter scales only with electron density, which is nearly the same in most tissue.

6-24. Answer = (c). The largest scatter angles result in the lowest retained energy for the Compton-scattered x-rays. However, the largest scatter angle is 180 degrees. An angle of 270 degrees is equal to 90 degrees, and 360 degrees is the same as 0 degrees.

6-25. Answer = (a). A generalization to remember is that the scattered radiation at 1 meter from the entrance surface is about 0.1% of the exposure level at the entrance surface. If a patient receives a fluoroscopy entrance surface exposure rate of 1 R per minute, the scattered radiation level at 1 meter away is about 1 mR per minute.

6-26. Answer = (d). The ejected electron energy is the incident photon energy minus the binding energy of the K-shell of the target material. In this case, it is 100 keV minus 20 keV, which equals 80 keV.

6-27. Answer = (e). Contrast media can be barium or iodine, which have higher density and higher atomic number than tissue. Air can also be used as a contrast medium; the low density of air makes it different from tissue.

6-28. Answer = (b). X-ray transmission is an exponential process.

6-29. Answer = (d). Following the photoelectric effect, there is a vacancy in the K-shell orbital electrons of the target atom. When the electrons rearrange themselves to fill the K-shell vacancy, a characteristic x-ray is emitted.

6-30. Answer = (a). Higher energy x-rays are more penetrating. Low kVp and less filtration produce lower energy x-rays. mAs affects only the number of x-rays and not the energy of the x-rays. With more x-rays, there are more x-rays penetrating the target; however, the percent transmission is the same so long as the energy is the same.

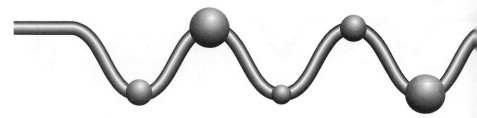

CHAPTER SEVEN

X-ray Filters

A. Basic Concepts

1. X-ray beam filters include any materials in the path of the x-rays (generated inside the x-ray tube) that must pass through the glass tube, housing, and collimator.

2. There are two basic types of filters:

- *Inherent filters* are materials that cannot be removed from the x-ray beam. These inherent filters include the glass wall of the x-ray tube, the oil inside the x-ray tube housing, and the mirror in the collimator. Typically, inherent filters have the equivalence of 0.5 to 1.5 mm of aluminum.

- *Added filters* are materials that can be removed from the x-ray beam. Added filters are usually metals such as aluminum or copper in radiographic and fluoroscopic x-ray tubes or molybdenum or rhodium in mammography tubes. In radiographic x-ray tubes, the added filters are typically 0.0 to 3.0 mm of aluminum. In cardiac and angiography x-ray tubes, the added filtration is more; these x-ray tubes can have up to 0.9 mm of copper filtration.

3. Filters affect both the *quantity* and *quality* of the x-ray beam.

- *Quantity* is the energy in the x-ray beam (number of x-rays and energies), and it is usually expressed as the measured exposure in mR or coulombs/kg.

- *Quality* is the penetration of the x-ray beam, and it is expressed by its half-value layer (HVL) in millimeters of aluminum.

4. The basic purpose of filters is to remove preferentially more of the low-energy x-rays than the high-energy x-rays (which reduces the patient's radiation dose). See the accompanying graph.

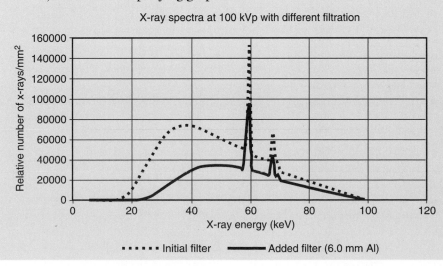

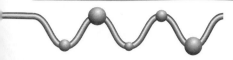

5. The remaining x-rays are more penetrating, and the radiation dose to the patient is reduced because fewer incident x-rays are required to get the necessary radiation to the image receptor.

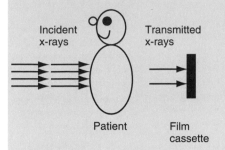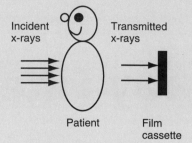

Lower filtration x-rays are less penetrating and more incident x-rays are required to have adequate x-rays at film cassette

High filtration x-rays are more penetrating. A smaller number of incident x-rays can be used to get the same number of x-rays onto the film cassette.

6. The effects of added filtration on the x-ray beam are the following:

   ● There are fewer x-rays in the x-ray beam because the filter absorbs or scatters x-rays, or both.

   ● More low-energy than high-energy x-rays are removed.

   ● Thus, the average energy of all the remaining x-rays is increased.

   ● The maximum energy is always controlled by and numerically equal to the kVp.

   $E_{max} = kVp$

   ● Average x-ray energy = E_{aver} = 1/3 to 1/2 $E_{max.}$

   ● The average x-ray energy is higher after more filtration.

   ● The minimum x-ray energy is higher because the lowest energy x-rays, which are not very penetrating, have been eliminated. The longest wavelength (lowest energy) is now slightly shorter.

   ● The remaining x-rays are more penetrating and have a longer HVL.

   ● Because x-rays are removed by the filters, fewer x-rays remain, which may necessitate the usage of more mAs.

   ● Because of the aforementioned loss of x-rays and more mAs, the exposure time required for clinical images may increase, resulting in more motion blur.

   ● More mAs means more x-ray tube heating effects. The reduced number of x-rays and greater mAs needed to produce images with filtration reduce tube life.

7. The effects of added filtration on the patient and radiographic image are the following:

   ● Added filtration reduces the patient's radiation dose by 30% to 60% because the remaining x-rays are more penetrating and fewer incident x-rays can be used.

   ● Added filtration causes a decrease in subject contrast by removing the lower energy x-rays, which interact primarily by means of the photoelectric effect.

   ● The higher energy x-rays that remain after filtration interact mostly by means of Compton scatter, and the scattered x-rays degrade subject contrast.

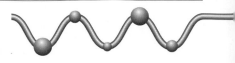

- Image quality is degraded because of the aforementioned effects.
- The absorption efficiency of the image receptor decreases because of the greater penetration of the high-energy photons.

8. The HVL increases with added filtration of the x-ray beam. It is usually measured in the thickness of aluminum required to reduce the radiation exposure to exactly 50%. The HVL of diagnostic x-rays is usually 2.5 to 8.0 mm of aluminum.

   - Measured HVL is greater with increasing kVp.
   - Measured HVL is greater with more x-ray tube filtration material.
   - Measured HVL is **not** the same value as the actual amount of material in the x-ray beam.
   - The measurement conditions for HVL require a narrowly collimated x-ray beam, placement of the detector far from the aluminum sheets used to measure the HVL to eliminate inclusion of scattered photons, pure aluminum sheets, and a radiation detector that has a relatively uniform response to different x-ray energies.

9. Federal requirements for filtration can be specified in two different ways: the minimum measured HVL allowed or the minimum amount of material allowed in the x-ray beam.

10. The purpose of these limits is to ensure adequate filtration in the x-ray beam to remove the lowest energy x-rays, which contribute significantly to the patient's radiation dose. These lowest energy x-rays do not have adequate energy to penetrate through the patient to reach the image receptor.

11. Federal requirements for HVL limits are the following:

    - Mammography:

      $HVL > (kVp/100) + 0.03$ in mm Al eq

      $HVL < (kVp/100) + C$ in mm Al eq

      where $C = 0.12$ for Mo/Mo, 0.19 Mo/Rh, and 0.21 for Rh/Rh.

    - Diagnostic above 71 kVp:

      $HVL > (2.2)(kVp/100) + 0.56$ in mm Al eq

12. Federal requirements for the minimum amount of material to be placed in the path of an x-ray beam:

    - Below 30 kVp: total filtration > 0.3 mm Al eq
    - Between 30 and 50 kVp: total filtration > 0.5 mm Al eq
    - Between 50 and 70 kVp: total filtration > 1.5 mm Al eq
    - Above 70 kVp: total filtration > 2.5 mm Al eq

13. For tissue, the HVL for mammography x-ray beams is about 1 cm of compressed tissue. For diagnostic x-ray beams, the HVL in tissue depends on the kVp used for the examination; however, the HVL is typically between 3.0 and 5.0 cm of tissue. Therefore, a 24-cm-thick patient is about 6 HVL, and only 1% to 5% of the incident x-rays actually pass through the patient.

14. **Summary:** Too little filtration results in a high radiation dose to the patient because of inclusion of many low-energy x-rays that cannot penetrate through the patient. Too much filtration results in degraded image quality because high-energy x-rays produce less subject contrast and more Compton-scattered x-rays.

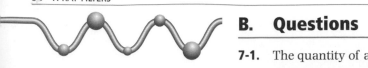

B. Questions

7-1. The quantity of an x-ray beam is usually measured in units of _____.

(a) Number of photons   (b) Coul/kg of air   (c) keV
(d) mm Al eq   (e) dB

7-2. Added filtration to an x-ray beam _____ the quantity of the x-rays.

(a) Does not change   (b) Increases   (c) Decreases
(d) Cannot be determined

7-3. The quality of an x-ray beam is usually measured in units of _____.

(a) Number of photons   (b) Coul/kg of air   (c) keV
(d) mm Al eq   (e) dB

7-4. The quality of an x-ray beam increases with an increase in _____.

(a) kVp only   (b) kVp and mA only   (c) kVp, mA, and time
(d) kVp and filtration   (e) kVp, filtration, and ripple

7-5. The quantity of an x-ray beam increases with an increase in _____.

(a) kVp only   (b) kVp and mA only   (c) kVp, mA, and time
(d) kVp and filtration   (e) kVp, filtration, and ripple

7-6. Good geometry for HVL measurements requires all of the following, *except* _____.

(a) Narrow x-ray beam   (b) Detector close to aluminum sheets
(c) Air gap   (d) Small detector size
(e) Detector with uniform energy response

7-7. If 6% of the incident x-rays pass through a portion of the patient's anatomy that is 20 cm thick, the HVL of that tissue is about _____. (Neglect beam hardening.)

(a) 2 cm   (b) 3 cm   (c) 4 cm   (d) 5 cm   (e) 6 cm

7-8. The typical value of HVL for an 80-kVp x-ray beam is about _____ mm Al eq.

(a) 20 μm   (b) 0.4 mm   (c) 0.35 cm   (d) 0.07 m   (e) 0.05 inch

7-9. The typical HVL in lead of a normally filtered 100-kVp x-ray beam is about _____ mm.

(a) 0.02   (b) 0.10   (c) 0.25   (d) 0.5   (e) 1.0

7-10. A 0.5-mm leaded radiation protection apron transmits about _____ of the incident x-rays.

(a) 25%   (b) 10%   (c) 5%   (d) 1%   (e) 0.25%

7-11. X-ray beams with low HVL values generally result in _____ radiation dose to the patient and _____ image subject contrast.

(a) Increased, increased   (b) Increased, decreased   (c) Decreased, increased
(d) Decreased, decreased   (e) Decreased, no change in

7-12. Increased x-ray beam HVLs generally result in _____ quantity and _____ quality.

(a) Increased, increased   (b) Increased, decreased   (c) Decreased, increased
(d) Decreased, decreased   (e) Decreased, no change in

7-13. Regulatory agencies specify that the filtration of an x-ray beam used clinically at 71 kVp must have a measured HVL of at least _____ mm of aluminum equivalent.

(a) 1.0   (b) 1.5   (c) 2.1   (d) 2.7   (e) 3.3

7-14. The reason for the regulatory limits on minimum measured HVL is to
_____.

(a) Decrease motion blur   (b) Reduce patient's radiation dose
(c) Decrease focal spot size   (d) Improve subject contrast
(e) Reduce anode heating

7-15. Detrimental effects of added x-ray beam filtration include all of the following,
except _____.

(a) Increased image unsharpness   (b) Reduction of contrast
(c) Reduction of x-ray tube life   (d) More scattered photons
(e) Latent image fading

7-16. For mammography with a molybdenum anode and filter, regulations require
the measured HVL at 27 kVp to be at least _____ mm of aluminum
equivalent.

(a) 0.10   (b) 0.30   (c) 0.50   (d) 1.0   (e) 1.5

7-17. Mammography regulations specify lower measured HVL values for the x-ray
beam for all of the following reasons, *except* _____.

(a) Lower kVp values are used   (b) Anatomic thickness is less
(c) Subject contrast is needed   (d) Breast radiation dose sensitivity is low
(e) Motion blur concerns exist

7-18. K-edge filters refer to _____.

(a) Greater and discontinuous attenuation at K-shell binding energy of the filter
(b) Characteristic x-rays of the anode
(c) Potassium-based x-ray filters
(d) Artifacts at the edge of the collimator
(e) Different copper alloys

7-19. Added filters degrade image contrast because _____.

(a) Characteristic x-rays are emitted from the filter
(b) Average x-ray energies into the Compton region are higher
(c) Average x-ray energies are lower into photoelectric region
(d) Filters make grids ineffective
(e) Filters reduce image receptor efficiency

7-20. The shortest wavelength x-rays are affected primarily by the _____.

(a) Filtration   (b) Ripple   (c) kVp   (d) mA   (e) Focal spot size

7-21. The longest wavelength x-rays (emerging from the x-ray tube and collimator)
are affected primarily by the _____.

(a) Filtration   (b) Ripple   (c) kVp   (d) mA   (e) Focal spot size

7-22. The average energy of an x-ray spectrum is affected by all of the following,
except _____.

(a) Filtration   (b) Ripple   (c) kVp   (d) mA   (e) Anode material

7-23. Lower energy x-rays are preferentially absorbed in metallic filters because
_____ occurs more often at low energies.

(a) Coherent scatter   (b) Photoelectric effect   (c) Compton scatter
(d) Pair production   (e) Inverse square effect

7-24. The following materials have all been used as filtration in diagnostic x-ray
beams, *except* _____.

(a) Aluminum   (b) Copper   (c) Molybdenum   (d) Rhodium   (e) Lead

7-25. The average energy of a 100-kVp beam is about _____ keV.

(a) 10   (b) 25   (c) 40   (d) 69.5   (e) 77.7

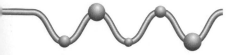

C. Answers

7-1. Answer = (b). Quantity is measured by the effect of the x-rays on air in terms of exposure in units of either milliroentgens (mR) or coulombs per kg of air. Quantity increases with: higher kVp, more mAs, or less filtration.

7-2. Answer = (c). The filters preferentially remove the low-energy x-rays, leaving the higher energy x-rays. The average energy increases; however, the total number of x-rays is smaller because a significant number of low-energy x-rays are removed by the filter.

7-3. Answer = (d). The quality is the measure of the penetration of the x-ray beam. It is usually given as the HVL of the beam in mm of aluminum. As the penetration increases, more mm of aluminum are required to reduce the x-rays to 50% of the unattenuated value.

7-4. Answer = (d). Increasing the kVp results in an increase in both the maximum x-ray energy (which is equal numerically to the kVp) and the average x-ray energy. Greater filtration removes the lower energy x-rays so that the remaining x-rays have a higher average energy. The product of mA and time is the mAs, which increases only the number of x-rays; the distribution of x-ray energies is unchanged. Greater ripple in the x-ray tube voltage results in the x-rays having a lower average energy.

7-5. Answer = (c). The quantity is related to the total number of x-rays. mAs increases the number of x-rays without changing their energy distribution. Greater kVp increases both the number of x-rays and their average/maximum energy. More filtration results in fewer x-rays with a higher average energy and with greater penetration. More ripple produces fewer x-rays with a lower average energy.

7-6. Answer = (b). Measurement of HVL requires that any scatter resulting from interactions in the aluminum sheets be excluded from detection by the dosimeter. This requires an air gap and a small detector to allow the scatter to miss the detector. A narrow x-ray beam minimizes the amount of scatter. A uniform energy response allows the detector to measure all energies equally well.

7-7. Answer = (d). The first HVL reduces the intensity to 50%. The second HVL reduces the beam to 25%. The third HVL reduces the intensity to 12.5%. The fourth HVL reduces the beam to 6.25%. If four HVLs have a thickness of 20 cm, one HVL would be about 5 cm in thickness.

7-8. Answer = (c). At 80 kVp with routine filtration, the HVL is typically 2.4 to 4.5 mm of aluminum equivalent. Test questions can use different set of units; 3.5 mm of aluminum is equal to 0.35 cm of aluminum.

7-9. Answer = (b). A normally filtered 100-kVp beam has an HVL of 0.10 mm of lead, and a highly filtered beam (such as leakage radiation) has an HVL of about 0.24 mm of lead.

7-10. Answer = (c). If the normally filtered 100-kVp x-ray beam has an HVL of 0.10 mm of lead and a standard protective apron has 0.50 mm of lead, the protective apron has about five HVLs. A five-HVL thickness reduces the intensity to 3%. The measured value in published literature is about 4% to 6%.

7-11. Answer = (a). Low HVLs mean that the x-ray beam is lightly filtered. The average x-ray energy is low. Hence, the lower energy x-rays do not penetrate well and radiation doses are high. Low-energy x-rays have more photoelectric effect interactions in matter, which improve image contrast.

7-12. Answer = (c). If the increased HVL is due to more filtration of the x-rays, the number of x-rays decreases because of removal of low-energy x-rays, and the penetration of the remaining x-rays is greater. However, if the increased HVL is due to higher kVp, both the number of x-rays and the penetration are increased. Thus, the answer for higher kVp would be (a).

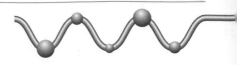

7-13. Answer = (c). Using the equation provided, specified HVL = 2.2(71/100) + 0.56 = 1.54 + 0.56 = 2.10 mm aluminum equivalent.

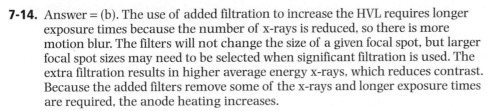

7-14. Answer = (b). The use of added filtration to increase the HVL requires longer exposure times because the number of x-rays is reduced, so there is more motion blur. The filters will not change the size of a given focal spot, but larger focal spot sizes may need to be selected when significant filtration is used. The extra filtration results in higher average energy x-rays, which reduces contrast. Because the added filters remove some of the x-rays and longer exposure times are required, the anode heating increases.

7-15. Answer = (e). Added filtration requires longer x-ray exposures and thus more motion blur (unsharpness). The higher energy x-rays produce more scatter (more Compton interactions) and reduced image contrast (less photoelectric interactions). Because of longer x-ray exposures and increased anode heating, the tube life is decreased. Latent image fading occurs when film-screen cassettes are processed much later than the x-ray exposure.

7-16. Answer = (b). For mammography with a molybdenum anode, the equation for minimum HVL is (kVp/100) + 0.03 = (27/100) + 0.03 = 0.30 mm Al eq.

7-17. Answer = (d). Lower kVp values are used in mammography to enhance subject contrast. This results in lower HVLs. Fortunately, the thickness of the compressed breast is only a few centimeters; otherwise, the radiation doses would be very high because of the lack of penetration. Minimum HVLs are specified so that the radiation dose does not become excessive; this is important because the breast tissue is sensitive to cancer risk as a result of the radiation. More filtration (to obtain higher HVLs) could result in longer exposure time and more motion blur.

7-18. Answer = (a). When the energy of the incident x-rays is less than the K-shell binding energy of the attenuation material, the photoelectric interaction can occur only with the L-shell, M-shell, and so on. At energies just above the K-shell binding energy, the interactions include the K-shell electrons, and the attenuation coefficient increases discontinuously at this point.

7-19. Answer = (b). Filters do not affect grid efficiency much. The higher energy x-rays do slightly decrease image receptor efficiency, but this has little effect on the image contrast. There are also some characteristic x-rays from the filters, but the air gap results in little effect on image contrast. The higher average x-ray energy from added filtration results in a greater portion of Compton interactions, which in turn reduces the contrast.

7-20. Answer = (c). The shortest wavelength x-rays are the highest energy x-rays. These x-rays are directly related to the kVp used. The mA affects the total number of x-rays produced; it does not affect the energy. Focal spot size affects spatial resolution, anode heating, and maximum mA that can be used.

7-21. Answer = (a). The longest wavelength x-rays are the lowest energy x-rays. The x-ray beam filtration removes many of the lower energy x-rays; thus, it controls the minimum x-ray energy emerging from the collimator.

7-22. Answer = (d). kVp controls the maximum and average energy. The filters eliminate the lowest energy x-rays so that the remaining x-rays have a higher average energy. Higher ripple in the kVp waveform reduces the average x-ray energy. The anode material determines the energy of the characteristic x-ray produced. The mA controls only the total number of x-rays, not the x-ray energy.

7-23. Answer = (b). Coherent scatter interactions affect only a small percentage of all x-ray interactions. Compton scatter interactions occur at higher x-ray energies, and pair production requires greater than 1.02 MeV. Inverse square effect is related to distance and not x-ray energy.

7-24. Answer = (e). Lead is too attenuating for most x-ray beam filtration. It is used primarily as a radiation shielding material. Be aware that special plastics with some lead content are used as "shaped filters" for scoliosis, orthopedic leg, and cardiac studies.

7-25. Answer = (c). The average energy is about 0.33 to 0.50 of the kVp; hence, the average energy for 100-kVp x-rays would be about 33 to 50 keV. For most x-ray beams, the average energy is closer to 0.5 times the kVp than to 0.33 times the kVp. The best answer in this range is 40 keV.

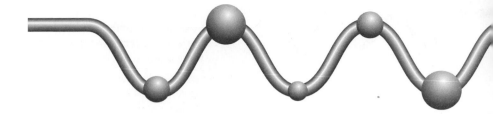

CHAPTER EIGHT

Collimators and Grids

A. Collimators

1. The **major functions of collimators** are to:

    - Prevent the irradiation of unnecessary parts of a patient's anatomy
    - Restrict x-rays so that they image only areas of clinical interest
    - Reduce scatter radiation by using a smaller field of view (FoV)
    - Improve image contrast by means of scatter reduction

2. **Types of collimation devices** include the following:

    - **Fixed aperture,** which have rectangular holes cut into metal diaphragms. These devices have been used in mammography units and linear tomography units.
    - **Cones,** which are cylinders attached to the x-ray tube to provide spacers. These devices have been used on dental units.
    - **Variable aperture,** which have two sets of orthogonal lead blades that can be adjusted to provide variable-size rectangular FoVs. These devices are the most common units used on most x-ray tubes.
    - **Iris,** which is a series of leaded blades that provide a circular FoV.

3. The number of scattered x-rays compared with unattenuated primary x-rays that pass through a patient's anatomy is called the **scatter-to-primary (S/P) ratio**.

    - S/P increases exponentially with a patient's thickness.
    - S/P increases with larger FoVs but levels out at about 1000 cm^2

    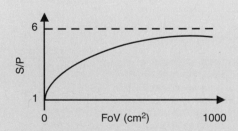

    - S/P increases with higher kVp because there is a larger percentage of Compton scatter interactions than photoelectric interactions.
    - S/P increases with greater added filtration because there is a larger percentage of Compton scatter interactions than photoelectric interactions.

4. A **positive beam limitation (PBL) device** is an automatic collimator that senses the size of the cassette and collimates the x-ray FoV to match the cassette.

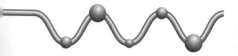

5. Federal regulations require the light and x-ray field to be congruent to within ±2% of the source-to-image receptor distance (SID) in any one orthogonal direction.

6. For *positive beam limitation* (PBL) systems, the errors in x-ray/light alignment must be less than 3% of SID in any one orthogonal direction, and the sum of errors in two orthogonal directions (without regard to positive or negative error) must be less than 4% of SID.

7. X-ray/light alignment is checked by placing pennies on the four sides of the light FoV and then taking a radiograph of the pennies to see the edges of the x-ray FoV. The distance between the edge of the pennies and the dark area on the film where the x-rays struck is measured on both sides and in two orthogonal directions. The errors on the left and right sides are added together as positive values. The summed error is divided by the SID and multiplied by 100%. The requirement is that this value be less than 2%.

B. Grids

1. The *major points regarding grids* are the following:

   - Grids remove x-rays that are scattered in the patient's body.

   - Scattered x-rays degrade the image contrast.

   - Grids tend to improve the image contrast by removing the scattered x-rays. (This reduces the S/P ratio.)

   - Unfortunately, by removing the scattered x-rays, grids results in fewer x-rays reaching the image receptor. Thus, the radiation dose to the patient must be increased to maintain the same image density for film-screen systems or the same relative noise (signal-to-noise ratio [SNR]) for digital systems.

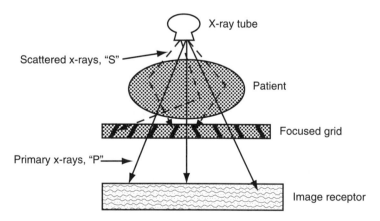

2. Grids consist of a sheet of thin lead strips spaced apart by some other material.

   - *Interspace material* is usually aluminum; however, carbon fiber is used on some grids because it attenuates less than aluminum and results in a smaller dose of radiation to the patient.

   - The ratio of the height, H, to the width between lead strips, W, is known as the grid ratio, r.

   - Grid ratios range from 6:1 up to 17:1.

   - Higher grid ratios remove more scattered x-rays, but they are sensitive to positioning errors.

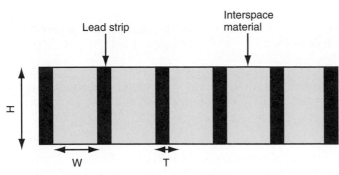

3. $r = H/W$.

4. The number of lead strips per cm, N, equals $1/(W + T)$. As N increases, the grid lines become less noticeable in the image (for grids that do not move).

5. Grids can be classified in several different ways:

   - *Focused grids*—lead strips point to the x-ray tube focal spot.
   - *Parallel grids*—lead strips are parallel.
   - *Crossed grids*—two sets of grids with grid lines perpendicular to each are sandwiched together. Their grid ratio is the sum of the grid ratios of the two grids: $r = r_1 + r_2$.
   - *Cellular grids*—instead of lead strips, grids are composed of little rectangular cells. (See the comparison drawing from the top view.) Cellular grids have been used in mammography units.

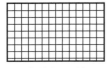

Cellular grid

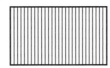

Standard linear grid

6. Grids are also classified by their motion:

   - *Bucky grids*—moving grids. Bucky grids do not show grid lines on the image because of the motion during exposure. However, these grids need slightly more radiation and longer exposure times to allow motion to blur grid lines.
   - *Stationary (or non-Bucky) grids*—grids that do not move. Generally, stationary grids are used (1) for chest x-rays, because short exposure times are used that do not allow enough time for motion, and (2) for some portable x-ray cassettes.

7. *Bucky factor* (patient's dose with grid/patient's dose without grid) = radiation transmitted through patient and incident upon the grid versus the portion of this radiation that passes through the grid to the image receptor. As the Bucky factor increases, the patient's radiation dose increases.

8. *Selectivity (Σ)*—ratio of the primary radiation transmitted through the grid divided by the scattered radiation transmitted through the grid.

   $\Sigma = T_P/T_S$

   - As the selectivity increases, more scattered x-rays are removed by the grid and the image contrast improves.

9. If C_0 is the contrast of an image with no scattered x-rays included, the contrast with scattered x-rays included (C') depends on the amount of scattered x-rays, defined by the scatter-to-primary x-ray ratio (S/P).

   $C' = C_0/[1 + (S/P)]$

   - As the amount of scattered x-rays increases (because of higher kVp or larger FoV collimation or thicker body anatomy), the S/P ratio increases and the inherent image contrast decreases.

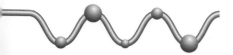

- A grid removes some of the scattered x-rays from the image as a result of its selectivity. Primary x-rays pass preferentially through the grid, whereas a significant portion of the scattered x-rays are attenuated.

$$C'' = C_0/[1 + (S/P)(1/\Sigma)]$$

- **_Contrast improvement factor (K)_**—ratio of the contrast with a grid divided by the contrast without a grid. The grid improves image contrast by removing scattered x-rays from the image.

$$K = C''/C'$$

- In general, as the grid ratio (r) increases, the selectivity (Σ) increases, the Bucky factor increases, the patient's radiation dose increases, the image contrast improves (K), and fewer scattered x-rays are used in the resultant image.

10. **_Grid cutoff_**—at a distance from the center of the grid, the grid design attenuates both scatter and primary x-rays from passing through it. Beyond this distance, film density (or digital value) is greatly diminished. For example, with parallel grids, there is a cutoff distance (d_C) from the center of the image receptor.

$$d_C = [SID/r]$$

- where SID = distance from focal spot (source) to image receptor and r = grid ratio.

- Parallel grids are designed to be operated with an x-ray source far from the grid (e.g., infinitely far away from the grid) so that incident x-rays are nearly parallel, like the lead strips in the grid.

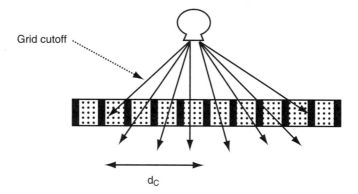

Grid cutoff

d_C

11. **_Reasons for cutoff with focused grids_** are the following:
    - Grid placed "upside down"—center dark and rest of image light
    - Distance decentering—density gradually decreases on both sides of center of image
    - Lateral decentering—image uniformly decreased in density or more radiation dose required to get equivalent density.
    - Combined lateral and distance decentering—dark on one side and light on other side of center of image

12. Moving grids (Bucky grids) require a larger dose to the patient and greater exposure time than stationary grids.

13. Recommendations:
    - Use r = 8:1 with less than 90 kVp or small anatomic thickness, or both
    - Use r = 12:1 with greater than 90 kVp or large anatomic thickness, or both

14. **_Focal distance_** is the distance at which the focused grid is intended to be used. It is the optimal distance from the focal spot of the x-ray tube to the grid surface. There is usually a range of distances in which cutoff is minimal.

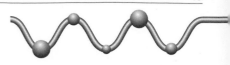

15. *Air gap techniques* can be used instead of a grid to reduce the number of scattered x-rays in the image. These techniques require an air gap between the patient's exit surface and the image receptor at least equal to the patient's thickness. Long SIDs are used to reduce geometric magnification of anatomy. Air gaps are more effective at lower kVp values.

C. Questions

8-1. The most commonly used type of x-ray beam collimation in diagnostic radiology is _____.

(a) Fixed aperture   (b) Cones   (c) Variable aperture
(d) Intensity-modulated radiation therapy (IMRT)   (e) Wedges

8-2. The most commonly used type of x-ray beam collimation in dental units is _____.

(a) Fixed aperture   (b) Cones   (c) Variable aperture
(d) IMRT   (e) Wedges

8-3. Mammography units use either _____ or _____ collimation devices.

(a) Fixed aperture   (b) Cone   (c) Variable aperture
(d) IMRT   (e) Wedge

8-4. Collimation beyond the edges of the cassette results in all of the following *except* _____.

(a) Increased number of scattered x-rays   (b) Degraded resolution
(c) Degraded contrast   (d) Greater biologic risk to the patient
(e) Higher radiation dose per gram of tissue

8-5. The automatic collimation system that tracks the cassette size and SID is called the _____.

(a) AEC   (b) ABC   (c) PBL   (d) SSD   (e) AoP

8-6. Regulations require the x-ray field and light alignment to be within ± ____% of the SID in both orthogonal directions.

(a) 0.5   (b) 1.0   (c) 2.0   (d) 3.0   (e) 4.0

8-7. For standard radiographic and fluoroscopic x-ray tubes, the collimator blades are composed of _____.

(a) Plastic   (b) Aluminum   (c) Copper   (d) Lead   (e) Uranium

8-8. The amount of scattered radiation increases with FoV and gradually levels out at about an FoV of _____ cm × _____cm.

(a) 10, 10   (b) 15, 15   (c) 20, 20   (d) 25, 25   (e) 30, 30

8-9. The scatter-to-primary (S/P) ratio is influenced by all of the following, *except* _____.

(a) kVp   (b) Focal spot size   (c) FoV   (d) Patient's thickness
(e) X-ray filtration

8-10. The S/P ratio for thick anatomy can be as large as _____.

(a) 0.5:1   (b) 1:1   (c) 2:1   (d) 5:1   (e) 10:1

8-11. The ideal source-to-image receptor distance (SID) for a parallel grid is _____.

(a) 100 cm   (b) 40 inches   (c) 72 inches   (d) 180 cm   (e) Infinity

8-12. Grid cutoff becomes more likely with _____.

(a) High line frequency   (b) Low lead content   (c) Low selectivity
(d) High grid ratios   (e) Low Bucky factors

8-13. Use of grids results in _____ radiation dose to the patient and _____ image contrast.

(a) Increased, improved   (b) Decreased, improved   (c) Increased, degraded
(d) Decreased, degraded   (e) The same, degraded

8-14. As grid selectivity increases, the Bucky factor _____ and scattered x-ray transmission _____.

(a) Increases, increases   (b) Increases, decreases   (c) Decreases, increases
(d) Decreases, decreases   (e) Stays the same, decreases

8-15. In comparison with a stationary grid, a moving (Bucky) grid requires _____.

(a) Higher kVp   (b) More radiation dose to the patient
(c) Shorter exposure times   (d) Longer SID   (e) Smaller FoV

8-16. The S/P ratio increases with _____.

(a) Larger FoV   (b) Higher kVp   (c) Thicker patient anatomy
(d) Denser body tissue   (e) All of the above

8-17. A grid problem that results in higher density on one side of the center of the image than the other side is due to _____.

(a) Upside-down grid   (b) Distance decentering   (c) Lateral decentering
(d) Distance and lateral decentering

8-18. A grid problem that results in the center of the image being dark and all other portions of the image being clear is due to_____.

(a) Upside-down grid   (b) Distance decentering   (c) Lateral decentering
(d) Distance and lateral decentering   (e) Tilted grid

8-19. A grid problem that results in a uniform reduction in the density everywhere in the image is due to _____.

(a) Upside-down grid   (b) Distance decentering   (c) Lateral decentering
(d) Distance and lateral decentering   (e) Tilted grid

8-20. A grid problem that results in the density gradually decreasing from the center of the image toward both edges is due to _____.

(a) Upside-down grid   (b) Distance decentering   (c) Lateral decentering
(d) Distance and lateral decentering   (e) Tilted grid

8-21. Another way to reduce the number of scattered x-rays that reach the image receptor without the use of grids is to use _____.

(a) Heavy filtration   (b) Small focal spot sizes   (c) Longer SIDs
(d) Air gaps   (e) Wedge filters

8-22. Grids can result in a contrast improvement factor of about _____.

(a) 0.5–1.0   (b) 1.0–2.0   (c) 2.0–3.0   (d) 4.0–6.0   (e) >10.0

8-23. The Bucky factor is the _____.

(a) Contrast with a grid divided by contrast without a grid
(b) Dose with a moving grid divided by dose with a stationary grid
(c) Dose with a grid divided by dose without a grid
(d) Density with a grid divided by density without a grid
(e) kVp used with a grid divided by kVp used without a grid

8-24. For a parallel grid with a 10:1 ratio used at an SID of 100 cm, the grid cutoff occurs with cassette sizes greater than _____ cm.

(a) 10   (b) 20   (c) 30   (d) 40   (e) 50

8-25. If two grids with a ratio of 6:1 are mounted as crossed grids, the effective grid ratio is _____.

(a) 1:1   (b) 6:1   (c) 8.5:1   (d) 12:1   (e) 36:1

8-26. Stationary grids are usually employed for radiographic images of the _____.

    (a) Breast   (b) Extremities   (c) Chest   (d) Skull   (e) Abdomen

8-27. When higher kVp values are used in radiographs, typically grids with _____ are employed.

    (a) Lower lead content   (b) Higher line frequency   (c) Longer SID range
    (d) Higher grid ratio   (e) Copper covers

8-28. For fluoroscopy of newborn infants, grids with the following ratio are employed:_____.

    (a) 2:1   (b) 5:1   (c) 8:1   (d) 12:1   (e) No grids are used

8-29. For routine mammography imaging, grids with the following ratio are employed:_____.

    (a) 2:1   (b) 5:1   (c) 8:1   (d) 12:1   (e) No grids are used

8-30. To reduce the patient's radiation dose, grids can be modified by using _____ for the interspace material.

    (a) Air   (b) Aluminum   (c) Carbon fiber   (d) Copper   (e) Paper

D.   Answers

8-1. Answer = (c). Collimators with adjustable knobs to limit the x-ray field in the longitudinal and transverse directions are called variable aperture collimators. Some mammography units use metal plates with rectangular holes cut into the plates called fixed apertures. Dental x-ray units use a cone to space the x-ray tube away from the skin to reduce the radiation dose to the patient. IMRT refers to ***intensity-modulated radiation therapy***, in which special multileaf collimators are used for radiation therapy. Wedges are leaded plastic plates that can be inserted to modulate the intensity of the x-rays at the edges of the body or near the lungs, where there is little attenuation of the x-rays.

8-2. Answer = (b). See explanation provide in Answer 8-1.

8-3. Answer = (a) for older units or (c) for newer units. See explanation provided in Answer 8-1.

8-4. Answer = (b). Collimation beyond the edge of the cassette results in radiation exposure of tissue that is not imaged. This increases the biologic risk of radiation exposure. Large FoVs result in an increase in scattered radiation. The excess scattered radiation decreases image contrast and increases the radiation dose a little. High contrast, spatial resolution is not affected by an increase in scattered radiation.

8-5. Answer = (c). AEC is automatic exposure control, or phototiming. ABC refers to automatic brightness control, which is the system that adjusts the kVp and mA to maintain the fluoroscopic television display brightness. SSD is source-to-skin distance. AoP refers to automatic optimization of parameters, which employs the automatic selection of kVp, mA, filter, and exposure duration in mammography. PBL is positive beam limitation, which is the automatic collimator adjustment system.

8-6. Answer = (c). See notes about regulatory requirements for collimator and light alignment accuracy (point 5 in section A).

8-7. Answer = (d). Aluminum fixed apertures are sometimes used in mammography. Uranium collimator blades are often used in radiation therapy accelerators. Plastic and copper are not used for collimator blades.

8-8. Answer = (e). The number of scattered x-rays increases with FoV up to a size of about 30 cm × 30 cm = 900 cm^2.

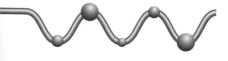

8-9. Answer = (b). Focal spot size affects image blur and thus spatial resolution. Higher kVp and added filters increase the average energy of the x-rays; higher energies mean more Compton scatter interactions. Thicker body anatomy results in fewer primary x-rays and more scatter interactions in the body. Large FoV, as stated, increases the number of scattered x-rays.

8-10. Answer = (d). Only very thin body parts, such as hands and feet, have a low S/P ratio of 1:1 or less. Abdomen radiographs of large adults can have a S/P ratio of 4:1 or more.

8-11. Answer = (e). Parallel grids require parallel incident x-rays to avoid cutoff. Large SIDs best produce parallel x-ray beams.

8-12. Answer = (d). High line frequencies result in the grid lines being less visible on stationary grids. Lead content affects the ability of x-rays to penetrate through the grid lead strips; high lead content is needed for high-kVp x-rays. Low selectivity and low Bucky factors mean low grid ratios. Selectivity is related to contrast improvement because it removes scattered x-rays. Bucky factor is the increase in radiation dose to the patient that results from using a grid.

8-13. Answer = (a). Grids remove scattered x-rays; to maintain density (or SNR for digital image receptors), more x-ray photons must be used to replace the scattered x-rays eliminated by the grid. Because many scattered photons are removed and not absorbed by the image receptor, there is less degradation of contrast due to the scattered x-rays.

8-14. Answer = (b). Increased selectivity results from higher grid ratios. High selectivity removes a considerable number of scattered x-rays, so that fewer x-rays are transmitted to the image receptor; thus, radiation must be increased to darken the image, which results in a larger radiation dose to the patient. The positive aspect is that the contrast in the image improves.

8-15. Answer = (b). Moving versus stationary grids are not influenced by kVp, SID, or FoV. However, because moving lead grid strips cover the entire image receptor instead of one fixed area, as do stationary grids, more radiation is required for moving grids. This increased radiation is usually produced by increasing the exposure time.

8-16. Answer = (e). All the listed factors increase the S/P ratio.

8-17. Answer = (d). See Grids section for grid problems.

8-18. Answer = (a). See Grids section for grid problems.

8-19. Answer = (c). See Grids section for grid problems.

8-20. Answer = (b). See Grids section for grid problems.

8-21. Answer = (d). Longer SIDs and smaller focal spots have no effect on the number of scattered x-rays. More filtration increases the energy of the x-rays, which results in more scattered x-rays, not less. Wedge filters are use in cardiac and angiographic rooms to block excess transmission at the edge of the body and in the lungs. An air gap allows the scattered x-rays to miss the image receptor.

8-22. Answer = (d). The contrast improvement depends on both the number of scattered x-rays (S/P) in the beam and the grid ratio. For thick anatomy, scattered x-rays severely degrade image contrast. A high-ratio grid can remove a significant number of the scattered x-rays and thus improve contrast over that seen without the grid.

8-23. Answer = (c). Self-explanatory.

8-24. Answer = (b). Size = $(2 \times d_C) = (2 \times SID)/r = (2 \times 100)/10 = 20$ cm.

8-25. Answer = (d). For crossed grids, add the grid ratios; $6 + 6 =$ an effective ratio of 12.

8-26. Answer = (c). To stop respiratory motion of the lungs, very short exposure times (of the order of 5–10 msec) are required. Moving grids not only cannot start but also completely blur the grid lines in this short x-ray exposure time. Hence, chest x-rays use stationary grids.

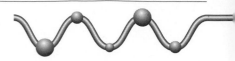

8-27. Answer = (d). For higher energy x-rays, either greater lead content or high grid ratios are used to prevent penetration through the lead strips of the grid.

8-28. Answer = (e). Because newborn babies are small, very few scattered x-rays are produced. Hence, no grid is necessary.

8-29. Answer = (b). Because of the low kVp and the thin anatomy of the compressed breast, there is only a moderate amount of scattered x-radiation. Hence, low-ratio grids are adequate to maintain acceptable image contrast.

8-30. Answer = (c). Air cannot be used because there is nothing to support physically the structure of the lead grid strips. Metals with a high atomic number attenuate too many of the primary x-rays. Paper and wood were used for interspace materials on some older grids; however, the paper and wood absorbed humidity from the air over time and became nonuniform. Hence, a material with low atomic number that is solid and nonhygroscopic, such as carbon fiber, is ideal.

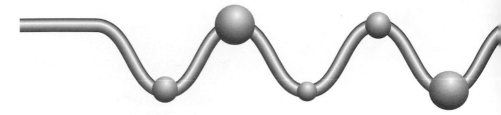

CHAPTER NINE

Intensifying Screens

A. Basic Concepts

1. The basic purpose of intensifying screens is to capture a large percentage of the x-rays that pass though the patient and grid and convert this radiation into light, which is then directed onto x-ray film.

   • The **advantage** of intensifying screens is that they reduce the amount of x-ray radiation to the patient in comparison with direct exposure of film without use of intensifying screens.

   • **Intensification factor** is the radiation required for direct exposure of film without intensifying screens divided by the radiation required with screens.

   • Intensification factors are usually greater than 40 to 50. This means that intensifying screens reduce the radiation dose to the patient by more than 50 times.

2. The **disadvantage** of intensifying screens is that the image quality is diminished. The reduction of the radiation dose results in increased image noise (quantum mottle), and light dispersion in the intensifying screens reduces the spatial resolution.

   • Thicker intensifying screens stop more of the x-rays and reduce the radiation dose to the patient.

   • In standard radiography, a cassette with two screens is used with a double-emulsion film. One screen is mounted to the front of the cassette, and the other is mounted to the back of the cassette.

   • The thicker screens result in more of the light diverging; thicker screens reduce spatial resolution more than thinner screens.

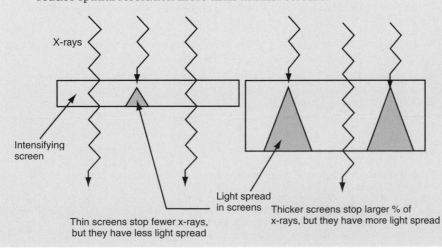

X-rays

Intensifying screen

Light spread in screens

Thin screens stop fewer x-rays, but they have less light spread

Thicker screens stop larger % of x-rays, but they have more light spread

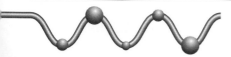

3. Two types of efficiency are associated with intensifying screens to produce the overall screen efficiency, ε.

   - ***Absorption efficiency***, α, is the fraction of x-rays that interact with the screen.

   - ***Conversion efficiency***, κ, is the fraction of the energy deposited in the intensifying screen that is converted in light.

     $\varepsilon = \alpha \times \kappa$

   - Typical values of α are 20% to 60%, dependent on screen composition material and thickness.

   - Typical values of κ are 5% in older calcium tungstate ($CaWO_4$) screens to 16% to 18% in newer rare-earth phosphor screens.

   - The overall speed of an intensifying screen depends on both good absorption of x-rays and good conversion of the energy deposited in the screens to light.

   - The patient's radiation dose is directly related to the speed of the intensifying screen, the film speed, and the film processing conditions.

   - As the speed of the film-screen combination increases, the patient's dose is reduced.

4. An intensifying screen is constructed of four different layers:

   - A plastic ***base material*** to act as a support structure.

   - A ***reflective layer*** (such as TiO_2) to reflect light back toward the film.

   - A ***phosphor layer*** of high atomic number (Z) material that stops the x-rays and converts the x-ray energy to light. It is the light that exposes the film.

   - Direct x-ray interactions with the film represent 1% to 5% of the total interaction with the film emulsion. More than 95% of the exposure is due to light from the intensifying screen.

   - A clear plastic ***protective coating*** prevents water and cleaning chemicals from affecting the phosphor crystals. Light from the phosphor crystal easily passes through the protective coating of screens.

5. The absorption efficiency of intensifying screens depends on the type of atomic elements in the phosphor material.

6. $CaWO_4$ has a K-edge where the x-ray absorption is greatest around 70 keV because of the tungsten material in the phosphor. It emits light in a continuous color (wavelength) spectrum in the blue region.

7. The most common rare earth phosphor is gadolinium oxysulfate (Gd_2O_2S), which emits light (blue, green, and yellow) in discrete wavelengths.

8. Other rare earth phosphors of intensifying screens include $La_2O_2S_7$ (blue), $LaOBr$ (blue), Y_2O_2S (blue), and Y_2TaO_4 (ultraviolet).

9. Many of the rare earth phosphors have an absorption efficiency that changes significantly with the kVp used to take the clinical images.

10. A number of factors affect the speed of intensifying screens:

    - The thickness of the phosphor layer in the screen is important.

    - Reflective layers use more of the light and are more efficient, but the light spread is greater, reducing spatial resolution.

    - Use of dyes to absorb light reduces light spread, improving spatial resolution, but it also requires a larger radiation dose to the patient because it is less efficient.

    - The conversion efficiency of the phosphor converting deposited x-ray energy to light is another factor in speed.

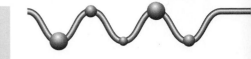

11. Use of intensifying screens can change the relative speed of the film-screen combination by about a factor of 32 from the slowest to the fastest. Films can double or halve the speed.

12. *Mottle (image noise)* is a result of variation in density for a uniform radiation exposure of the film-screen cassette. It has three components:

- *Screen mottle* is due to variation in the thickness and density of the screen from point to point.

- *Film (or grain) mottle* is due to variations in the silver grains from point to point on the film surface.

- *Quantum mottle* (QM) is due to statistical variations in the number of x-rays per mm^2 of the image surface.

- *QM is by far the most important* of the three types of mottle.

13. For film-screen combinations, the QM:

- Is higher for greater intensifying screen conversion efficiency (κ)

- *Does NOT depend on screen thickness* or absorption efficiency (α)

- If only the overall speed (S) is known, depends on S/α

- Is higher for faster film speed

- Is higher for faster processing because of higher temperature, greater developer concentration, and slower film transport speeds in the processor

14. *Film-screen contact* is important for uniformity and good spatial resolution.

- Dirt or nonuniform pressure causes "poor" film contact to the intensifying screen.

- Clean screens regularly: weekly for mammographic units and at least quarterly for radiographic units.

- Test contact with radiographs of uniform mesh on a cassette at a long focal spot–to-film distance (SID) that show blotches for nonuniform contact.

B. Questions

9-1. All of the following are typical intensifying screen phosphors, *except* _____.

(a) CaWO$_4$ (b) LiF   (c) Gd$_2$O$_2$S   (d) LaOBr   (e) Y$_2$TaO$_4$

9-2. The intensifying screen phosphor that emits both blue and green light in discrete color lines is _____.

(a) CaWO$_4$ (b) LiF   (c) Gd$_2$O$_2$S   (d) LaOBr   (e) Y$_2$TaO$_4$

9-3. The _____ is the intensifying screen phosphor that emits a nearly continuous light spectrum of primarily blue light without discrete lines of emission.

(a) CaWO$_4$ (b) LiF   (c) Gd$_2$O$_2$S   (d) LaOBr   (e) Y$_2$TaO$_4$

9-4. The _____ is the intensifying screen phosphor that emits discrete lines of emission primarily in the ultraviolet range.

(a) CaWO$_4$ (b) LiF   (c) Gd$_2$O$_2$S   (d) LaOBr   (e) Y$_2$TaO$_4$

9-5. The intensifying screen phosphors that are classified as rare earth screens include which of the following? (i) CaWO$_4$, (ii) LiF, (iii) Gd$_2$O$_2$S, (iv) LaOBr, (v) Y$_2$TaO$_4$

(a) i, ii, and iii   (b) ii, iii, and iv   (c) Only iii   (d) iii, iv, and v
(e) Only iii and iv

9-6. Standard radiographic cassettes have _____ intensifying screen(s), and mammography cassettes have _____ screen(s).

(a) 1, 2   (b) 2, 1   (c) 2, 2   (d) 1, 1   (e) 2, 0

9-7. Radiographic intensifying screens should be cleaned at least _____, and mammography intensifying screens should be cleaned at least _____.

(a) Weekly, daily   (b) Monthly, weekly   (c) Quarterly, weekly
(d) Quarterly, monthly   (e) Yearly, quarterly

9-8. Quality control tests that should be performed to evaluate film-screen cassettes include all of the following, *except* _____.

(a) Film-screen contact   (b) Uniformity   (c) Light leaks   (d) Dispersion
(e) Visual inspection of intensifying screens

9-9. Thicker intensifying screens result in _____.

(a) Degraded spatial resolution   (b) Slower speeds
(c) Less quantum mottle   (d) Higher radiation doses to the patient
(e) Greater conversion efficiency

9-10. The main purpose of intensifying screens is to _____.

(a) Improve resolution   (b) Reduce quantum mottle
(c) Reduce radiation dose to the patient   (d) Increase image contrast
(e) Increase financial cost

9-11. As kVp use is increased, the light production of the intensifying screens _____.

(a) Remains constant   (b) Increases   (c) Decreases
(d) Depends on phosphor material and kVp   (e) Is negligible

9-12. The QM for intensifying screens depends on _____.

(a) Geometric efficiency   (b) Absorption efficiency
(c) Conversion efficiency   (d) Screen thickness   (e) Screen pressure

9-13. To maximize the overall efficiency of a film-screen combination, it is important to match the _____ of the film to the screen phosphor.

(a) Contrast   (b) Color sensitivity   (c) Thickness   (d) Spatial resolution
(e) Elasticity

9-14. In comparison with an image receptor composed of film alone, an intensifying screen plus film combination reduces the patient's radiation by at least a factor of _____.

(a) 2   (b) 10   (c) 50   (d) 1000   (e) 5000

9-15. Behind the rear intensifying screen in a radiographic cassette is a layer of _____.

(a) Plastic   (b) Lead   (c) Copper   (d) Aluminum   (e) Paper

9-16. The intensifying screen selection can affect all of the following image quality parameters, *except* _____.

(a) Spatial resolution   (b) Patient's radiation dose   (c) Contrast
(d) QM   (e) Unsharpness

9-17. The amount of QM produced by intensifying screens depends on all of the following factors, *except* _____.

(a) Reflective layer   (b) Dyes added to intensifying screen
(c) Screen thickness   (d) Type of phosphor   (e) kVp used

9-18. The spatial resolution of a film-screen combination depends on _____.

(a) Film alone   (b) Screen alone   (c) Both film and screen
(d) Neither film nor screen   (e) Only x-ray tube focal spot

9-19. The image contrast of a film-screen combination depends on _____.

(a) Film alone   (b) Screen alone   (c) Both film and screen
(d) Neither film nor screen   (e) Only x-ray tube kVp

9-20. The radiation dose to the patient and the speed of a film-screen combination depend on _____.

(a) Film alone   (b) Screen alone   (c) Both film and screen
(d) Neither film nor screen   (e) Primarily the grid

9-21. The QM of a film-screen combination depends on ____.

(a) Film alone   (b) Screen alone   (c) Both film and screen
(d) Neither film nor screen   (e) Primarily x-ray filtration

9-22. The principal factor affecting the overall image noise (mottle) is the _____.

(a) Screen mottle   (b) Silver grain mottle   (c) Quantum mottle
(d) Filter mottle   (e) Dielectric mottle

9-23. Film-screen contact is tested using a _____.

(a) Uniform mesh screen   (b) Densitometer   (c) Penetrometer
(d) Step wedge   (e) Spinning top

9-24. If two intensifying screens have the same overall efficiency (speed) and screen X has a higher conversion efficiency than Y, the screen with the better spatial resolution is _____.

(a) X   (b) Y   (c) Neither; both are the same
(d) Unknown; not enough information provided
(e) Not important; question is irrelevant

9-25. If screen Y has 2.0 times the absorption efficiency and 0.5 times the conversion efficiency of screen X, _____ screen has the lower radiation dose to the patient and _____ screen has the lower quantum mottle.

(a) Neither, X   (b) Neither, Y   (c) X, neither   (d) Y, neither   (e) X, Y

C.   Answers

9-1. Answer = (b). $CaWO_4$ is an older type of intensifying screen phosphor that is *not* a rare earth metal. Gd_2O_2S, LaOBr, and Y_2TaO_4 are of the newer-type rare-earth phosphors that have a greater conversion efficiency and emit light in discrete wavelengths instead of continuous spectra. LiF is a crystal used for thermoluminescent dosimeters (TLDs), which are used in some personnel radiation badges.

9-2. Answer = (c). $CaWO_4$ emits in a continuous blue spectrum. LaOBr emits in discrete wavelengths (color lines) primarily in the blue region of the visible light spectrum. Y_2TaO_4 is a rare earth phosphor that emits discrete color lines primarily in the ultraviolet portion of the light spectrum.

9-3. Answer = (a). See answers to 9-1 and 9-2.

9-4. Answer = (e). See answers to 9-1 and 9-2.

9-5. Answer = (d). See notes in this chapter (**A7** and **A8**).

9-6. Answer = (b). Radiographic cassettes use front and rear intensifying screens with dual-emulsion film so that an emulsion layer faces each screen. The dual screens reduce the radiation dose to the patient. However, the quantum mottle (QM) is increased, and spatial resolution is degraded. In mammography, it is important to improve spatial resolution; thus, a single intensifying screen with a single-emulsion film is used despite the fact that the relative speed is less.

9-7. Answer = (c). Although the need to clean intensifying screens depends on usage, dirt, and other conditions, accreditation and regulatory programs specify that cleaning of mammography screens should take place weekly because small dust specks might create clinically unacceptable artifacts in the images. Quarterly cleaning of radiographic screens is usually the longest specified interval, and more frequent cleaning might be necessary, depending on conditions in any particular facility.

9-8. Answer = (d). Dispersion refers to the light spread in the screens, which is a function of design. Film-screen contact is the mesh test used to uncover warped cassettes and dirty screens. Uniformity is required for mammography film-screen cassettes to make sure that the AEC (phototimer) produces similar densities for the same phantom. Light leaks can occur with older cassettes in which fog is produced because of failure to prevent ambient light from leaking inside to the film. Visual inspection is performed to find damage to the protective coating and discoloration of the phosphor related to humidity, which causes the phosphors to change with age.

9-9. Answer = (a). Thicker screens have better absorption efficiency, which reduces the radiation dose to the patient and increases the speed of the system. The conversion efficiency is unaffected because it depends only on selection of the screen phosphor material. Because conversion efficiency is unchanged with screen thickness, the QM is not changed.

9-10. Answer = (c). Film (without intensifying screens) has better spatial resolution and less QM than film-screen systems. The film alone (of the film-screen combination) affects the image contrast; the screen has no effect on image contrast. Use of screens does increase costs, but this is not a goal, nor is it relevant to image quality.

9-11. Answer = (d). With all intensifying screens, the absorption efficiency depends on the K-edge of the material in the screen phosphor. With rare earth screens, the K-edge can occur at assorted energies between 17 and 50 keV, depending on the phosphor used. Moreover, the absorption efficiency changes significantly with kVp. AEC (phototimers) must have curves to compensate for this change in efficiency with kVp in order to maintain consistent film densities at all kVp values.

9-12. Answer = (c). Geometric efficiency is pertinent only to radiation detectors, not intensifying screens. Absorption efficiency depends on screen thickness but does not affect QM. Screen pressure is important to film-screen contact and spatial resolution and uniformity within a radiograph.

9-13. Answer = (b). Contrast, thickness, and spatial resolution of the film have no effect on the overall efficiency of the matching of the film to the screen. Elasticity of the film has nothing to do with speed or efficiency.

9-14. Answer = (c). A film-screen system of average speed would have an intensification factor of at least 50. A system with a relative speed of 400 would have a factor 4 times greater, or about 200. A value of 1000 or more is too high.

9-15. Answer = (b). In most radiographic cassettes, there is a thin lead layer intended to block any x-rays transmitted through the two intensifying screens of the cassette. This approach is acceptable because the AEC detector (phototimer) of radiographic units is located in front of the cassette. For mammography, this method cannot be used because the AEC detector is located behind the cassette; instead, the cassette holder assembly is shielded with a thin layer of lead.

9-16. Answer = (c). Contrast is controlled only by the film and film processing. Screen thickness affects light spread, unsharpness, spatial resolution, speed, and radiation dose to the patient. The selection of screen phosphor type affects the QM.

9-17. Answer = (c). Anything that affects the amount of light produced per x-ray interaction in the intensifying screen affects the QM. The reflective layer redirects the light and boosts the light utilization. Absorption dyes absorb some

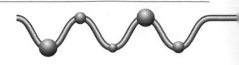

of the light produced to decrease the conversion efficiency. The change from calcium tungstate to rare earth screen phosphors results in an increase in the conversion efficiency. The kVp affects the absorption efficiency because of the K-edge of the phosphor. Also, higher energy x-rays that interact in the screen release more energy in the screen, producing more light per x-ray interaction, which increases the QM. Screen thickness affects only the absorption efficiency.

9-18. Answer = (b). The film resolution is much greater than the screen resolution, so that it has little influence on the overall spatial resolution. Although other things affect image spatial resolution, such as motion blur, parallax, and focal spot blur, the question asked specifically about film-screen resolution. Of these two items, the screen is the limitation.

9-19. Answer = (a). Although other things affect image contrast, such as filtration, kVp, and film processing, the question asked about film-screen contrast. Of the two items, the film is the component that affects the contrast; the screen does not affect the contrast.

9-20. Answer = (c). Although the grid ratio does affect the patient's radiation dose, the grid does not affect the film-screen speed. The film has an influence of about a factor of 3, and the intensifying screens can have a much greater effect on the speed and the radiation dose to the patient. Film processing also has a major influence on the speed and radiation dose; however, film processing is not one of the answer choices.

9-21. Answer = (c). The QM is affected by the intensifying screen conversion efficiency, the film speed, and the film processing conditions.

9-22. Answer = (c). Filter mottle and dielectric mottle are falsified terms. Of the three sources of mottle, quantum mottle is the most significant factor.

9-23. Answer = (a). The sensitometer and densitometer are used for film processor quality control, which is discussed in Chapter 10. A penetrometer is used to evaluate low contrast discrimination of fluoroscopic systems. A step wedge is a miniature aluminum staircase used to look at the contrast of film-screen systems. A spinning top can be used to measure exposure duration of some x-ray units.

9-24. Answer = (a). If the overall speeds are the same and X has the higher conversion efficiency, the absorption efficiency of screen X is less. If the absorption efficiency is less, screen X must be thinner. The thinner screen has the better spatial resolution.

9-25. Answer = (b). The product of absorption and conversion efficiencies is 1.0; hence, the patient's radiation doses are the same. A higher conversion efficiency means more quantum mottle and better spatial resolution for screen X.

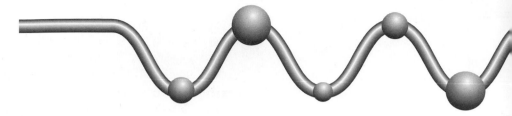

CHAPTER TEN

Film Characteristics, Film Processing, and Film Quality Control

A. Film Characteristics

1. Film composition is as follows:

- *Base* material of clear plastic (triacetate or polyester) to support the emulsion; it usually has a slight tint (blue or gray)

- *Adhesive layer* to hold the emulsion

- *Emulsion*, which is a mixture of gelatin plus silver halide grains

- A *supercoat* to protect the emulsion, which softens and allows chemicals to pass through during film processing

2. X-rays either interact with the intensifying screen to produce light, which affects the silver halide grains and rearranges their structure (95% to 99%), or interact directly with the silver halide crystals (about 1% to 5%).

- The rearranged silver halide crystals are *sensitivity specks*.

- During film processing, the sensitivity specks serve as centers where other silver ions gather and are oxidized.

- Oxidized silver atoms are black and block the light from the viewbox.

- The darker portions of the processed film are where the amount of light from the intensifying screen and direct interaction with emulsion are greatest. Where the interactions are few, this portion of the processed film is relatively clear and allows the most light from the viewbox to pass through the film.

- The film that has been exposed to x-rays but has not yet been run through the film processor is said to have a *latent image* that will appear after film processing.

- If there is a long delay between x-ray exposure and film processing, some of the affected silver grains can recombine with electrons and no longer act as sensitivity specks. Thus, long delays between x-ray exposure and film processing result in a film with fewer oxidized silver grains, producing a lighter film; this is called *latent image fading*.

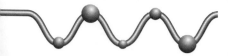

- When nearly all the silver halide grains have been affected by the x-rays, the processed film is the darkest that it can get. It blocks the most light from the viewbox. This maximum darkness of the film is called D_{MAX}. Additional x-ray exposure cannot make the film any darker.

3. **Density (D)** is defined as the logarithm (to the base 10) of the light incident upon the film from the viewbox (I_0) divided by the light transmitted through the exposed and processed x-ray film (I_T).

   $D = \log(I_0/I_T)$

4. For each 50% reduction in the amount of transmitted incident light from the viewbox, the density increases by the addition of another 0.30 optical density (OD) units.

(I_T/I_0)	DENSITY (OD)
1.0	0.0
0.5	0.30
0.25	0.60
0.125	0.90
0.0625	1.20

5. For each reduction in the amount of transmitted incident light from the viewbox by a factor of 10, the density increases by the addition of another 1.0 OD.

(I_T/I_0)	DENSITY (OD)
1.0	0.0
0.10	1.00
0.01	2.00
0.001	3.00
0.0001	4.00

6. Useful radiographic densities are usually defined to be in the range of 0.50 to about 2.5 OD because higher densities transmit too little light to be seen. However, in mammography, which uses viewboxes with a high light level and "hot lights," densities up to 3.5 may be seen.

7. Each film-screen combination has a distinctive **characteristic curve**, which plots the film density versus the logarithm of the radiation exposure used to obtain that density. This curve is also called the **H & D curve**.

   - The shape of the curve depends on the film selected, the intensifying screen selected, and the film processing conditions.

   - All curves have three different regions, called the toe, the linear portion, and the shoulder.

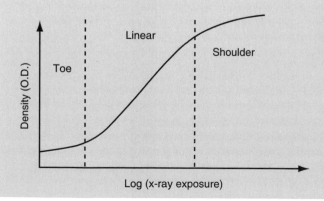

8. The ***toe*** is not a useful region because changes in the radiation exposure levels do not cause much of a change in film density. The ***shoulder*** is not a useful region because the film is so dark and most of the silver grains have been used. Additional radiation in the shoulder region does little to increase the density.

9. In the ***linear region***, every increase in radiation causes a linear increase in density. The slope at every portion of the characteristic curve is called the gamma (γ) and the average slope of the curve between densities of about 0.50 and 2.50 OD is called the average contrast gradient (γ).

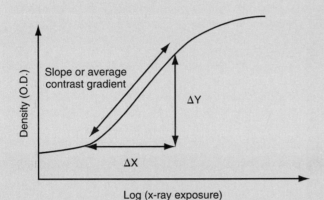

Log (x-ray exposure)

10. The change in density divided by the change in log (x-ray exposure) in the linear portion of the characteristic curve is the ***average contrast gradient*** of the film.

   ● Values < 2.50 are seen with ***latitude film***, which does not show much contrast.

   ● Values >3.0 are seen with ***contrast film***.

   ● ***The intensifying screen choice does not affect the average contrast gradient***.

   ● The film processing conditions do affect the average contrast gradient and can either increase or decrease the value.

11. ***Base + fog*** level is the density of the film in the toe region of the characteristic curve.

   ● The density is a combination of the tint of the film and the exposure to cosmic rays, background radiation, light leaks, and heat, which cause the film grains to change without direct x-ray exposure.

   ● Base + fog densities should be less than 0.25 OD for radiographic film and less than 0.20 OD for mammography film.

12. ***Speed*** is related to the radiation level required to darken a film-screen combination to a density of 1.0 OD greater than the base + fog density. For example, if the base + fog density is 0.20 OD, the speed is 1.0 divided by the radiation (in roentgens), which results in a density of 1.20 OD.

   ● This definition is ***absolute speed***.

   ● There is also ***relative speed***, which compares a film-screen combination with an older "par speed" film-screen system that is arbitrarily assigned a value of relative speed = 100.

   ● Other film-screen combinations that require less radiation to achieve a density of 1.0 OD above the base + fog level would have a relative speed proportionally greater than 100, and systems that require more radiation would have a relative speed proportionally less than 100.

   ● For example, a combination that requires 25% of the radiation of a par speed combination would have a relative speed of 400.

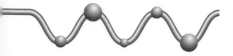

TYPE	EXPOSURE FOR 1.0 OD ABOVE BASE + FOG	ABSOLUTE SPEED	RELATIVE SPEED
Extremity	4.0 mR	250 R^{-1}	50
Par	2.0 mR	500 R^{-1}	100
Rare earth	0.5 mR = 0.0005 R	2000 R^{-1}	400

- *Higher speed values mean less radiation to the patient for equivalent film densities*.

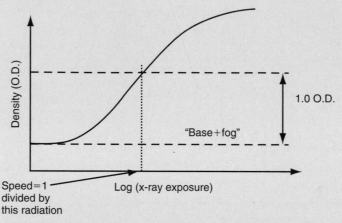

13. Differences in film types have only a minor influence on the overall film-screen speed—a factor of about two times or half the speed. The screen selection has the greatest impact on the overall speed of the combination.

14. The *spatial resolution* of plain film without an intensifying screen is very high, at about 50 to 100 line pairs per millimeter (LP/mm). Hence, it is the intensifying screen that limits the overall spatial resolution of the film-screen combination; the film selection does *not* limit the spatial resolution of the combination.

B. Film Processing

1. Film processing consists of four stages in automated units:
   - *Development* softens the supercoat and wets the film, then oxidizes the silver grains that have been exposed to light or x-rays but does not affect unexposed silver grains.
   - *Fixation* washes off unaltered and unoxidized silver grains and stops the development process.
   - *Washing* washes off the chemicals from the film.
   - *Drying* dries the film.

2. Problems with the developer section can affect the film speed, contrast gradient, and base + fog.

3. Problems with the fixer section can affect the archival storage. Incomplete fixing causes the film to darken with age of storage.

4. Problems with the wash section leave spots on the film.

5. Excessive heat in the dryer section causes the film to wrinkle, and too little heat results in wet films.

6. Too much heat in the developer section (or slow transport speed or chemicals that are too concentrated) results in more base + fog density, a higher average contrast gradient, and a faster speed. A low temperature of the developer solution (or fast transport speed or low chemical specific gravity) results in low

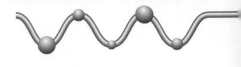

base + fog density and lower average contrast gradient and requires more radiation to darken the film (low film speed).

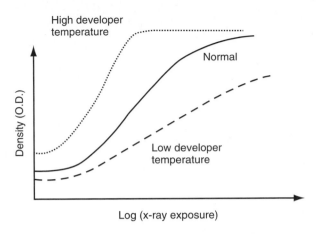

7. Typical developer temperatures range from 92° F to 95° F (34.0° C).

8. Silver removed from the film goes into the fixer solution. Because silver is toxic and valuable, it is then usually electrolytically **reclaimed** from the solution.

9. Automated film processors often measure the amount of film being processed and add a small amount of chemical in the developer and fixer to replace the amount being depleted. This is called **replenishment.**

C. Film Processor Quality Control

1. A **sensitometer** is an electronic device that exposes a QC film to 21 different levels of light to produce a latent image with 21 different levels of density.

2. A **densitometer** is an electronic device that measures and digitally displays the darkness of a processed film in units of OD (optical density).

3. Once a film processor as been optimized and stabilized, a sensitometer is used to expose a film from a QC control box, and the film is processed.

   - The density step closest to 1.20 OD is selected as a **speed step** to be monitored on a daily basis. This density must be within ±0.15 OD of the established aim value.

   - The density step that is closest to 2.2 OD above base + fog is selected as the high-density (HD) step. The density step that is closest to 0.4 OD but greater than 0.4 OD is selected as the low-density (LD) step. The density of these steps is measured daily. The difference in density between HD and LD steps is calculated; this is called the **contrast index**. It is determined daily and should be within ±0.15 OD of the established value.

   - The density of the **base + fog** level on the daily QC film is also measured. The base + fog density must be less than the values listed.

   - A digital thermometer is used to measure the **developer temperature**, which should be within ±1.0° F of the recommended value.

4. **Darkroom fog** of film related to light leaks must be assessed. A sensitometer is used to expose a film on both edges. Half the film is covered and placed in the darkroom for 2 minutes. It is then processed, and the density of the speed step is measured on both sides of the film. The uncovered speed step should not be more than +0.05 OD higher than the covered speed step. If the density exceeds this level, methods to lessen light leaks in the darkroom must be employed.

5. Film can be sensitive to different wavelengths (colors) of visible light. Standard silver halide film is sensitive to blue light. To obtain sensitivity to green light,

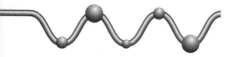

orthochromatic film is needed. Special dyes are used to improve sensitivity to other wavelengths of light. Panchromatic film is sensitive to even longer wavelength visible light.

D. Questions

10-1. An exposed and developed radiographic film that transmits only 3% of the incident viewbox light has a density of _____ OD.

(a) 0.5   (b) 1.0   (c) 1.5   (d) 2.0   (e) 2.5

10-2. The range of exposure values that produce acceptable densities of the exposed and processed film is called the _____.

(a) Speed   (b) Base + fog   (c) Average contrast gradient
(d) D_{MAX} (e) Latitude

10-3. The _____ is equal to 1.0 divided by the radiation in roentgens needed to produce a density of 1.0 OD above the background levels of the unexposed and developed film.

(a) Speed   (b) Base + fog   (c) Average contrast gradient
(d) D_{MAX} (e) Latitude

10-4. The density of an unexposed and processed film is called _____.

(a) Speed   (b) Base + fog   (c) Average contrast gradient
(d) D_{MAX} (e) Latitude

10-5. The _____ is the highest density that can be obtained on an exposed and processed film.

(a) Speed   (b) Base + fog   (c) Average contrast gradient
(d) D_{MAX} (e) Latitude

10-6. The average slope of a film characteristic curve is called the _____.

(a) Speed   (b) Base + fog   (c) Average contrast gradient
(d) D_{MAX} (e) Latitude

10-7. If the film is not sensitive to the wavelength (color) of light emitted from the phosphors in the intensifying screens, the _____ decreases.

(a) Spatial resolution   (b) Speed   (c) Contrast   (d) Latitude
(e) Exposure time

10-8. The selection of the film can affect all of the following imaging quality parameters, *except* _____.

(a) Patient's radiation dose   (b) Image contrast   (c) Spatial resolution
(d) Quantum mottle (noise)   (e) Base + fog levels

10-9. Increasing the developer temperature in the film processor can cause all image changes, *except* _____.

(a) Increased quantum mottle (noise)   (b) Increased base + fog
(c) Greater average contrast gradient
(d) Reduced radiation dose to the patient   (e) Improved latitude

10-10. The ideal film processor developer temperature for most radiographic film, chemicals, and processors is approximately _____ .

(a) 85° F   (b) 90° F   (c) 95° F   (d) 100° F   (e) 105° F

10-11. Film processor performance is monitored by QC systems that use a(n) _____.

(a) Dosimeter   (b) Sensitometer   (c) Photometer   (d) Strain gauge
(e) Interferometer

10-12. The parameters typically measured in most film processor QC programs include all of the following items, *except* _____.

(a) Temperature (b) Speed point (c) pH levels (d) Contrast index
(e) Base + fog densities

10-13. Parameters that can affect film processor performance include all of the following, *except* _____.

(a) Developer temperature (b) Replenishment rates
(c) Specific gravity of chemistry (d) Fixer temperature
(e) Bromine content

10-14. The darkroom-light fog levels should cause the speed point density to increase less than _____ OD for a 2-minute exposure.

(a) 0.02 (b) 0.05 (c) 0.10 (d) 0.15 (e) 0.20

10-15. The base + fog level for radiographic film should be less than _____ OD.

(a) 0.05 (b) 0.10 (c) 0.15 (d) 0.20 (e) 0.25

10-16. The useful density range for most radiographic film is usually considered to be between _____OD and _____ OD.

(a) 0.2, 1.2 (b) 0.3, 1.8 (c) 0.4, 2.2 (d) 0.5, 2.5 (e) 0.6, 3.0

10-17. In the linear portion of a film characteristic curve, a density increase from 1.2 to 1.8 OD (for an average contrast gradient of 3.0) requires a radiation increase of about _____ %.

(a) 20 (b) 40 (c) 60 (d) 80 (e) 100

10-18. A film-screen combination has a density of 1.50 OD for an incident radiation level of 1.0 mR. If the incident radiation is increased to 2.0 mR, the density increases to 2.31 OD. The average contrast gradient of this film-screen combination is _____.

(a) 2.00 (b) 2.35 (c) 2.70 (d) 3.00 (e) 3.33

10-19. All of the following improvements to film have contributed to better image quality, *except* _____.

(a) Tabular silver grains (b) Activator dyes (c) Anticrossover layers
(d) Asymmetrical emulsion layers (e) Thicker supercoats

10-20. Delays in the processing of exposed film cause _____.

(a) Increased contrast (b) Loss of film density (c) Increased base + fog
(d) More scatter radiation (e) No effect at all

10-21. Long-term archival storage of exposed and developed film depends on _____.

(a) Proper development temperature (b) Adequate fixing
(c) Proper washing (d) Proper film dryer temperatures
(e) Flood replenishment

10-22. In matching a film with an intensifying screen cassette, one should consider all the following characteristics of the film, *except* _____.

(a) Contrast (b) Color sensitivity (c) Speed (d) Spatial resolution
(e) Tint

10-23. The film characteristic curve (H & D) plots _____ versus _____.

(a) Radiation, contrast (b) Contrast, latitude (c) Density, resolution
(d) Density, log (exposure) (e) Speed, temperature

10-24. The speed point step of most film processor QC programs is usually chosen around a density of _____ OD.

(a) 0.50 (b) 1.00 (c) 1.20 (d) 1.50 (e) 2.00

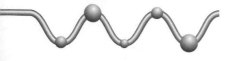

10-25. Film processor QC programs usually require both the speed point and the contrast index to vary less than ±_____ OD from the established aim values.

(a) 0.05   (b) 0.10   (c) 0.15   (d) 0.20   (e) 0.30

E.   Answers

10-1. Answer = (c). Each reduction of one half in light intensity adds a density of 0.30 OD. Hence, 50% = 0.30 OD; 25% = 0.30 + 0.30 = 0.60 OD; 12.5% = 0.30 + 0.30 + 0.30 = 0.90 OD; 6.25% = 0.30 + 0.30 + 0.30 + 0.30 = 1.20 OD; and 3.125% = 0.30 + 0.30 + 0.30 + 0.30 + 0.30 = 1.50 OD.

10-2. Answer = (e). The latitude of the film is the range of exposures that produce acceptable film densities. Also, latitude refers to a film that is the opposite of a contrast film; the film shows more shades of gray rather than a sharp difference of dark and clear densities.

10-3. Answer = (a). This is the definition of the absolute speed of a film-screen combination.

10-4. Answer = (b). An unexposed and processed film has density related to the film base tint and silver grains that have been affected by cosmic rays, background radiation, light leaks (such as darkroom fog), and thermal effects.

10-5. Answer = (d). When almost all the silver grains are oxidized, the highest density is obtained, which is called density maximum (D_{MAX}).

10-6. Answer = (c). See the definition of average contrast gradient (point 9 under "Film Characteristics").

10-7. Answer = (b). The spatial resolution, contrast, and latitude do not change when the film and intensifying screen are color mismatched. The mismatch results in more light being required to create a sensitivity speck because the light is not of the optimal wavelength (color) to transfer its energy to the silver grains. Hence, more light and more radiation are required. The radiation dose to the patient and the exposure time also increase.

10-8. Answer = (c). The film selection affects the overall film-screen speed (although not as much as the intensifying screen), the contrast, the latitude, the base + fog level, and the D_{MAX}. Because the spatial resolution of film is about 10 times better than that of the intensifying screen, the film does not affect the overall resolution of the combination. The intensifying screen is the "weak link" that dominates the overall spatial resolution.

10-9. Answer = (e). Higher developer temperatures increase the speed, contrast gradient, and base + fog levels. The higher speed of the system means that the patient's radiation dose is less. Moreover, the higher speed is equivalent to a more efficient film-screen system, which increases the quantum mottle. Because contrast and latitude are opposites, increasing contrast reduces latitude.

10-10. Answer = (c). The ideal temperature for most developer solutions is between 92° F and 95° F, with 95° F being the most common temperature.

10-11. Answer = (b). A dosimeter is used to measure radiation exposure levels. A photometer is used to measure light intensity levels. A strain gauge is used to measure mechanical pressures and forces. An interferometer is used to measure small distance differences according to shifts in wavelengths of light. Film processor QC is done with a sensitometer to expose the film to difference steps of light intensity, and a densitometer is used to measure the density differences on the processed film.

10-12. Answer = (c). Although the pH of the developer solution does have an effect on film processing, the relation is complex and depends on many other factors.

Moreover, pH is difficult to measure properly. Hence, pH is usually not included in the QC program.

10-13. Answer = (d). Developer temperature directly affects the chemical reaction rates and film density. Fixer solution affects only archival storage of the film. Replenishment is needed to replace depleted chemicals as the film interacts with the solutions. Specific gravity determines whether the chemical is diluted with water, which reduces its potency. Although not mentioned in the notes, bromine content is important to the reaction rates of the development process. In any event, the correct answer could have been narrowed to (d) or (e) by eliminating the answers known to be incorrect.

10-14. Answer = (b). The darkroom fog caused by stray light must be less than an increase of 0.05 OD in 2 minutes, as stated in the notes.

10-15. Answer = (e). Base + fog on radiographic film should be less than 0.25 OD, and less than 0.20 OD for mammography film.

10-16. Answer = (d). Film densities of less than 0.5 OD are in the toe of the characteristic film curves, with diminished contrast, and are too light to use. Film densities of more than 2.5 OD transmit less than 0.25% of the incident light. Unless the film is linear in this region, the viewbox has high-intensity light, and the viewing room is very dark, it would be difficult to visualize details on the film because of the low light transmission through this level of film darkness.

10-17. Answer = (c). In the linear portion of the characteristic curve, the density (D) is related to the radiation exposure (Ex) by the average contrast gradient (γ).

$$D = \gamma \log(Ex) + (B + F)$$

This equation can be rearranged to solve for density differences, $\Delta D = D_2 - D_1$.

$$\Delta D = \gamma \log(Ex_2/Ex_1)$$

$$[Ex_2/Ex_1] = 10^{+(\Delta D/\gamma)}$$

A simple generalization usually gives approximate answers for normal film with an average contrast gradient of about 3.0. ***The rule is that each 0.10 OD change requires about a 10% change in radiation exposure to the film-screen cassette.***

10-18. Answer = (c). The radiation is double, and log (2.0) = 0.30. The difference in film density is 0.81 OD. Average contrast gradient is the difference in density divided by the log of the ratio of the radiation exposures: 0.81/0.30 = 2.70.

10-19. Answer = (e). Tabular silver grains are flat and allow better packing and coverage of the film surface. Activator dyes enable the incident light from the intensifying screens to be better absorbed by the film and to transfer the energy to the silver grains. Anticrossover layer is a special light-absorbing coating that is placed behind the silver grain layer; it prevents light from the front screen from passing through the adjacent silver emulsion layer of film and exposing the rear film emulsion layer on double-emulsion-layer film. Because of the divergence of light from the screen and parallax of front and rear emulsion layers, crossover degrades image quality by making edges of objects unsharp. Asymmetrical coating of a different front and rear emulsion layer permits the film characteristic layer to be shaped with a dual slope that is useful for certain clinical studies (e.g., chest radiographs). Thicker supercoats on the film would allow more light divergence and light scattering, which would reduce spatial resolution and make edges unsharp.

10-20. Answer = (b). Delays in the processing of exposed film cassettes or even computed radiography (CR) cassettes for periods of time of 60 minutes or longer cause the densities on the processed image to be less. This is known as ***latent image fading***. With film, the delays allow the ions created by the x-ray exposure to migrate and repair the latent specks.

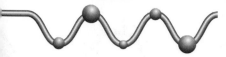

10-21. Answer = (b). Developer temperature affects the speed, contrast, and density of the film. Failure to wash film properly can leave spots and a white coating on the film. Too high a dryer temperature causes the film to wrinkle, and too low a temperature leaves a wet film. Flood replenishment constantly adds small amounts of chemical to the developer and fixer tank; it is used in film processors that process very few films per day. Chemicals not only are lost in processing the films but also deteriorate because of heat, evaporation, and oxidation after being unused for long periods of times. Fixer is supposed to remove unexposed silver grains; dilute fixer solution leaves the unexposed silver grains on the film, which then change because of the heat and ambient light over long periods of time. Thus, films that are not properly fixed darken over time.

10-22. Answer = (d). It is important to select film that provides the proper contrast, radiation dose to the patient (speed), and tint needed for clinical studies. To utilize the light from the intensifying screens efficiently, the film should be sensitive to the same color of light as emitted by the intensifying screens. Because the spatial resolution of almost all film is much greater than that of the intensifying screens, film selection does not affect spatial resolution limitations.

10-23. Answer = (d). See the graphs on pages 78 and 79.

10-24. Answer = (c). Traditionally, the speed point is usually 1.0 OD above the base + fog density (which is usually 0.15 to 0.25 OD). The useful range of film densities is between 0.50 and 2.5 OD and is also the linear range. Hence, a density of 1.20 OD is near the center of this range.

10-25. Answer = (c). See the notes and state and local regulatory requirements as well as American College of Radiology accreditation requirements.

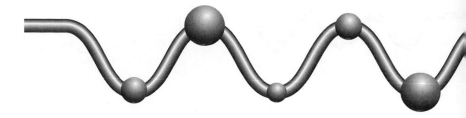

CHAPTER ELEVEN

Computers in Radiology

A. Basic Concepts

1. Computers use binary arithmetic.

- Electrical signals that have a voltage (usually 5 volts) are counted as a "1."
- Electrical signals with zero voltage are counted as a "0."
- Electrical noise is ignored because the signals are close to cither 1 or 0.
- The electrical signal shown in the figure has a binary number equivalent of 10101011.

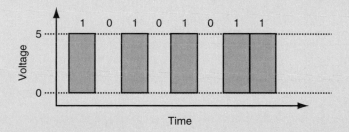

2. The interpretation of the binary signal is that each position represents 2 to a power.

- The first number to the right is $2^0 = 1$.
- The second number from the right is $2^1 = 2$.
- Similarly, for the other positions, see the table.

Binary	1	0	1	0	1	0	1	1
Power of 2^N	2^7	2^6	2^5	2^4	2^3	2^2	2^1	2^0
Equivalent number of 2^N power	128	64	32	16	8	4	2	1
Conversion of binary number	128	0	32	0	8	0	2	1

- The binary number 10101011 converts to $128 + 0 + 32 + 0 + 8 + 0 + 2 + 1 = 171$.
- If the last digit is a 1, the number is odd.
- If the last digit is a 0, the number is even.
- If all eight digits are 1, the number is 255.

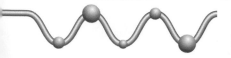

- If the left digit of an eight-digit binary is 1, the number is greater than 128.

3. Each 0 or 1 in a binary number is called a bit (b).

4. Each group of eight binary bits is called a byte (B).

5. *1 MB* = 1 megabyte = 1,000,000 bytes = 8,000,000 bits.

6. The pixel value of computed radiography (CR), digital radiography (DR), computed tomography (CT) images, and magnetic resonance imaging (MRI) scans may cover a large range of values. For example, CT images cover values from −1000 HU to +3000 HU.

7. *A range of 4096 levels* requires a binary number with 12 bits. However, because computers store numbers in bytes, two bytes would be required even though *only 12 bits are necessary*.

8. The rate at which data can be transmitted is listed in bits per second, which is called *baud*. A transmission rate of 1000 bits per second is called a kilobaud.

   - Personal *computer modems* transmit data over *telephone lines* (plain old telephone service, or POTS) at 56 kilobaud (Kbps).

   - An *integrated services digital network (ISDN)*, such as two telephone lines, transmits data at 128 kbps.

   - *Dedicated service lines (DSLs)* and coaxial cable lines (T1) transmit data at 1.5 Mbps.

   - Cable television lines transmit data at <10 Mbps.

   - Fiber-optic cable (backbone) lines transmit data at a rate of 100 Mbps.

   - Satellite links transmit data at <200 Mbps.

9. Computer calculation speed is measured in *millions of instructions per second (MIPS)*. Modern personal computers operate at frequencies of 3 to 10 GHz.

10. Computer components are classified into *input devices (I)* that feed data into the computer; *output devices (O)* that send out data from memory; and *memory devices*.

    - Input devices include: keyboard, floppy disk (and other disks), magnetic tapes, and modems.

    - A modem is a device that connects to a telephone to convert digital numbers to a signal for the telephone line and convert it back again to a digital number to be read by another computer at the other end of the telephone line.

    - Output devices include a video monitor (video display terminal, or VDT), printer, various memory disks, hard memory inside the computer, and a modem.

11. Memory components for a computer include the following:

    - *CPU (central processing unit)* is the device in a computer that performs the calculations. It executes instructions (the program) and performs operations on data.

    - *RAM (random access memory)* is a type of temporary memory in a computer used to run programs, process images, and store information temporarily. The size of the RAM on personal computers is typically 64 to 512 MB. Information stored in RAM is lost when the computer is turned off.

    - A computer also has a *hard memory*, which is retained when the computer is turned off. This is a magnetic/optical (M/O) memory. For personal computers, the hard memory is around 20 to 100 gigabytes (GB).

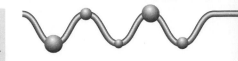

- **ROM (read only memory)** is used to store certain instructions and programs such as the **BIOS (basic input/output system)** and the **POST (power on self test)**. ROMs are electronic circuit chips that are permanently programmed.

- Dual-sided **floppy disks** hold 1.44 MB of data.

- **Zip disks** hold 100 MB of memory.

- *CDs* are **compact disks**, which come in two varieties: CD-R, on which data can be written but not erased, and CD-R/W, on which data can be written and erased for reuse. CDs typically hold 650 MB of data.

- **Jaz disks** hold 1000 to 2000 MB of memory.

- **Optical disks** can hold 2 to 8 GB. These are called **WORM (write once, read many)** disks. A laser writes by burning holes in a plastic substrate, which is permanent and can be read many times without erasing the information.

- **Digital archival tapes (DATs)** can hold 70 GB of data.

12. The electronic system in a computer is based on transistor circuits called flip-flops. Flip-flops change state from 0 to 1 and back with every input voltage pulse.

    - The logic system is called Boolean algebra and consists of various gates.

    - **And gate** requires both A and B pulses to be 1 to produce an output of 1. For all other possible inputs, the output is 0.

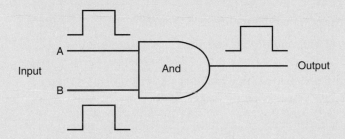

    - **Or gate** requires either A or B (or both) pulses to be 1 to produce an output of 1; if both A and B are 0, the output is 0.

    - **Nand gate** requires both A and B pulses to be 1 to produce an output of 0. For all other possible inputs, the output is 1.

    - **Nor gate** requires neither A nor B pulses to be 1 to produce an output of 1.

    - Similar gate circuits are used to add, subtract, multiply, and divide.

13. **Microprocessors** are combinations of many transistors in one or more small solid-state electronic chips called **integrated circuits** that perform assigned functions in the computer.

14. Computers need software instructions, which determine the manner in which given data are stored at different address locations and in which mathematical operations are performed. These instructions are called the **disk operating system (DOS)**.

15. **Bus** refers to the connection between various parts of the computer that carries the signals and data between these sections.

    - **Serial port** (e.g., RS-232) is an input/output connector for many peripheral devices, such as a mouse, modem, and electronic digital instruments. The signals are sent sequentially. The advantage is less cross-talk (interference), but the data transmission is slow.

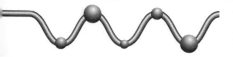

- *Parallel port* (e.g., Centronics) is an input/output connector for most computer printers. Signals are sent in parallel over several cables. The advantage is a much higher data transmission speed, but there is more cross-talk (interference) between adjacent cable wires.

16. *Flatbed scanners* use a small, high-intensity light beam to scan pictures or word documents and convert them into electronic data.

   - The scanned data can be in the form of a bitmap or various types of compressed data, such as joint picture experts group (JPEG) files, wavelet transforms, and TREE software.

   - For lossless (not clinically noticeable or significant) data compression, no more than 2:1 compression is currently used, even though higher levels of compression (up to 10:1) show little degradation.

   - Optical character recognition (OCR) software is used to make certain that the scanners properly interpret alphabetic symbols.

17. Networks connect two or more computers in order to share software and information. Connections can be via either *local area networks (LANs)* or the *World Wide Web (WWW)*, which connects facilities that are far apart.

18. *Analog-to-digital conversion (ADC)* devices convert continuously varying signals to digital signals with discrete steps of voltage.

B.   Questions

11-1.   The system of counting used by computers is called _____ system.

(a) Octal   (b) Hexadecimal   (c) Decimal   (d) Quadratic
(e) Binary

11-2.   The computer number 100111 is equal to a value of _____.

(a) 4   (b) 25   (c) 31   (d) 39   (e) 46

11-3.   A disk that has a larger memory size than a CD-ROM is called a _____.

(a) Modem   (b) USB   (c) Buffer   (d) HTML   (e) DVD

11-4.   A device that converts digital information to signals that can be transmitted through a telephone line to another computer is called a _____.

(a) Modem   (b) USB   (c) Buffer   (d) HTML   (e) DVD

11-5.   An electrical connection port in a computer that can accept serial data from an external device such as a digital camera or a flatbed scanner is called a _____.

(a) Modem   (b) USB   (c) Buffer   (d) HTML   (e) DVD

11-6.   Computer software that enables various computer programs to be linked together in a multitasking manner is called a _____.

(a) Modem   (b) USB   (c) Buffer   (d) HTML   (e) DVD

11-7.   A temporary data storage component that allows rapid information transfer is called a _____.

(a) Modem   (b) USB   (c) Buffer   (d) HTML   (e) DVD

11-8.   One would list computer transfer data links in order from slowest to fastest as follows: _____.

(a) ISDBN, POTS, T1, and satellite
(b) POTS, satellite, ISDN, and T1
(c) Satellite, POTS, ISDN, and T1

(d) T1, ISDN, POTS, and satellite

(e) POTS, ISDN, T1, and satellite

11-9. The number of 256×256 MRI images that can be stored on a CD-ROM disk without any data compression is _____.

(a) 1000   (b) 2500   (c) 5000   (d) 7500   (c) 9000

11-10. The number of 512×512 CT images that can be stored on a CD-ROM disk with 2:1 compression of data is _____.

(a) 1000   (b) 2500   (c) 5000   (d) 7500   (c) 9000

11-11. All of the following can be a part of the LAN, *except* _____.

(a) File server   (b) Firewall   (c) UPS   (d) Token ring   (e) Node

11-12. A mouse is usually connected to a computer with _____.

(a) A serial port   (b) A parallel port   (c) Both ports   (d) Neither port
(e) A multiplexer

11-13. A computer printer is usually connected to the computer with _____.

(a) A serial port   (b) A parallel port   (c) Both ports   (d) Neither port
(e) A multiplexer

11-14. The slowest data transmission is with a(n) _____.

(a) RS-232   (b) Centronics connection   (c) Multiplexer
(d) RF wireless connection   (e) Trionic switch

11-15. The temporary computer memory that can be accessed randomly is a type of memory classified as _____.

(a) BIOS   (b) R/W   (c) DOS   (d) WORM   (e) RAM

11-16. The hardware device that activates start-up of a computer and initiates the connection to internal subsystems and software is called the _____.

(a) BIOS   (b) R/W   (c) DOS   (d) WORM   (e) RAM

11-17. The _____ is the software that converts digital numbers into computer operations and must be loaded into the computer before anything can be used.

(a) BIOS   (b) R/W   (c) DOS   (d) WORM   (e) RAM

11-18. The long-term memory that cannot be erased, as on some types of optical disks, is designated as _____.

(a) BIOS   (b) R/W   (c) DOS   (d) WORM   (e) RAM

11-19. A method of data compression is called _____.

(a) JPEG   (b) VDT   (c) Facsimile (fax)   (d) POST   (e) Flip-flop

11-20. All of the following are types of printers for computer output, *except* ___.

(a) Bubble jet   (b) Dot matrix   (c) Xonix   (d) Thermal contact
(e) Laser matrix

11-21. The type of logical operations used by the electronic circuits inside a computer is called _____.

(a) Fuzzy logic   (b) Iterative operators   (c) Inverse matrix
(d) Boolean algebra   (e) Speculative calculus

11-22. A _____ consists of the individual 0 and 1 digits that make up the language of computers.

(a) MIPS   (b) Baud   (c) Byte   (d) Bit   (e) Icon

11-23. The speed at which computer operations can be performed by a computer is measured in units of _____.

(a) MIPS   (b) Baud   (c) Byte   (d) Bit   (e) Icon

11-24. The rate at which computer data can be transmitted over a link is measured in terms of bits per second or _____.

(a) MIPS   (b) Baud   (c) Byte   (d) Bit   (e) Icon

11-25. _____ is a group of eight computer digits.

(a) MIPS   (b) Baud   (c) Byte   (d) Bit   (e) Icon

11-26. _____ is a computer symbol that is used to select computer operations.

(a) MIPS   (b) Baud   (c) Byte   (d) Bit   (e) Icon

11-27. _____ represents the ranking of digital storage devices from the smallest capacity to the largest capacity.

(a) Jaz, Zip, DAT, CD, floppy   (b) Floppy, Zip, CD, Jaz, DAT
(c) DAT, Jaz, Zip, floppy, CD   (d) CD, floppy, Jaz, Zip, DAT
(e) Floppy, CD, Zip, Zap, DAT

11-28. The two classifications of different types of personal computers are _____ and _____.

(a) CRT, plasma   (b) Acute, somatic   (c) PC, Mac
(d) Remote, hardwire   (e) DOS, Windows

11-29. The internal electrical conductors that connect various internal component subsystems with the computer are called the _____.

(a) EPROM   (b) Bus   (c) Flip-flops   (d) 12 DIP   (e) Zener diode

11-30. All of the following are types of computer display screens, *except* _____.

(a) LCD   (b) Plasma   (c) CRT   (d) LED   (e) EPI

C.   Answers

11-1. Answer = (e). The octal system uses binary bits, but it groups the binary bits in a base of 8. The hexadecimal system groups the binary bits in the base 10 counting system. The decimal system is our conventional counting system, in which each digit represents the number 10 to a different power. For example, the number 23 means 2 of 10^1 plus 3 of 10^0. The decimal system is not used directly in computers. The binary system is used because it is relatively insensitive to electronic noise. The binary numbers are then reconverted to decimal numbers for output. Quadratic describes the relationship between a dependent variable and the square of an independent variable; it is not a counting system.

11-2. Answer = (d). This answer can be quickly determined. The sixth digit is a 1, so that the value must be greater than $2^{N-1} = 2^{6-1} = 2^5 = 2 \times 2 \times 2 \times 2 \times 2 = 32$. Hence, answers (a), (b), and (c) can be eliminated because they are less than 32. The last binary digit is a 1; thus, the number must be an odd number such as 1, 3, 5, or 7. Because answer (e) is even, it is eliminated, leaving only one correct answer. More meticulously, the binary bits mean $32 + 0 + 0 + 4 + 2 + 1 = 39$.

11-3. Answer = (e). A CD-ROM has a memory size of 650 MB, and a digital video disk (DVD) has a memory size of many gigabytes. A modem is used to convert binary computer data to signals that can be transmitted from the computer over telephone lines to another computer. Modems are used when the WWW is used. USB stands for universal serial bus, which is an electrical connector system that allows digital cameras, flatbed scanners, and other peripheral devices to be connected to a computer. A buffer is a piece of computer hardware used to allow input of data into temporary storage at higher speeds than computers can normally handle; then the data are retrieved at a slower rate and processed by the computer. HTML is short for HyperText Markup Language, the authoring language used to create documents on the World Wide Web.

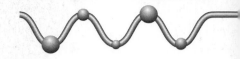

The software programs allow computers to do many things simultaneously (multitasking) and share information from various computer programs and other computers.

11-4. Answer = (a). See answer to Question 11-3.

11-5. Answer = (b). See answer to Question 11-3.

11-6. Answer = (d). See answer to Question 11-3.

11-7. Answer = (c). See answer to Question 11-3.

11-8. Answer = (e). To rank the choices, identify the slowest or the fastest means to eliminate several of the answers. The slowest transfer rate is provided by plain old telephone service (POTS), which has a rate of 56 kilobaud. This eliminates (a), (c), and (d) as potential answers. The fastest transfer rates are with T1 or fiber-optic lines, at rates of 1 to 3 and 100 megabaud, respectively. ISDN has a data transfer rate of 128 Kbps (kilobaud), and satellite has a rate of about 200 Mbps.

11-9. Answer = (c). A CD-ROM has a memory size of 650 MB. A single MRI image has $256 \times 256 \times 2$ bytes, or 131,072 B (0.131072 MB). Dividing the memory size by the data in a single MRI image yields an answer of 4959, or about 5000.

11-10. Answer = (b). A CT image has double the amount of data in each of the horizontal and vertical directions. Hence, the data for a 512×512 CT image should be $2 \times 2 = 4$ times more than for a 256×256 MRI image. However, the data compression of 2:1 reduces the size by a factor of 2, so the CT image should be only two times larger than the MRI image. Because the CT images contain more data, fewer can be stored on a CD. This eliminates answers (c), (d), and (e). Half of the answer to Question 11-9 is 2500 images. Most storage units for CT scanners use optical disks with capacities of 4 or more GB so that more images can be stored on a single disk.

11-11. Answer = (c). A UPS is a universal power supply, which is an electrical power filter used to remove electrical spikes and drops and to provide a constant voltage. Computers and other digital systems can use these to prevent computer failure related to rapid electrical fluctuations. However, UPS devices are not specifically parts of computer networks. File servers are computers used in networks to direct traffic and transfer data from the main memory source to individual computers on a network, which are called nodes. Firewalls are security devices that are designed to prevent unauthorized users ("hackers") from gaining access to the network and its data.

There are several ways to connect computers together into a network. One method is a token ring, which sequentially transfers data from one computer in the network to another until it reaches the intended recipient. Another connection scheme that allows direct transfer from the source to the destination is called an ethernet.

11-12. Answer = (a). A multiplexer is a device that frequency-encodes signals so than many different signals can be sent simultaneously over a single cable.

11-13. Answer = (b). Although some modern printers allow newer USB or "fire wire" serial connections, most current printers use a multiple-cable parallel scheme to speed up the data transfer process.

11-14. Answer = (a). An RS-232 is a serial port. A Centronics is a faster parallel port. A multiplexer was described in Answer 11-12. RF and optical wireless connections are fast. A trionics switch is a nonsensical phrase that is not real.

11-15. Answer = (e). BIOS is the boot-up input output system, which starts up computers and establishes the connections for the various devices and software. R/W means read/write; it pertains to the ability to place data on a memory device and then erase the data to reuse the device. An example is the CD-R/W, which can be reused many times. DOS is the disk operating system, which can convert the instructions in digital signals, perform the operations, and convert

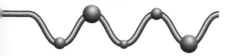

the data into usable output. Similar modern systems include Windows and others. WORM means write once, read many times. Optical disks can be burned by a laser to record data that can be permanently encoded. The data can then be read many times without being changed. RAM means random access memory. RAM is temporary memory that is erased when the computer is turned off. If one types a letter on a computer and fails to save it to the hard memory disk or an external memory device, the letter disappears when the computer is turned off.

11-16. Answer = (a). See answer to Question 11-15.

11-17. Answer = (c). See answer to Question 11-15.

11-18. Answer = (d). See answer to Question 11-15.

11-19. Answer = (a). JPEG stands for joint picture expert group, which is the organization that developed the compression software. VDT is the video display terminal, or the computer monitor. Facsimile (fax) is a system that can scan documents, convert them into signals for transmission over the telephone line, and convert the signals back through a printer into a document. POST is the hardware device in a computer that does the power-on and start-up tests to make certain that all components are functioning properly. Flip-flop is the basic component of most computer logic devices that function like "and gates" and "or gates."

11-20. Answer = (c). Xonix is a nonsense word that does not represent any type of printer.

11-21. Answer = (d). Fuzzy logic is used in digital still cameras and video cameras to focus the lens automatically based on the images. Iterative operations can be used to reconstruct images for CT scanner data or similar data sets. Inverse matrix is a mathematical method used to solve matrix problems. Speculative calculus is a nonsensical term based on the mathematics of calculus.

11-22. Answer = (d). MIPS is millions of instructions per second, and it is a measure of the rate at which a computer can do operations such as addition, subtraction, and changing locations of data. A bit (b) is the 1 or 0 of the binary numbers used by a computer. A group of 8 bits (which can form a number up to 255 in value) is called a byte (B). Baud is the measure of data transmission through links; a rate of 1 bit per second is equal to a baud. An icon is a pictorial symbol that is used to represent a computer operation. For example, a picture of an open folder is used to designate the operation of opening stored computer files.

11-23. Answer = (a). See the answer to Question 11-22.

11-24. Answer = (b). See the answer to Question 11-22.

11-25. Answer = (c). See the answer to Question 11-22.

11-26. Answer = (e). See the answer to Question 11-22.

11-27. Answer = (b). Again, the best way to eliminate potential answers is to pick the lowest and highest capacity memory storage devices. A floppy disk holds the lowest capacity of data, at 1.44 MB (about 1.5 MB), and a DAT (digital archival tape or digital audio tape) has the highest capacity at 70 GB. Thus, answers (a), (c), and (d) can be eliminated. A zip disk holds 100 MB of data, a CD holds 650 MB, and a jaz disk holds 1 to 2 GB.

11-28. Answer = (c). Plasma and CRT are two different types of display monitors. Acute describes immediate medical symptoms that occur suddenly versus long-term, chronic effects. Remote and hardwire refer to two ways of connecting peripheral components to a computer. Hardwire connections use a cable, and remote connections transfer data by RF waves or optical signals from a distance. DOS and Windows are two types of computer operating software.

11-29. Answer = (b). EPROM (erasable programmable read-only memory) is an electrical hardwired logic component that does a certain computer operation that can *not* be changed. Flip-flops are the basic electronic circuit that

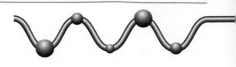

compose the structure for Boolean algebraic decisions, such as "and gates" and "or gates." A 12 DIP is a socket that has 12 dual in-line pins; it is used for the insertion of integrated circuit chips. A zener diode is a solid-state device used in power supplies for electrical devices to help provide a constant voltage.

11-30. Answer = (e). LCD is a liquid crystal display, which is a flat-type monitor. A plasma display is found on many new, flat-screen television sets. CRT is a cathode ray tube that is deep because of the electron gun of the tube. An LED is light-emitting diode. EPI (echo planar imaging) is a type of pulse sequence used in MRI.

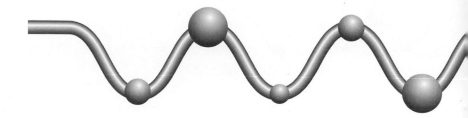

CHAPTER TWELVE

Computed Radiography, Digital Radiography, and Picture Archiving, Communications, and Storage

A. Computed Radiography (CR)

1. CR is computed radiography.

- It uses cassettes externally similar to film-screen cassettes.
- These cassettes can be used with existing x-ray equipment in a similar manner to film-screen cassettes.
- Inside the light-tight carbon fiber cassettes are plates that are composed of barium fluorohalides (BaFBr).
- A special reader is required to read the phosphor and erase it electronically.

2. X-ray radiation causes ionization in the plates, which results in electrons being trapped in excited energy states.

3. The readout unit opens the cassette and removes the plate. The plate is placed on a conveyor belt. A laser scans the plate one line at a time (fast direction). The conveyor belt then moves the cassette mechanically to the next line (slow direction).

4. The laser light adds energy to the electrons trapped in the excited state. These trapped electrons eventually fall to the ground energy level, emitting light in the process. The light is of a higher frequency than the light of the laser. This process is called *photostimulated phosphor emission (PSP)*.

5. An optical filter separates the intensity of the laser light from the PSP light. The PSP light is then measured by a light detector, such as a *photomultiplier tube (PMT)*.

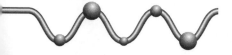

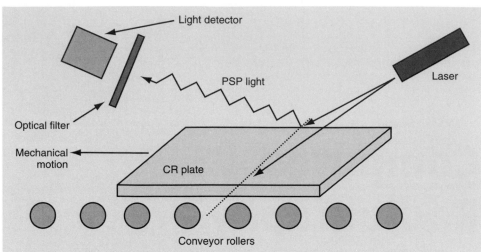

6. Where more x-rays strike the phosphor of the cassette, more PSP light is produced. The measured light is converted to an electrical signal with amplitude directly related to the intensity of the x-rays hitting the cassette at that location.

7. A bright light source flashes the PSP plate to erase it. It is then reinserted into the cassette.

8. Advantages of CR include the following:

   - A large dynamic range—12 bits or 4096 levels of radiation can be recorded; this compares with about 8 bits or 256 levels for film-screen cassettes

   - Ability to record radiation levels from 0.01 to 100 mR incident on the cassette

   - Multiple image display formats with different software postprocessing

   - Easy distribution of images electronically

   - No lost films and better long-term storage and retrieval

   - Better low-contrast image quality and discrimination

   - More compact image storage

9. Disadvantages of CR include the following:

   - Radiation doses are about double those of 400-relative-speed film-screen systems.

   - Spatial resolution is lower than in film-screen systems: CR has a limit of about 3.0 to 3.5 LP/mm, and film-screen systems have spatial resolution of about 6.0 to 10.0 LP/mm.

   - The electronics are complex and expensive.

   - The support staff must be highly skilled to maintain the electronics.

   - Technologic obsolescence increases costs; system must be upgraded often.

   - Additional network costs are incurred to transmit and receive images.

   - Latent image fades during the first 10 to 20 minutes.

10. The spatial resolution limit equals the number of pixels in the image divided by [2 × FoV (mm)].

    - Because the same matrix size is often used for all FoVs in some systems, large cassettes have worse spatial resolution than smaller cassettes.

    - For 2500 pixels and a 14 × 17-inch cassette (35 × 43 cm), spatial resolution is 2500/[2 × 430 mm] = 2.9 LP/mm.

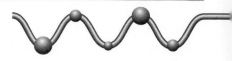

11. The average amount of radiation incident upon the CR cassette to form an image is measured by an exposure index number (EI#).

$$EI\# = 1000 \times \log_{10} [\text{exposure in mR}] + 2000 \text{ (Kodak system)}$$

- This ranges from an exposure level of 0.01 mR with EI# = 0.0.
- It ranges to an exposure level of 100.0 mR with EI# = 4000.
- Darkness is a log scale display.
- Different software displays are available, such as high contrast, edge enhancement, and black and white reversed.

12. Sources of digital images include CR, DR, MRI, CT, ultrasonography, angiography, and digital subtraction angiography.

13. Typical data sizes of some digital images can be calculated using the formula [matrix width × matrix length × depth in bytes]. Values are listed in the table.

MATRIX SIZE	NUMBER OF PIXELS	BIT DEPTH	IMAGE SIZE (MBYTES)
CR or DR 1024 × 1024	1,048,576	8	1
CR or DR 2048 × 2048	4,194,304	12	6
MRI 256 × 256	65,536	12	0.13
Ultrasound 512 × 512	262,144	8	0.26 (gray)
			0.78 (color)
CT 512 × 512	262,144	12	0.52
Digital mammography 3000 × 3625	10,875,000	12	21.8

B. Digital Radiography (DR)

1. DR is digital radiography.

- DR requires specialized equipment that replaces the cassette tray with a specialized digital detector system.
- This detector is fragile. If the system design requires modification or the detector is damaged, replacement of the entire x-ray unit is required.
- The systems are of two different designs: direct and indirect.
- Data from the detector are directly digitized and sent out to a picture archiving, communications, and storage (PACS) system.

2. *Direct DR* is usually composed of an array of amorphous selenium detectors that capture the ionizations created in the detectors and measure the charge deposited directly.

3. *Indirect DR* usually has a scintillator such as cesium iodide (CsI) coated over an array of light-sensing solid-state devices, such as a charge-coupled device (CCD) or photodiode transistor-transistor logic (TTL) chips, as shown in the figure.

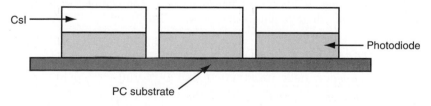

4. The *pitch* refers to the sides of each detector element of a DR array.

5. The *area of a detector* is equal to the product of pitch × pitch.

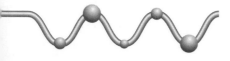

6. Not all of the area of a detector array is usable to detect x-rays. Some of the area is occupied by readout switches and printed circuit leads.

7. The usable area for detection divided by the total area of each detector, expressed as a percentage, is called the ***fill factor***.

8. High fill factors result in use of more of the radiation, which reduces the patient's entrance radiation doses. Typical values for the fill factor range from 55% to about 85%.

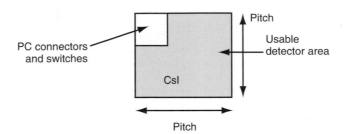

9. Other losses of incident x-ray energy occur by penetration through the detectors, light losses in the detector, and failure to convert deposited energy into light. The overall efficiency of the system in using the incident x-ray energy is called the ***detected quantum efficiency (DQE)***.

10. Most DR systems use detector pitch sizes of 150 to 200 microns, or 0.15 to 0.20 mm. The exception is mammography DR detectors, which have pitch sizes of 0.025 to 0.10 mm, depending on the manufacturer and the design of the detector.

11. Both CR and DR systems are associated with worse spatial resolution than the film-screen cassette; however, the increased dynamic range, the adjustable display contrast (with window width and level adjustment), the software image processing features, and the capability for digital archiving seem to outweigh the loss in resolution.

12. DR requires much less time to acquire and distribute images than the CR systems. This feature increases patient throughput.

13. The main disadvantage is the high cost of installing DR systems. Each room must have its own DR equipment. In contrast, CR cassettes can be used in multiple rooms, and the x-ray equipment does not require any modification to be able to use CR cassettes instead of film-screen cassettes.

C. Picture Archiving, Communications, and Storage (PACS)

1. *PACS* stands for picture archiving, communications, and storage. Imaging data from this modality are in the digital image communication format of ***Digital Imaging and Communications in Medicine (DICOM)*** so that it can be recognized by all vendors.

2. Sources of digital images include CR, DR, magnetic resonance imaging (MRI), computed tomography (CT), ultrasonography, angiography and cardiac systems, fluoroscopy systems, digital mammography, and film digitizers.

3. The systems can be grouped in a local area network (LAN) or on the World Wide Web (WWW). The following are elements of PACS systems:

   ● Token ring: a sequentially linked system that must transfer data from one terminal to the next in order

   ● Ethernet: a system in which communications can go directly from the source to the recipient

   ● Node: each connection on the network

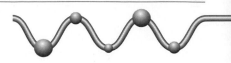

- Servers: computers that act as traffic control to receive a request, direct images to proper storage, and retrieve and transmit images
- Short-term image storage
- Long-term archival storage

4. Short-term image storage (RAID)

- RAID = redundant array of individual disks
- Each RAID consists of multiple (24 or more) disk drives.
- Each disk drive can store tens of gigabytes of image data.
- The total capacity of one RAID is hundreds of gigabytes.
- Typical short-term storage may consist of multiple RAIDs capable of storing a few TB (terabytes). This is the typical amount of image data produced annually at a small hospital.

5. Long-term storage can consist of DAT or DLT (types of digital archival tapes).

- Each DAT or DLT = 70 GB.
- A library consists of hundreds of DLTs allowing storage of tens of TB (terabytes) of image data.
- Data are typically stored with 2:1 lossless compression.

6. The storage capacity depends on the type and number of examinations performed. *Typical study sizes* are listed in the table.

IMAGING PROCEDURE	MATRIX SIZE	NUMBER OF IMAGES	DATA SIZE* (Mbytes)
CT (body)	512×512	100	52
MRI (head)	256×256	120	16
CR (extremity)	2048×2500	5	51
CR (chest)	2048×2500	2	21
Digital mammography	3000×3625	5	109

*Uncompressed images

- Digital mammography image data require so much data storage that they are often handled separately.
- Although CT images consist of only about 0.5 MB (uncompressed) per image, the large number of images results in significant image storage space.

7. The speed at which images can be transferred over a PACS depends on the type of connection.

TYPE OF CONNECTION	SPEED (Kbits/sec)	SPEED (sec/MB)	TIME TO TRANSMIT 6 MB IMAGE
56 K modem	56	143	858 sec = 14.3 min
ISDN line	128	62.5	375 sec = 6.25 min
T1 line	1,540	5.2	31.2 sec = 0.52 min
Optical fiber	100,000	0.08	0.48 sec

- **Backbone**: the main wire or fiber-optic cable connecting nodes. The main network connection is usually a T1 line or optical fiber because of speed demands.

8. Readout monitors for a PACS system need to be of good quality with a long-range gray scale and a display of at least 2000×2000.

- **SMPTE pattern**: The SMPTE (Society of Motion Picture and Television Engineers) pattern is used to check the monitors for consistent gray scale, low-contrast visibility, high-contrast resolution, and distortion.
- Light intensity of monitors is important for good image quality; 200 to 400 Cd/m^2 light output is desirable.

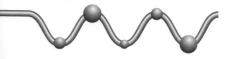

- Uniformity of monitor light intensity is also important.
- Because of high light intensity, monitor life may be limited to 1 to 3 years.

D. Questions

12-1. A PACS system includes all of the following components, *except* _____.

(a) Servers   (b) Transmission lines   (c) Display systems
(d) Redundant storage devices   (e) Image acquisition devices

12-2. A major difference between CR and DR acquisition devices is _____.

(a) Patient throughput   (b) Detector type   (c) Patient radiation dose
(d) Compatibility with film-screen systems   (e) All of the above

12-3. The detector of a CR system is a _____ and the detector of a DR system is _____.

(a) NaI, CaWO$_4$ (b) BaFBr, CsI   (c) GdO$_2$S$_2$, BGO   (d) LaOBr, LiF
(e) Xenon, ceramic crystal

12-4. _____ is the system in which x-ray radiation causes excitation energy to be stored in electron traps in crystals and released by a readout laser.

(a) PSP   (b) TLD   (c) Scintillation process   (d) Ionization chamber
(e) PMT

12-5. The largest amount of information (in bytes) is contained in a single _____ image.

(a) CT   (b) MRI   (c) Gray scale ultrasound   (d) Digital mammography
(e) CR extremity

12-6. The largest amount of information (in bytes) contained in all the images in a patient's examination occurs with a(n) _____.

(a) Nuclear camera   (b) Gray scale ultrasound   (c) DR of the chest
(d) CT of the abdomen and pelvis   (e) MRI of the head

12-7. A major advantage of a CR system over a film-screen system is improved _____.

(a) Spatial resolution   (b) Dynamic range   (c) Radiation dose to the patient   (d) Scatter rejection   (e) All of the above

12-8. The major disadvantage of a CR system in comparison with a film-screen system is degraded _____.

(a) Spatial resolution   (b) Image latitude
(c) Low-contrast discrimination   (d) Repeat rate   (e) Image distortion

12-9. A major problem with DR image receptors is _____.

(a) Temperature stability   (b) "Bad" pixels   (c) Low fill factor
(d) Image persistence   (e) All of the above

12-10. The time required to transmit 100 CT images over a fiber-optic PACS network is about ____ seconds.

(a) 5   (b) 25   (c) 100   (d) 200   (e) 500

12-11. List in order of increasing speed the following types of PACS network links: (i) ISDN (ii) DSL (iii) POTS (iv) Satellites

(a) i, ii, iii, iv   (b) iii, ii, i, iv   (c) ii, iii, i, iv   (d) iii, i, ii, iv   (e) i, ii, iv, iii

12-12. An intermediate image storage device on a PACS system could consist of a group of _____.

(a) DLT drives   (b) RAIDs   (c) MOD disks   (d) Zip disks
(e) Dual deck DVDs

12-13. Long-term image storage on a PACS system could consist of one or more libraries of _____.

(a) DLT drives   (b) RAIDs   (c) MOD disks   (d) Zip disks
(e) Dual deck DVDs

12-14. An individual image display station on a PACS network might be called a(n) _____.

(a) Mole   (b) Modem   (c) Node   (d) Cell   (e) MCA

12-15. The device that directs the storage and retrieval of information in a PACS system is called a(n) _____.

(a) PHA   (b) Transducer   (c) Server   (d) Translator
(e) Encryptor

12-16. A device that protects a PACS network from intrusion by "hackers" is called a(n) _____.

(a) Decimator   (b) Firewall   (c) USB   (d) Condenser   (e) ADC

12-17. Video monitors in a PACS network can be evaluated using a(n) _____ pattern.

(a) Holography   (b) NEMA   (c) SMPTE   (d) JPEG
(e) NCRP

12-18. The overall efficiency of a digital image receptor in using incident radiation for image formation is called the _____.

(a) MTF   (b) CNR   (c) RSD   (d) DQE   (e) PSP

12-19. The pitch for radiography DR systems is about _____ microns, and the pitch for mammography DR systems is about _____ microns.

(a) 200, 100   (b) 100, 50   (c) 50, 25   (d) 20, 10
(e) 2, 1

12-20. The two categories of DR detectors are _____ and _____.

(a) Liquid, solid   (b) Direct, indirect   (c) Optical, chemical
(d) Coupled, distributed   (e) Resilient, disseminated

12-21. If a DLT tape can store 1300 body CT examinations, it would be expected to hold _____ MRI examinations.

(a) 650   (b) 1300   (c) 2600   (d) 5200   (e) 10,800

12-22. A radiologist has an ISDN line installed at home and wants to send a CT study with 100 images compressed 2:1 to the home computer. The time required for this transmission would be about _____ minutes.

(a) 5   (b) 10   (c) 25   (d) 50   (e) 100

12-23. A chest radiograph is taken on a DR unit with a 17×17-inch detector that has 200 microns of spatial resolution, and the image is displayed on a monitor with a 1200×1500 matrix with edge enhancement software. The factor limiting the spatial resolution most is the _____.

(a) Focal spot blur   (b) Software   (c) Detector size
(d) Display matrix   (e) Motion blur

12-24. The same image storage device can store about _____ as many gray scale ultrasound images as MRI images.

(a) 25%   (b) 50%   (c) 100%   (d) 2 times   (e) 4 times

12-25. The spatial resolution of CR or DR systems is about _____ LP/mm, and the spatial resolution of standard radiography film-screen systems is about _____ LP/mm.

(a) 1.5, 3   (b) 3, 7   (c) 6, 12   (d) 10, 5   (e) 20, 10

E. Answers

12-1. Answer = (e). The image acquisition devices, such as a CT scanner and CR units, are not considered part of the PACS system. The system consists of hardware for the transmission, reception, storage, retrieval, and display of clinical images. Usually, redundant storage is used in case the storage unit is damaged by fire, flood, or other accident or fails electronically.

12-2. Answer = (e). Because the CR cassettes must be taken to a reader and individually processed, the CR systems have much slower patient throughput than DR systems. As described in the notes for this chapter, the detectors for CR and DR are different in design. CR is usually equivalent to a 200-relative-speed film-screen system, and DR is usually faster than a 400-relative-speed system. CR systems can be used with film-screen x-ray equipment, and the CR cassette is exposed in the same Bucky tray. However, the CR cassette must be taken to a special CR plate reader to process the image. The DR system requires replacement of the Bucky tray with a dedicated image receptor, and the images are electronically obtained from the detector and transmitted to the PACS system.

12-3. Answer = (b). See notes in this chapter (**A1** and **B3**).

12-4. Answer = (a). The description is for a CR system. The phosphor material is called a photostimulated phosphor. The laser (photo or light) stimulates the trapped electrons from x-ray irradiation to fall to ground energy level, releasing light of a different wavelength from the laser light. TLD is a thermoluminescent dosimeter, which also works with trapped electrons that are released by heating the crystals to emit light; TLDs are used as personnel dosimeters. Scintillation crystals emit light (with no stimulation) immediately after irradiation. Ionization chambers measure the charge created in air by the passage of radiation through the air. PMT is a photomultiplier tube used in nuclear medicine radiation detectors.

12-5. Answer = (d). The largest image matrix with the largest number of bits per pixel produces the image with the largest data size. Digital mammography units use 12 to 14 bits per pixel and have a matrix size ranging from 1800×2400 to 7200×9600. The next largest matrix sizes are for CR and DR and are typically 2000×2500. CT has a matrix of only 512×512, and MRI has half the matrix size at 256×256 (or less).

12-6. Answer = (d). Nuclear medicine matrix sizes are about the same as those of MRI, or less. A study with a large amount of data requires both a large matrix and many images. Although CR of the chest involves a large matrix, there are typically only two images in a chest study. MRI and CT examinations typically have around 100 images each; however, the CT matrix is four times the size (twice in each orthogonal direction) of an MRI matrix.

12-7. Answer = (b). A CR image typically has a spatial resolution of about 2 to 3.5 LP/mm, whereas a film-screen image receptor has a spatial resolution of about 4 to 8 LP/mm. The dynamic range is the ratio of the highest usable radiation level necessary to form an image divided by the lowest usable radiation level. For CR, the dynamic range is equal to [100 mR/0.01 mR] = 10,000. For film-screen systems, the dynamic range is around 10 to 50 at most. CR is equivalent to a 200-relative-speed film-screen system, whereas most clinical film-screens have a 400 or greater relative speed. Hence, CR delivers a greater radiation dose to the patient than a typical film-screen system. Both CR and film-screen systems are sensitive to scattered radiation.

12-8. Answer = (a). As explained in the answer to Question 12-7, CR has less spatial resolution than typical film-screen systems. Because of the large dynamic range and the ability to window and level, CR and DR have large latitude and the ability to demonstrate low-contrast objects. Other than error in the patient's positioning, there are usually low repeat rates with CR and DR systems. Because of the alignment of detectors and readout elements, spatial distortion with CR, DR, or film-screen systems is minimal.

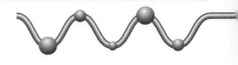

12-9. Answer = (e). DR systems usually have a coolant circulating through a heat sink plate to maintain a constant detector temperature. Manufacture of sheets with a matrix of DR detectors is subject to inoperable ("bad") detectors because of dust settling on the detector or minor flaws in the construction of the miniature solid-state devices. Because of a need to include electrical leads and switches in very small matrix elements, the fill factor on many DR systems is about 60% to 80%. DR detectors can have ghost images because of high radiation doses, resulting in image persistence.

12-10. Answer = (a). From data in the notes of this chapter, 100 uncompressed CT images would have 52 MB of data. The transmission time would be

[52 MB × (8 bits/byte)]/100 Mbps = 4.16 seconds

12-11. Answer = (d). POTS is plain old telephone service, which has a transmission rate of 56 Kbps. ISDN stands for independent service dedicated network (two-telephone line to carry data), with a rate of 128 Kbps. DSL (dedicated service line), which is a T1 line, has a rate of around 1.5 Mbps. Satellite and microwave links can approach a data rate of 200 Mbps.

12-12. Answer = (b). RAIDs typically have multiple disks that each have a memory storage capacity of tens of gigabytes for a total capacity of about hundreds of gigabytes. DLTs are long-term storage devices that have a capacity of 70 GB each; libraries can contain 200 DLT tapes. MODs, which are magneto-optical disks, can have a capacity of 2 to 10 GB; a single MOD does not have enough data storage for intermediate storage. Zip disks are small disks that hold only 100 MB each; zip disks have too small a capacity for intermediate storage. DVDs hold 4 to 10 GB each; two DVDs do not have enough capacity.

12-13. Answer = (a). See answer to Question 12-12.

12-14. Answer = (c). Mole is not applicable to the question. A modem is used to send and receive computer data over telephone lines. A cell could refer to one module in the matrix or one detector element in a DR matrix. MCA is a multichannel analyzer, which is used in nuclear medicine measurements.

12-15. Answer = (c). PHA is a pulse height analyzer, which is used to measure radioisotope spectra. A transducer is an ultrasound transmitter and receiver. A translator may be used to convert a data stream into a message. An encryptor uses a program to scramble a data stream into a code that cannot easily be translated into a message.

12-16. Answer = (b). Decimator is a fictitious term. USB stands for a universal serial bus, which is a connector for cables to be used for computer output. A condenser is the same as an electronic component called a capacitor. ADC is an analog-to-digital converter, which changes analog signals to digital signals.

12-17. Answer = (c). Holography is the use of phased laser beams to create a three-dimensional image that can be seen on some credit cards. NEMA stands for National Electronic Manufacturers' Association, which certifies the safety of electrical devices. JPEG is a software scheme for data compression of images. NCRP is the National Council on Radiation Protection, which issues documents that provide guidance for appropriate radiation safety.

12-18. Answer = (d). MTF is the modulation transfer function, which is used to measure the spatial resolution of an imaging system. CNR is the contrast-to-noise ratio, which is used to evaluate low-contrast visibility. RSD is relative standard deviation, which is a measure of statistical fluctuation or image noise. PSP is photostimulated phosphor, or the CR imaging phosphor method.

12-19. Answer = (a). The pitch for radiographic DR image receptors must be larger to cover larger size cassettes. Radiographic DR image receptors have a pitch of 150 to 200 microns, and mammographic DR image receptors have a pitch of 25 to 100 microns.

12-20. Answer = (b). See notes in this chapter (**B2** and **B3**). The other choices have no relationship to CR, DR, or PACS.

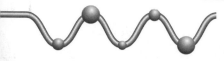

12-21. Answer = (d). A typical MRI image is a 256×256 matrix, whereas a CT image is a 512×512 matrix. Thus, in general, a CT image has four times more data than an MRI image. Thus, the DLT tape should hold about four times more MRI images, or 4×1300 CT images = 5200 MRI images.

12-22. Answer = (c). The CT data size is $512 \times 512 \times 2$ bytes $\times 8$ bits/byte $\times 100$ images $\times 0.5$ for compression = 210 Mbits. The ISDN transmits data at 128,000 bps. The amount of data is divided by the transmission rate and divided by 60 seconds/minute = 27.3 minutes.

12-23. Answer = (d). The matrix size is equal to [17 inches $\times 25.4$ mm/inch/ 0.200 mm] = 2159. So the detector resolution is better than the display matrix resolution. Focal spot blur for chest x-rays is minimal. Edge enhancement software improves spatial resolution and does not degrade it. Chest x-rays have short exposure times of about 5 to 20 milliseconds; thus, there is insufficient time to have motion blur.

12-24. Answer = (b). From the notes in this chapter, an ultrasound image has 0.25 MB of data and a MRI image has 0.13 MB of data, uncompressed. Thus, because ultrasound images are larger, fewer can be stored on an archival device.

12-25. Answer = (b). CR and DR have lower spatial resolution than film-screen systems. From previous notes, film-screen resolution for a standard radiograph is about 4 to 8 LP/mm.

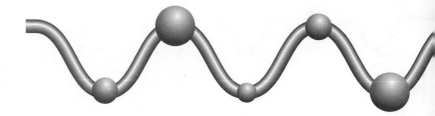

CHAPTER THIRTEEN

Image Quality

A. Basic Concepts

1. There are six basic descriptors of image quality:

   - *Density*—the overall darkness of the image

   - *Spatial resolution*—the ability to see small high-contrast objects or fine details

   - *Contrast*—the difference in darkness (density) between adjacent areas

   - *Latitude*—the ability to display many different gray scales in density for the various portions of the anatomy imaged *or* the size of the range in radiation levels transmitted through the body that appear as a shade of gray without becoming too light or too dark

   - *Unsharpness*—blur at the edges of structures

   - *Noise (or mottle)*—random variation in the background darkness (density)

2. *Contrast and latitude are opposites*. If contrast increases, latitude must decrease. If latitude increases, contrast must decrease.

   - A latitude image has a gray-looking appearance with little difference in darkness between adjacent structures in the anatomy.

   - An image with a great deal of contrast is nearly black versus white for different parts of the anatomy.

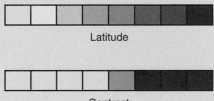

3. Image contrast (also called radiographic contrast) is the combined effect of both subject contrast and image receptor contrast.

4. Subject contrast is the difference in the number of x-rays that pass through the various parts of the body and impinge on the film (analog) or digital receptor (computed radiography [CR]/digital radiography [DR] cassette).

5. Subject contrast depends on the following factors:

   - Thickness differences in the anatomic structures

   - Density differences in the anatomic structures

   - Differences in the atomic number (Z) in the tissues

   - Introduction of "contrast media" such as iodine, barium, or air

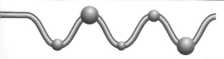

- The energy of the x-rays controlled by the kVp and x-ray beam filtration
- Effect of grids removing scattered x-rays

6. High-energy x-rays have less photoelectric effect and more Compton interactions with the tissues, which reduces the inherent subject contrast and results in more scattered x-rays, subsequently further decreasing the subject contrast.

7. ***Image receptor contrast for a film-screen system*** depends on the following factors:

   - The selection of the film, which affects the characteristic curve contrast
   - The film processing conditions—temperature, developer concentration, and so forth
   - Light and background fog of the film
   - The density of the film, which controls the contrast gradient—which is highest in the linear region of the characteristic curve and much lower in the toe and shoulder of the curve

   Type of intensifying screen does *not* affect the contrast.

8. ***Film fog*** is affected by:

   - Improper film storage
   - Film processing conditions (e.g., high temperature)
   - Light leaks

9. Image receptor contrast for a CR/DR system depends on:

   - Window and level settings for the display
   - Software processing of the data, such as smoothing and edge enhancement
   - Display monitor contrast gradient

10. Unsharpness or blur depends on:

    - Geometric unsharpness or focal spot blur
    - Motion unsharpness or voluntary and involuntary motion of the patient
    - Intensifying screen unsharpness or thickness of screens, affecting light dispersion
    - Absorption unsharpness of anatomic organs, which can have tapered edges
    - Parallax unsharpness related to dual-emulsion film with opposite sides displaced

11. ***Focal spot blur*** is due to the fact that the focal spot has a dimension (F) and to the fact that magnification of the image (M) occurs because of the divergence of the x-rays and the displacement of the anatomy away from the image receptor.

    - M, magnification, equals SID/SOD, where SID = distance from focal spot to image receptor and SOD = distance from focal spot to anatomy.
    - P, penumbra or blur, equals $(M - 1) \times F$.
    - If a part of the anatomy is directly against the image receptor, M = 1.0, and there is no magnification.
    - Blur increases with larger focal spots and greater magnification (see figure shown on next page).

12. ***Unsharpness and spatial resolution are related***. As unsharpness increases, edges of objects become blurry and spatial resolution deteriorates!

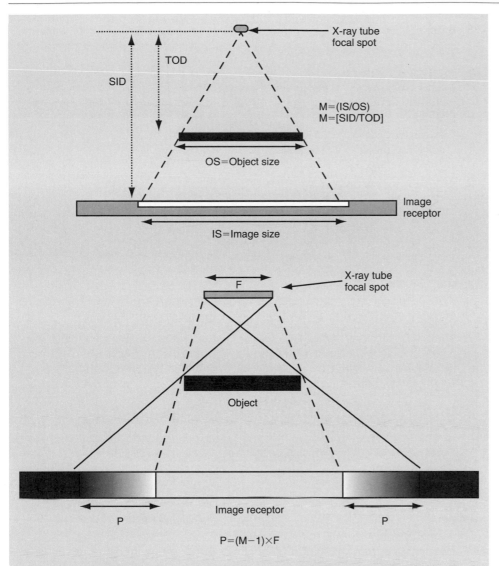

$M=(IS/OS)$
$M=[SID/TOD]$

OS=Object size

IS=Image size

$P=(M-1)\times F$

13. **Spatial resolution** can be measured in several different but related ways.

- Smallest diameter circular hole in an object that can be seen.

- Largest number of **line pairs per mm (LP/mm)** in a bar pattern that can be visualized.

- Best **modulation transfer function** graph.

14. Bar pattern with **no edge unsharpness** in LP/mm is shown below.

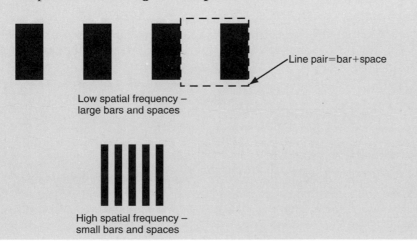

Line pair=bar+space

Low spatial frequency – large bars and spaces

High spatial frequency – small bars and spaces

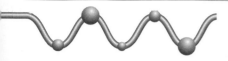

15. Bar patterns with edge unsharpness demonstrate that edge unsharpness limits spatial resolution for small bars and spaces; however, edge unsharpness has little effect on the spatial resolution of large objects.

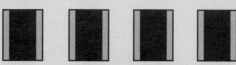

Low spatial frequency with edge unsharpness

High spatial frequency with edge unsharpness

16. With small bars and spaces, the blur fills the space between the bars and reduces the contrast between the bars and spaces until the bars merge together and cannot be distinguished. At this point, spatial resolution is lost.

17. *Modulation transfer function (MTF)* evaluates edge unsharpness in a different fashion. For a very thin bar, the bar plus the unsharpness related to just the image receptor is scanned by a densitometer to yield a distance versus density plot.

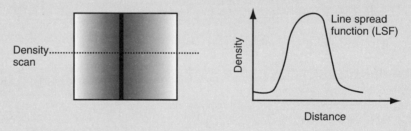

18. The density scan of the blur of a thin line taken from an image receptor (after it is converted to intensity) is called the line spread function (LSF). Wide LSF plots mean significant blur and degraded spatial resolution.

19. Next, a mathematical operation called a Fourier transform is performed on the LSF to convert the plot into a new graph of MTF value versus spatial frequency in LP/mm.

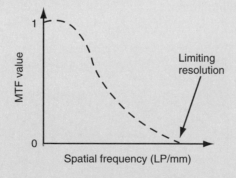

20. The axes of the MTF graph have the following meaning.

- The vertical axis (MTF value) indicates the fraction of the image contrast that is preserved.

- A value of 1 means that the imaging system does not degrade the contrast at all.

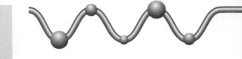

- A value of 0 means that all the contrast is blurred to 0 by the imaging system. In the absence of image noise, a reduction in the MTF of an object with 100% contrast is the limiting spatial resolution of the image receptor.

- The horizontal axis (spatial frequency) is related to the size of the object being imaged. Large objects are at low frequencies, and small objects are at high frequencies.

- The highest MTF curve represents the best imaging system. Hence, in the accompanying graph, imaging system C is best, imaging system B is second, and imaging system A is the worst.

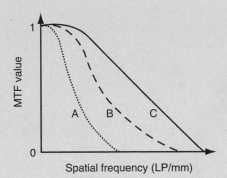

21. If image noise is present, the limiting spatial resolution for an object with 100% contrast is at the point where the MTF graph degrades the image contrast to the noise level. (The actual situation is worse in that the image contrast must be several times greater than the noise level to be clearly visible.)

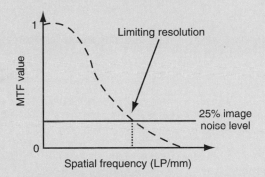

22. If there is 25% image noise and the contrast of the object is only 50%, an MTF of 0.50 reduces the image contrast to half its initial value (25%); at this point (or actually with even less degradation), the image contrast is at the noise level and cannot be seen.

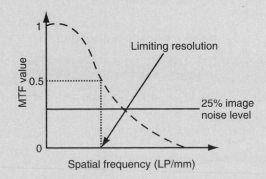

23. For an imaging system with many different components, such as an image intensifier, an optical lens, and a television camera, each component has its

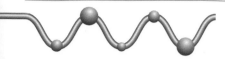

own MTF graph. The overall MTF for the composite system is the product of the MTFs of the individual components.

$$MTF_{SYSTEM} = MTF_1 \times MTF_2 \times MTF_3 \times ...$$

24. Radiographic mottle comprises the following:

- **Quantum mottle,** or number of x-rays per mm² used to form the image
- **Screen mottle,** or random variation in thickness and structure of the screen
- **Grain mottle,** or random variations in the coating of film with silver grains
- Quantum mottle (QM) dominates the others.
- QM is proportional to $100\%/(N)^{0.5}$ where N is the number of x-rays per unit area forming the image.
- To reduce the QM by half, the amount of radiation used to form the image must be four times greater.

B. Questions

13-1. Unsharpness in film-screen images can be caused by all of the following factors, *except* _____.

(a) Focal spot penumbra   (b) Screen light dispersion   (c) Parallax
(d) Motion blur   (e) Film grain size

13-2. All of the following represent methods of measuring the effective x-ray tube focal spot size, *except* _____.

(a) Slit camera   (b) Pinhole camera   (c) Scanning microdensitometer
(d) Line pair pattern   (e) Star pattern

13-3. The best way to reduce motion unsharpness is by use of_____.

(a) Mechanical restraints   (b) Higher kVp   (c) Muscle relaxants
(d) Shorter exposure times   (e) Lower mA settings

13-4. Intensifying screen blur can be reduced by _____.

(a) Adding a reflective layer   (b) Using thin screens
(c) Removing the anticrossover layer   (d) Using higher kVp values
(e) Using high-ratio grids

13-5. Magnification of anatomic structures (by moving the body parts away from the image receptor) _____ the spatial resolution.

(a) Always improves   (b) Always degrades   (c) Has no effect on
(d) Improves to a given magnification and then degrades
(e) Has a synergistic impact on

13-6. For a film-screen system, _____ can degrade the subject contrast.

(a) Low developer temperatures   (b) Thick intensifying screens
(c) Adding x-ray filtration   (d) Large focal spots   (e) Low kVp values

13-7. Increasing kVp while maintaining constant film-screen density will_____.

(a) Increase the radiation dose to the patient   (b) Increase motion blur
(c) Reduce quantum mottle   (d) Increase latitude   (e) Improve image contrast

13-8. Changing the intensifying screen phosphor from $CaWO_4$ to Gd_2O_2S will _____.

(a) Increase the radiation dose to the patient   (b) Improve spatial resolution
(c) Increase quantum mottle   (d) Reduce scatter radiation
(e) Reduce parallax

13-9. The MTF describes the _____ as a function of spatial resolution.

(a) FWHM   (b) LSF   (c) Loss of contrast   (d) QM
(e) Log (exposure)

13-10. If the MTFs of two components in an imaging system are known, the overall MTF of the two components combined is the _____ the two MTF curves.

(a) Sum of   (b) Difference between   (c) Product of   (d) Ratio of
(e) Square root of the sum of the squares of

13-11. Increasing the x-ray beam filtration will _____.

(a) Increase image contrast   (b) Increase exposure times
(c) Increase patient's dose   (d) Reduce the spatial resolution
(e) Decrease the mAs used

13-12. The edge unsharpnesses related to several different components of the imaging system are known. The width of combined blurs is equal to the _____ the individual blurs.

(a) Sum of   (b) Difference between   (c) Product of   (d) Ratio of
(e) Square root of the sum of the squares of

13-13. If an imaging system has a limiting spatial resolution of 8 LP/mm, the smallest detectable object is about _____ micron(s).

(a) 1.0   (b) 11   (c) 120   (d) 1300   (e) 14,000

13-14. Screen A has twice the conversion efficiency of screen B. Film B is 25% faster than film A. However, film-screen combinations A and B have the same overall speed. The film-screen combination with the best spatial resolution _____.

(a) Is film-screen A   (b) Is film-screen B   (c) Is the same for both
(d) Cannot be determined

13-15. Screen A has twice the conversion efficiency of screen B. Film B is 25% faster than film A. However, film-screen combinations A and B have the same overall speed. The film-screen combination that produces images with the most quantum mottle _____.

(a) Is film-screen A   (b) Is film-screen B   (c) Is the same for both
(d) Cannot be determined

13-16. Screen A has twice the conversion efficiency of screen B. Film B is 25% faster than film A. However, film-screen combinations A and B have the same overall speed. The film-screen combination that produces images with the least amount of motion blur _____.

(a) Is film-screen A   (b) Is film-screen B   (c) Is the same for both
(d) Cannot be determined

13-17. Screen A has twice the conversion efficiency of screen B. Film B is 25% faster than film A. However, film-screen combinations A and B have the same overall speed. The film-screen combination that produces images with the greatest radiographic contrast _____.

(a) Is film-screen A   (b) Is film-screen B   (c) Is the same for both
(d) Cannot be determined

13-18. Screen A has twice the conversion efficiency of screen B. Film B is 25% faster than film A. However, film-screen combinations A and B have the same overall speed. The film-screen combination with the lowest radiation doses to patients _____.

(a) Is film-screen A   (b) Is film-screen B   (c) Is the same for both
(d) Cannot be determined

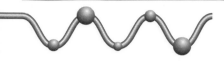

13-19. Screen A has twice the conversion efficiency of screen B. Film B is 25% faster than film A. However, film-screen combinations A and B have the same overall speed. The film-screen combination that is relatively insensitive to kVp changes _____.

(a) Is film-screen A   (b) Is film-screen B   (c) Is the same for both
(d) Cannot be determined

13-20. Quantum mottle strongly depends on all of the following factors, *except* _____.

(a) Screen conversion efficiency   (b) Film speed
(c) Film processing conditions   (d) Phosphor material
(e) Film grain differences

13-21. Low-contrast visibility (or discrimination) is primarily affected by _____.

(a) Screen unsharpness   (b) Quantum mottle   (c) Focal spot size
(d) Absorption unsharpness   (e) Parallax unsharpness

13-22. The effectiveness of imaging systems is sometimes expressed by the _____, which equals (TP + TN)/(TP + FP + TN + FN), where TP = true positives, TN = true negatives, FP = false positives, and FN = false negatives.

(a) Specificity   (b) Accuracy   (c) Sensitivity
(d) ROC (receiver operating characteristic)   (e) C-D diagram

13-23. The effectiveness of imaging systems is sometimes expressed by the _____, which equals (TP)/(TP + FN), where TP = true positives, TN = true negatives, FP = false positives, and FN = false negatives.

(a) Specificity   (b) Accuracy   (c) Sensitivity   (d) ROC
(e) C-D diagram

13-24. The effectiveness of imaging systems is sometimes expressed by the _____, which equals (TN)/(TN + FP), where TP = true positives, TN = true negatives, FP = false positives, and FN = false negatives.

(a) Specificity   (b) Accuracy   (c) Sensitivity   (d) ROC
(e) C-D diagram

13-25. The effectiveness of imaging systems is sometimes expressed by the _____, which is a graph of TP as a function of FN, where TP = true positives, TN = true negatives, FP = false positives, and FN = false negatives.

(a) Specificity   (b) Accuracy   (c) Sensitivity   (d) ROC
(e) C-D diagram

13-26. The effectiveness of imaging systems is sometimes expressed by the _____, which is a graph of the smallest detectable object diameters at various image contrast levels.

(a) Specificity   (b) Accuracy   (c) Sensitivity   (d) ROC
(e) C-D diagram

13-27. Image receptor contrast for a film-screen system can be affected by all of the following factors, *except* _____.

(a) Developer chemistry concentration   (b) Immersion time
(c) Developer temperature   (d) Fixer concentration
(e) Film type selection

13-28. Subject contrast can be enhanced by all of the following factors, *except* _____.

(a) Low kVp values   (b) Reduced x-ray filtration   (c) High-ratio grids
(d) Use of compression of patient   (e) Film type selection

13-29. If the image latitude is increased, the _____ will decrease.

(a) Speed   (b) Base + fog   (c) Spatial resolution
(d) Contrast   (e) Quantum mottle

13-30. The clinical film-screen combinations used for _____ have the most latitude.

(a) Extremity imaging   (b) Gastrointestinal imaging
(c) Intravenous pyelography   (d) Chest radiography
(e) Breast imaging

13-31. The latitude of an imaging system can be increased by all of the following factors, *except* _____.

(a) Higher kVp values   (b) Adding x-ray filtration   (c) Screen selection
(d) Film selection   (e) Lower developer temperatures

13-32. The highest spatial resolution in clinical imaging is provided with _____.

(a) CR   (b) Ultrasonography   (c) Film-screen mammography
(d) Film-screen extremity radiography   (e) Film-screen chest radiography
(f) CT scanning

13-33. The largest dynamic range (or latitude) is provided by _____ images.

(a) Mammographic   (b) Abdominal   (c) CR   (d) Extremity
(e) Chest

13-34. List the imaging modalities in order from the lowest spatial resolution to the best spatial resolution, using the following definitions: (i) CT (ii) Film-screen chest radiography (iii) Positron emission tomography (iv) DR.

(a) i, ii, iii, iv   (b) iii, iv, ii, i   (c) iv, iii, ii, i   (d) ii, i, iv, iii   (e) iii, i, iv, ii

13-35. The spatial resolution of an imaging system can be measured by all of the following devices, *except* _____.

(a) Mesh test tool   (b) Bar line pattern   (c) Aluminum penetrometer
(d) LSF tool   (e) Thin wire in CT phantoms

13-36. Geometric unsharpness increases with _____.

(a) Higher kVp   (b) Greater magnification   (c) Thicker screens
(d) Faster speed screens   (e) Round anatomic organs

13-37. Long delays in time before processing an exposed CR or film-screen cassette causes _____.

(a) Light fog   (b) Reciprocity law failure   (c) Latent imaging fading
(d) Recombination losses   (e) Dead time losses

13-38. For CR and DR images, the displayed contrast can be changed by _____.

(a) Changing monitor brightness   (b) Using higher radiation doses
(c) Changing refresh rates   (d) Adjusting window and level
(e) Altering pixel size

13-39. For the following MTF graphs, the best imaging system for large objects is _____ and the best imaging system for the smallest objects is _____.

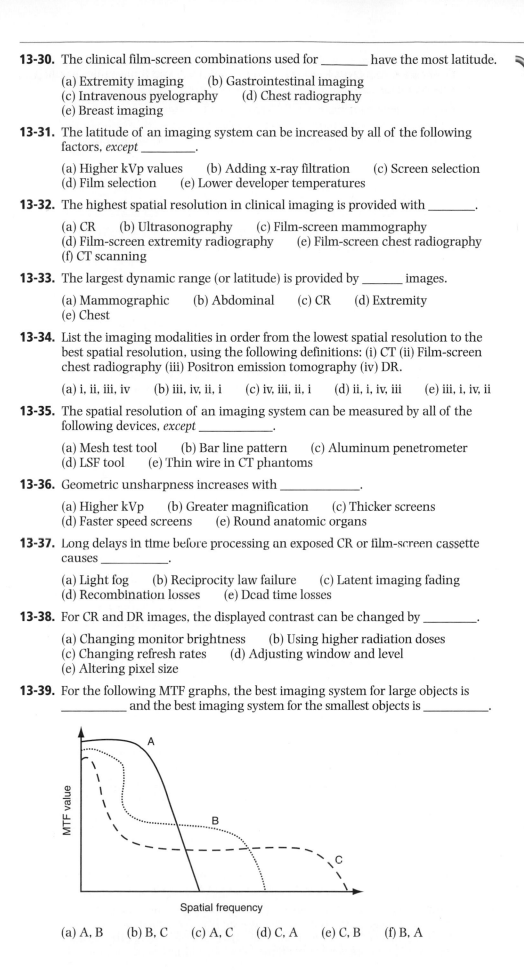

(a) A, B   (b) B, C   (c) A, C   (d) C, A   (e) C, B   (f) B, A

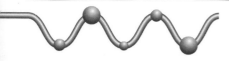

13-40. For a CR imaging system, the radiation dose used to image a uniform plastic phantom is increased by a factor of 4. The quantum mottles would be expected to _____.

(a) Increase by four times   (b) Increase by two times
(c) Decrease to one half of the previous value
(d) Decrease to one fourth of the previous value   (e) Remain the same

C.   Answers

13-1. Answer = (e). Film grain is so small that it causes negligible reduction in spatial resolution in comparison with all the other factors that limit resolution. If film alone (no screen) is used, its limiting spatial resolution is about 50 to 100 LP/mm, versus 4 to 10 LP/mm for most film-screen combinations.

13-2. Answer = (c). In slit and pinhole cameras, there is a small hole or slit in a metal plate that allows an image of the focal spot to be obtained by placing a film at a distance on the other side of the metal. The star pattern and line pair patterns follow the principle that for a given magnification, the penumbra causes spatial resolution to blur completely at a frequency that is directly related to focal spot size. By measuring the frequency at which the bar pattern disappears, one can infer the focal spot of the x-ray tube used in the imaging. A microdensitometer scans the darkness of the film as a function of the distance. It can be used to measure the line spread function (LSF), but it does not directly measure resolution.

13-3. Answer = (d). The best way to reduce motion unsharpness is to use short exposure times, which limit the amount of movement during the imaging process. Mechanical restraints and muscle relaxants can stop voluntary motion, but they cannot significantly alter involuntary motion such as breathing, cardiac contractions, and peristalsis. Lower mA produces increased exposure times, which results in more motion blur. Higher kVp indirectly reduces exposure times because the higher energy x-rays penetrate better and fewer x-rays are necessary. The better, more direct answer is shorter times.

13-4. Answer = (b). A reflective layer increases the light spread in the screen. The anticrossover layer refers to special film and does not apply to screens. The kVp values have no relationship to the spatial resolution of the screen. Grids are designed to remove scattered x-rays and should not have much impact on spatial resolution.

13-5. Answer = (d). Magnification improves the spatial resolution only at first because the effective size of the anatomic structure increases beyond the limits of the imaging system at higher magnification. At this higher magnification, focal spot blur increases steadily until it dominates and degrades the image resolution. Optimal magnification (M_{OPT}) occurs at $1 + [1/Fv_L]$, where F = focal spot size in mm and v_L = limiting resolution of the image receptor in LP/mm.

13-6. Answer = (c). Subject contrast refers to the differential attenuation of x-rays by different body tissues. Anything to do with the film, screen, and film processing is not involved in subject contrast; these are related to image receptor contrast. Screen thickness affects spatial resolution, speed, and radiation dose to the patient; it does not affect subject contrast. Focal spot size affects spatial resolution and image unsharpness, but it does not affect subject contrast. Adding filters increases the average energy of the x-rays, which degrades subject contrast. The kVp also affects subject contrast. Lower kVp values result in lower energy x-rays, which increase subject contrast.

13-7. Answer = (d). In an AEC (phototimed) system, higher kVp produces more penetrating x-rays, so that fewer x-rays are needed. The system shortens the exposure times, which reduces the motion blur. The effect is a reduction in radiation dose to the patient; for every increase of 10 kVp, the mAs is decreased by about 50%, which means a net reduction of radiation dose of about 30% to 40%. Higher kVp values have little impact on quantum mottle. High kVp means more Compton interactions and fewer photoelectric effect interactions; this reduces subject contrast. Contrast and latitude are inversely related. If contrast decreases, latitude increases.

13-8. Answer = (c). Changing the intensifying screen phosphor from calcium tungstate to a rare earth phosphor increases the conversion efficiency of the screen. Nothing is stated about the thickness of the screen. If the screen thickness does not change, the spatial resolution is the same. If the screen thickness is the same and the conversion efficiency is greater, the speed increases and the radiation dose to the patient decreases. Quantum mottle increases with higher conversion efficiency of the screens. With less radiation used, there are also fewer scattered x-rays. There is no change in parallax.

13-9. Answer = (c). The horizontal axis of the MTF graph is the spatial frequency measured in LP/mm. The vertical axis is the fraction of the original object contrast that is retained by the imaging system. MTF = 1.0 means that 100% of the object contrast is retained in the image. MTF = 0.0 means that the object contrast is totally lost because of image blur. FWHM is full width at half maximum, which is a measure of the blur.

13-10. Answer = (c). See note in this chapter (**A23**).

13-11. Answer = (b). Increasing the x-ray beam filtration results in fewer x-rays of higher energy. The higher energy x-rays decrease contrast and increase the latitude. Because there are fewer x-rays, more mAs and longer exposure times are needed to maintain the same film density. Radiation dose decreases because of the better penetration of the higher energy x-rays. There is no effect on the spatial resolution.

13-12. Answer = (e). Width of blurs sums like sides of a right triangle to obtain the length of the hypotenuse.

13-13. Answer = (c). Spatial resolution and the minimum detectable object size are related.

$(1/2v_L) < D_{MIN} < (1/v_L)$

Hence, $1/(8 \text{ LP/mm}) = 0.125$ mm or 125 microns.

13-14. Answer = (a). The overall speed is the product of absorption efficiency, conversion efficiency, and film speed. Absorption efficiency is related to screen thickness, which is not stated in this problem. For combination A, the overall efficiency is α_1(absorption efficiency) × 2(conversion efficiency) × 1(film speed). For combination B, the overall efficiency is α_2(absorption efficiency) × 1(conversion efficiency) × 1.25(film speed). Because the overall speeds for A and B are the same, $\alpha_1 = 0.625\alpha_2$. In other words, the absorption efficiency of screen A is only 62.5% of the absorption efficiency of screen B. Because combination A has an absorption efficiency 63% that of B, screen A must be much thinner. Thinner screens have the best spatial resolution.

13-15. Answer = (a). The screen conversion efficiency and film speed both affect the amount of QM. However, the conversion efficiency of A is a factor of 2, and the increased film speed of B is only 1.25 times greater. Even though both have increased QM, the larger number dominates.

13-16. Answer = (c). Because the overall speeds are the same for both A and B, the exposure times would be the same, and the motion blur would be the same.

13-17. Answer = (d). The contrast is affected by the film and not the screen. Nothing is stated about the average contrast gradient of each film. Moreover, nothing is stated about the film processing conditions.

13-18. Answer = (c). If the overall speeds are the same for both A and B, the radiation doses to the patient are the same.

13-19. Answer = (d). The speed of rare earth screens varies more with changes in kVp than does the speed of calcium tungstate screens. However, nothing is stated about the phosphors used for the screens.

13-20. Answer = (e). Although mottle depends on quantum mottle, screen mottle, and grain mottles, the main factor is the QM. Screen mottle and grain mottle make very limited contributions to the quantum mottle.

13-21. Answer = (b). Various types of unsharpness and focal spot blur primarily affect high-contrast spatial resolution. Low-contrast visibility is limited by the amount of image noise (or mottle). As the mottle increases in the image, objects must be of either greater contrast or larger size to be easily detected. The mottle is predominantly determined by the number of x-ray photons used to form the image. The QM is related to $100\%/(N)^{0.5}$. As the number of x-rays (N) used to form the image increases, the percentage of mottle decreases.

13-22. Answer = (b). There are several statistical methods of comparing the relative quality of different imaging systems. One method is to use a decision matrix of true positives, false positives, true negatives, and false negatives to evaluate image performance. The system should identify correctly a large portion of the true positives and true negatives compared with all choices; this is called accuracy.

13-23. Answer = (c). There are several statistical methods of comparing the relative quality of different imaging systems. One method is to use a decision matrix of true positives (TP), false positives, true negatives, and false negatives (FN) to evaluate image performance. The ability of the system to identify correctly those who have a disease is the number of TP divided by all with the disease (TP + FN); this is called sensitivity.

13-24. Answer = (a). There are several statistical methods of comparing the relative quality of different imaging systems. One method is to use a decision matrix of true positives, false positives (FP), true negatives (TN), and false negatives to evaluate image performance. It is also important for an imaging system to avoid diagnosis of normal individuals incorrectly as persons with a disease. This specificity is the fraction who are diagnosed as normal (TN) divided by all the results that are actually normal (TN + FP).

13-25. Answer = (d). A pure random guess would produce a graph showing an equal number of correct results (TP) and incorrect results (FP). This would be a 45-degree line on an ROC graph with TP on the y-axis and FP on the x-axis. Good imaging systems would produce many more TPs with few FPs. See the accompanying graph.

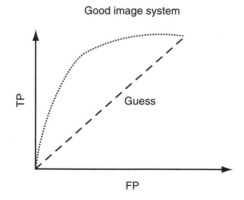

13-26. Answer = (e). As the contrast of an object decreases, the object size must be larger in diameter to be detected. Another way to improve performance is to use more radiation to form the image. With more x-ray photons used to form the image, the quantum mottle (image noise) decreases, and smaller diameter low-contrast objects become visible. See the accompanying graph (see figure shown in next page).

13-27. Answer = (d). The fixer concentration controls the number of unexposed silver grains removed from the film. Failure to remove these grains allows them to oxidize with time and darken the film. This process reduces the archival storage duration of film. It does not affect the initial contrast related to the image receptor.

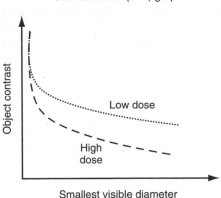

Contrast-detail (C-D) graph

Object contrast

Low dose

High dose

Smallest visible diameter

13-28. Answer = (e). Subject contrast is due to the differential transmission of x-rays through the body. Hence, subject contrast is affected by kVp, filtration, atomic number of the tissue, density of the tissue, thickness differences, and the grid. Film selection affects image receptor contrast. Both subject contrast and image receptor contrast influence the overall radiographic (image) contrast.

13-29. Answer = (d). Contrast and latitude are opposites. When contrast increases, latitude decreases, and vice versa.

13-30. Answer = (d). The clinical films with the most contrast are mammography films, which have an average contrast gradient of about 3.5 to 4.0. However, in general, extremity, gastrointestinal, and intravenous pyelography films are also contrast films, with an average contrast gradient of about 3.0. Chest radiography films typically have average contrast gradients of 2.0 to 2.7 and are labeled latitude films.

13-31. Answer = (c). Screen selection affects spatial resolution, speed, radiation dose to the patient, and quantum mottle. It does not affect the image contrast.

13-32. Answer = (c). Ultrasonography, MRI, and CT have similar spatial resolutions, around 1.0 LP/mm, with the resolution of CT and MRI being slightly better than that of ultrasonography. CR has a spatial resolution of about 3.0 to 3.5 LP/mm. Extremity films and chest films have spatial resolutions of about 8 to 10 LP/mm. Mammography film-screen systems have a spatial resolution of about 15 to 20 LP/mm.

13-33. Answer = (c). Digital systems such as CT, MRI, CR, and DR have a dynamic range much greater than that of any film system. In general, the range of radiation levels that can be recorded is usually 12 bits, or 4096 levels.

13-34. Answer = (e). One should try to identify the lowest and highest spatial resolution systems first to eliminate incorrect answers. Positron emission tomography, with a spatial resolution of about 0.75 to 1.0 cm, or 0.1 LP/mm, has the lowest resolution. CT is next lowest, with a resolution of about 1.0 LP/mm. CR has a resolution of about 3.0 to 3.5 LP/mm. The best spatial resolution of the items listed is that of chest radiography, with a value of 8 to 10 LP/mm.

13-35. Answer = (c). An aluminum penetrometer consists of two blocks of 0.75-inch-thick aluminum with a thin 1/32-inch aluminum plate with five large holes of different sizes drilled through the thin plate. It is used to measure typical radiation doses to patients and to look at fluoroscopic low-contrast visibility. A mesh tool is a series of different window screens with smaller and smaller mesh sizes and is used to measure spatial resolution. The bar pattern is the standard lead plus air bars of different sizes and is also used to measure spatial resolution. The LSF tool was described in the notes section. The thin wire in CT phantoms is used to measure the point spread function (PSF), from which the MTF can be determined.

13-36. Answer = (b). Geometric unsharpness is the same as focal spot unsharpness. It depends on both the focal spot size and the magnification in the image (obtained by displacing the objects away from the image receptor). Geometric unsharpness increases directly with the magnification and the focal spot size.

13-37. Answer = (c). Light fog can increase if the cassettes are damaged and allow light leakage inside the cassette; this does not normally occur in undamaged cassettes. In reciprocity failure, more mAs is required for very short and/or very long exposure times in order to maintain constant film density. It should be the same for any combination of mA and time which have the same mAs; an example of a film-screen that demonstrates this effect is a mammography combination. Recombination losses occur in radiation detectors that are operated at low voltages. Dead-time losses also occur in some radiation detectors that are operated at a very high count rate that the system electronics cannot handle.

13-38. Answer = (d). Although monitor brightness can affect the clinical image quality, it does not change the contrast. A higher dose rate affects the visibility of low-contrast objects by influencing the background quantum mottle, but it does not affect the image contrast. The refresh rate affects moving structures and can affect temporal resolution. Pixel size of the display could limit high-contrast spatial resolution. Although the measured values of digital images are fixed, the adjustment of window width and level can affect the apparent contrast on the display. It is an image receptor contrast parameter for digital images.

13-39. Answer = (c). Large objects are associated with a lower spatial frequency, and small objects are associated with the highest spatial frequencies. The best spatial resolution is seen with imaging systems with the highest vertical value (MTF value) on the graph.

13-40. Answer = (c). The relative QM is related to the number of photons (N) used to create the image. For digital systems, this is directly related to the radiation dose. QM is related to $100\%/(\text{rad dose})^{0.5}$. Therefore, if rad dose increases 4 times, the QM decreases by $100\%/(4)^{0.5} = 100\%/2.0 = 50\%$.

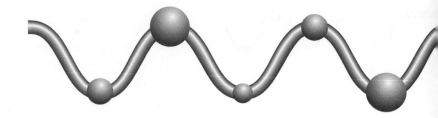

CHAPTER FOURTEEN

Radiation Doses and Safety

A. Basic Concepts

1. **Exposure (exp)** is defined only for x-rays and gamma rays with energies of less than 3 MeV and is measured only in air at standard temperature and pressure (STP). It is the amount of ionization created in air per unit volume of air as the x-ray radiation passes through the air.

   - **Old unit**: 1 roentgen (R) = $2.08 \times 10^{+9}$ ion pairs per cubic centimeter of air at STP
   - **New unit**: 1 coulomb per kilogram of air
   - **Conversion of units**: 1 R = 2.58×10^{-4} coul/kg

2. **Absorbed dose (AD)** is the amount of radiation energy deposited per unit of mass of material. It applies to all types of radiation with any energy in any material.

   - AD = [Δenergy/Δmass]
   - **Old unit**: 1 rad = 100 erg/g
   - **New unit**: 1 gray (Gy) = 1 Joule/kg
   - **Conversion of units**: 1 Gy = 100 rad
   - **Calculation process**: AD (cGy[centigray]) = f-factor × exp(R)
   - f-factor = $0.872 \times (\mu/\rho)_X/(\mu/\rho)_{AIR}$
   - The f-factor for diagnostic x-rays is typically 0.90 to 0.96 for most tissues in the body.
   - The f-factor for bone is about three to four times the tissue value at diagnostic x-ray energies.
   - The f-factor for adipose tissue (fat) is about half the tissue value at low kVp values and approaches the same value as tissue at higher kVp values.
   - Numerically, 1 R ~ 1 rad, within ±10%, or 1 R ~ 1 cGy ~ 0.01 Gy.

3. **Dose equivalent (DE)** corrects for the fact that some types of radiation (such as neutrons, protons, and alpha particles) are more damaging than x-rays and gamma rays. It also corrects for energy effects and differences in tissue type. Thus, for a certain number of DE radiation units, the same extent of biologic damage would be obtained regardless of type of radiation, energy level, or kind of tissue.

   - **Old unit**: 1 rem
   - **New unit**: 1 sievert (Sv)

- *Conversion of units*: 1 Sv = 100 rem
- *Calculation process*: DE = QF × AD
- *Quality factor (QF)* = relative damage with different types of radiation
- QF = 1.0 for x-rays, 0.9 for high-energy gamma rays, 10 for slow neutrons, 20 for fast neutrons, and 20 for alpha particles

4. *Effective dose equivalent (H_E)* multiplies the average radiation absorbed dose (D_j) in each organ group by a factor that represents the relative risk of fatal cancer and severe first-generation hereditary effects in that organ compared to the risk of exposure of all organs in the body. The multiplying factors are called weighting factors; in calculating effective dose equivalent, seven different groups of organs are used. The sum of all the weighting factors is equal to 1.0.

   - *Old unit*: 1 rem
   - *New unit*: 1 sievert (Sv)
   - *Conversion of units*: 1 Sv = 100 rem
   - Although the units are the same, they have a different meaning. The idea is to estimate the risk if only part of the body receives radiation, in comparison with a situation in which the entire body is exposed to radiation.
   - *Calculation process*: $H_E = \Sigma W_{Tj} \times D_j$
   - W_{Tj} = the weighting factor for the relative risk of fatal cancer and severe hereditary effects for each of the seven organ groups; factors for all organs total 1.00.

Table of Weighting Factors for H_E

ORGAN GROUP	W_T
Gonads	0.25
Breast	0.15
Red marrow	0.12
Lung	0.12
Thyroid	0.03
Bone surface	0.03
Remainder	0.30

5. *Effective dose (E)* multiplies the average absorbed dose in each organ group to assess the relative risks of all cancers (fatal and nonfatal) and all genetic effects in that organ group as well as life-shortening effects in comparison to exposure of all other organs of the body. The multiplying factors are called weighting factors; for effective dose, there are considered to be 13 different groups of organs. The sum of all the weighting factors is equal to 1.0.

   - *Old unit*: 1 rem
   - *New unit*: 1 sievert (Sv)
   - *Conversion of units*: 1 Sv = 100 rem
   - *Calculation process*: $E = \Sigma \omega_{Tj} \times D_j$
   - ω_{Tj} = the weighting factor for the relative risk of all cancers and all hereditary effects for each of the 13 organ groups; factors for all organs total 1.00.

Table of Weighting Factors for E

ORGAN GROUP	ω_T
Gonads	0.20
Breast	0.05
Red marrow	0.12
Lung	0.12

ORGAN GROUP	ω_T
Thyroid	0.05
Bone surface	0.01
Liver	0.05
Skin	0.01
Colon	0.12
Bladder	0.05
Stomach	0.12
Esophagus	0.05
Remainder	0.05

6. The risk factors for both effective dose equivalent and effective dose calculations are about 0.04 to 0.05 per Sv for fatal cancers, 0.01 per Sv for nonfatal cancers, and 0.01 per Sv for all severe hereditary effects. The total risk is about 0.06 to 0.07 per Sv. Therefore, if a group of individuals all receive an effective dose equivalent or effective dose of 1 Sv, the risk to the population is a 4% to 5% chance of developing fatal cancer.

7. If only a portion of the body is irradiated, the effective dose equivalent or the effective dose can be calculated to determine the needed dose adjustment. In this way, one can assess the risk of this nonuniform exposure, which would be less than a whole-body exposure at the same radiation level.

8. *Air kerma* describes the amount of energy released into a material by the radiation beam. Some of that energy may not be deposited locally with use of very high energy radiation in the MeV range, or a buildup depth may be needed to reach peak values. This measurement is similar to that of AD.

9. Combined units:
   - *Surface integral (area) dose* (mGy-cm^2) attempts to relate the radiation dose to its potential biologic impact more accurately by incorporating the amount of tissue that was irradiated. Newer fluoroscopy systems calculate this value for each clinical patient's study by monitoring collimator positions to measure the dose-area product (DAP).
   - *Integral (volume) dose* (Gy-g) adds up the dose per gram to all tissue irradiated, again to estimate better the impact of the radiation in regard to its biologic effects. This is difficult to do because most radiation doses are not uniform in magnitude in the body. For conventional x-rays, the radiation dose decreases exponentially from the entrance surface to the exit point.

10. *Triple 100 dose estimation*: For 100 kVp and 100 mAs at 100 cm from the focal spot, the *entrance skin exposure (ESE)* is about 1000 mR, or about 1 rad (cGy).

11. *Patients' radiation doses* can be calculated approximately by the following formula:

    $$ESD \text{ (mGy)} = 0.1 \times (\# \text{ kVp}/100)^2 \times (\text{mAs}) \times [100 \text{ cm}/d \text{ (cm)}]^2$$

    where d = distance and ESD = entrance skin dose.
    - This equation also works for fluoroscopy units that are not heavily filtered.
    - This calculated value is about four to five times too high for fluoroscopic units with significant copper x-ray beam filtration (> 0.2 mm Cu).

12. The following are typical clinical radiation doses at skin level (ESD):
    - Posteroanterior (PA) chest computed radiography (CR) = 0.40 mSv per image
    - Extremity CR = 1 to 2 mSv per image
    - Anteroposterior (AP) abdomen CR = 5 to 8 mSv per image
    - Lateral lumbosacral CR = 8 to 10 mSv per image
    - 1 minute of gastrointestinal fluoroscopy = 20 to 40 mSv per minute
    - 1 minute of cardiac cine = 200 to 400 mSv per minute

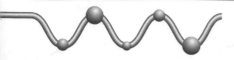

- Four digital subtraction angiography images = 20 to 40 mSv
- Head computed tomography (CT) scan = 40 to 60 mSv
- Body CT scan = 20 to 40 mSv
- Mammography (ESD) = 8 to 15 mSv per image
- Ultrasonography (US) and magnetic resonance imaging (MRI) = not applicable

13. Natural sources of radiation:
    - Cosmic rays at sea level = 0.26 mSv per year
    - Cosmic rays in airplane = 0.005 mSv per hour of flight
    - Terrestrial sources = 0.28 mSv per year
    - Radon = 2.0 mSv per year
    - Isotopes in the body = 0.15 to 0.27 mSv per year
    - All natural sources except radon = 1.0 mSv per year
    - Radon is the largest component of natural sources.

14. Human-made sources of radiation (average values):
    - Diagnostic radiology = 0.39 mSv per year
    - Nuclear medicine = 0.14 mSv per year
    - Consumer products = 0.05 to 0.13 mSv per year
    - Occupational sources = 0.01 mSv per year

15. How to reduce radiation dose to the patient:
    - Use higher kVp values.
    - Use more x-ray tube filtration.
    - Reduce fluoroscopy times.
    - Keep image receptor close to patient.
    - Regulate mAs for digital systems to reasonable levels.

16. ***Maximum permissible doses (MPDs)*** for radiation workers older than 18 years are shown in the table.

EXPOSED BODY PART	RADIATION WORKERS	PUBLIC AT LARGE	PATIENTS
Effective dose of whole body	50 mSv/yr (5000 mrem/yr)	1 mSv/yr*	Benefit vs. risk ratio
Eyes	150 mSv/yr (15,000 mrem/yr)	15 mSv/yr	Benefit vs. risk ratio
Fetus of pregnant woman	0.5 mSv/month (50 mrem/month)	Not specifically stated	Benefit vs. risk ratio
All other organs	500 mSv/yr (50,000 mrem/yr)	50 mSv/yr	Benefit vs. risk ratio

*Frequently exposed individuals; 5 mSv/yr infrequent.

17. ***Radiation badges*** worn by radiation workers can be used to calculate the effective dose equivalent (H_E) for occupationally exposed persons.
    - For one radiation badge worn outside the leaded apron,

      (BR_{OUT}): $H_E = 0.3 \times (BR_{OUT})$

    - For two radiation badges, where one is worn outside the leaded apron (BR_{OUT}) and one is worn under the leaded apron at the thorax,

      (BR_{IN}): $H_E = [0.04 \times (BR_{OUT})] + [1.5 \times (BR_{IN})]$

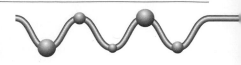

18. To shield radiation involving charged particles:

- All charged particles have a range. The ***range*** (R) is the thickness of a specified material that stops every charged particle.

- The range is dependent on the type of charged particle and its energy.

- For ***electrons***,

  $R_e = 0.530\,E - 0.106$ in cm of tissue

  where E = energy in MeV and 1 MeV < E < 20 MeV.

- For ***protons***,

  $R_p = 0.100[E/9.3]^{1.8}$ in cm of tissue

  where E = energy in MeV and 10 MeV < E < 200 MeV.

- For ***alpha*** particles,

  $R_\alpha = 0.001\,E$ in cm of tissue

  where E = energy in MeV and 0.5 MeV < E < 10 MeV.

- For the same particle in different materials,

  $R_X/R_{TISSUE} = \rho_{TISSUE}/\rho_X$

- In the shielding of charged particles, one should avoid materials with high atomic number (Z) to limit the production of bremsstrahlung x-rays during deceleration of the charged particles.

19. To shield radiation involving x-ray radiation:

- Remember that x-rays are never completely stopped by shielding materials.

- Shielding material is intended to limit the number of transmitted x-rays to a small fraction of the incident radiation levels.

- The half-value layer (HVL) is the thickness of a material that is required to reduce radiation levels to one half (0.5) of their incident value.

- Approximate first HVLs of some materials are listed in the table.

kVp	HVL (AIR)	HVL (TISSUE)	HVL (ALUMINUM)	HVL (LEAD)
60	10 m	1.2 cm	1.1 mm	0.02 mm
100	18 m	2.2 cm	3.0 mm	0.08 mm
140	24 m	2.9 cm	> 6.0 mm	0.18 mm

- Standard protective leaded aprons with 0.50-lead-equivalent thickness attenuate 94% to 96% of scattered x-rays for kVp of less than 100.

- There are three components of x-ray radiation that must be considered in shielding calculations: primary, leakage, and scattered.

- A generalization states that ***scattered radiation*** is about 0.1% (0.001) of the patient's entrance exposure at a distance of 1 meter from the patient.

- ***Leakage radiation*** penetrating through the x-ray tube housing is limited by law to less than 100 mR per hour at 1 meter from the tube when operated at maximum continuous mA and maximum kVp.

- Shielding calculations to determine necessary lead thickness (XLt) in the walls of an x-ray procedure room must consider at least the factors shown in the following table.

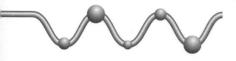

PARAMETER SYMBOL	DESCRIPTION	UNITS	EFFECT ON XLt
P	Permissible radiation level	R/wk	As P increases, XLt decreases
W	Workload	(mA – min)/wk	As W increases, XLt increases
U	Use factor	0 < value < 1.0	As U increases, XLt increases
T	Occupancy	0 < value < 1.0	As T increases, XLt increases
D	Distance	Meters	As D increases, XLt decreases
B	Attenuation	0 < value < 1.0	B is related to the XLt
α	Scatter fraction	About 0.001	As α increases, XLt increases

- Typical shielding in the walls of a fluoroscopic x-ray room is about 1.5 mm (1/16 inch) of lead thickness to a height of 7.0 feet.

B. Questions

14-1. _____ is used to assess the risk of fatal and nonfatal cancers as well as long-term genetic effects and shortened life.

(a) Exposure   (b) Absorbed dose   (c) Dose equivalent   (d) Effective dose
(e) Effective dose equivalent

14-2. _____ is a measure of air ionization per cubic centimeter or coul/kg.

(a) Exposure   (b) Absorbed dose   (c) Dose equivalent   (d) Effective dose
(e) Effective dose equivalent

14-3. _____ is a measure of radiation energy deposited per unit mass of material and does not account for type of radiation or type of tissue.

(a) Exposure   (b) Absorbed dose   (c) Dose equivalent   (d) Effective dose
(e) Effective dose equivalent

14-4. _____ is used to assess the risk of only fatal cancers and first-generation acute hereditary effects using seven different body organ groups.

(a) Exposure   (b) Absorbed dose   (c) Dose equivalent   (d) Effective dose
(e) Effective dose equivalent

14-5. _____ uses a QF to account for the relative damage caused by different types and energies of radiation in different types of tissue.

(a) Exposure   (b) Absorbed dose   (c) Dose equivalent   (d) Effective dose
(e) Effective dose equivalent

14-6. The QF for fast neutrons is _____ compared with the QF of x-rays, which is about _____.

(a) 1, 5   (b) 5, 1   (c) 10, 2   (d) 3, 4   (e) 20, 1   (f) 3.3, 0.9

14-7. The f-factor is used to convert exposure to _____.

(a) Absorbed dose   (c) Dose equivalent   (c) Effective dose
(d) Effective dose equivalent   (e) Surface integral dose   (f) Volume dose

14-8. The lowest surface dose from the following listed radiologic procedures is associated with _____ radiographs.

(a) Extremity   (b) Abdomen   (c) Breast (mammographic)
(d) Chest   (e) Skull

14-9. If the surface exposure in air at the skin of a patient is 3 R, the amount of absorbed dose to tissue at this location is expected to be about _____ mGy.

(a) 1   (b) 3   (c) 18   (d) 28   (e) 39   (f) 50   (g) 100

14-10. The general public, who may be in corridors or waiting rooms near an x-ray room, is permitted by regulations to receive less than _____ of radiation per year.

(a) 50 mrem   (b) 1 mSv   (c) 25 µGy   (d) 0.005 mSv
(e) 0. 010 rem

14-11. The MPD for radiation workers is limited to an effective radiation dose equal to or less than _____ per month.

(a) 50 mrem   (b) 4.17 mSv   (c) 5 cGy   (d) 0.001 Sv
(e) 200 mrad

14-12. According to regulations, the fetus of a pregnant radiation worker is allowed to receive a radiation dose equal to or less than _____ per month.

(a) 50 mrem   (b) 1 mSv   (c) 0.25 mGy   (d) 1.5 mSv   (e) 2 mR

14-13. For occupationally exposed persons, regulations limit the permissible radiation doses to less than _____ mSv per year for the eyes and less than _____ mSv per year for the thyroid.

(a) 50, 150   (b) 50, 50   (c) 150, 50   (d) 150, 500   (e) 1000, 2000

14-14. The risk of a fatal cancer or first-generation hereditary effects is about _____ % for a radiation dose of 10 cGy.

(a) 0.01   (b) 0.07   (c) 0.5   (d) 1.0   (e) 4.0

14-15. For scattered and leakage radiation, the usage (U) factor in shielding calculations is equal to _____.

(a) 0.0   (b) 0.25   (c) 0.50   (d) 0.75   (e) 1.0

14-16. Regulations specify that the leakage radiation from x-ray tubes at a distance of 1 meter should never exceed _____ mR per hour.

(a) 1.0   (b) 50   (c) 100   (d) 500   (e) 1000

14-17. If the entrance dose rate for a fluoroscopy patient is 3.0 cGy per minute, the expected scattered radiation level at the edge of the table (0.5 meter from the patient) would be about _____ mGy per hour.

(a) 0.03   (b) 0.5   (c) 7.2   (d) 29   (e) 100

14-18. If a protective apron with an equivalent thickness of 0.50 mm of lead attenuates 96% of the incident scattered radiation, a 0.25-mm leaded apron would be expected to attenuate ____ % of the radiation.

(a) 24   (b) 43   (c) 66   (d) 80   (e) 91

14-19. The ideal shielding material for beta particles would be _____.

(a) Plastic   (b) Aluminum   (c) Copper   (d) Lead   (e) Tungsten

14-20. The conversion factor that is used to calculate dose equivalent from absorbed dose is called the _____.

(a) QF   (b) f-factor   (c) Planck's constant   (d) LET   (e) MPD

14-21. The f-factor has dimensional units of _____.

(a) coul/kg   (b) cGy/R   (c) rem/rad   (d) risk/rem   (e) R/mAs

14-22. Order the following types of clinical radiography according to the associated radiation dose, from the lowest to the highest: (i) Extremity (ii) Chest (iii) Head CT scan (iv) Mammography.

(a) iv, ii, iii, i   (b) ii, i, iv, iii   (c) i, ii, iv, iii   (d) iii, i, ii, iv   (e) ii, iv, i, iii

14-23. The typical annual radiation dose from all natural sources to a person in the United States is about _____ mSv.

(a) 1.0   (b) 2.0   (c) 3.0   (d) 4.0   (e) 5.0

14-24. The major contributor to the annual radiation dose from natural sources is _____.

(a) Cosmic rays   (b) Solar flares   (c) Sources in the body
(d) Radon   (e) Nuclear power plants

14-25. If mammography examinations deliver an average glandular breast dose of radiation of 4 mSv, the expected incidence of fatal cancers induced by the examinations per 1 million patients is about _____ cases.

(a) 1   (b) 3   (c) 6   (d) 12   (e) 24   (f) 48   (g) 100

14-26. The HVL of 100-kVp x-rays in tissue is about _____.

(a) 0.1 cm   (b) 0.5 cm   (c) 1.0 cm   (d) 2.2 cm   (e) 7.0 cm

14-27. The expected skin entrance dose to a patient for an exposure taken at 90 kVp, 50 mAs, and 50 cm is about _____ mGy.

(a) 4   (b) 8   (c) 16   (d) 32   (e) 64   (f) 128

14-28. A typical barium enema examination entails about 5 minutes of fluoroscopy and 12 digital spot images of the abdomen. The skin entrance dose from the examination is about _____ mSv or _____ cGy (rads).

(a) 30, 3.0   (b) 65, 6.5   (c) 125, 12.5   (d) 240, 24   (e) 500, 50

14-29. A 2.0-MeV beta particle has a range of about 1 cm in tissue. The range of this particle in air would be about _____ cm.

(a) 0.8   (b) 8   (c) 80   (d) 800   (e) 8,000

14-30. By regulation, the maximum effective dose allowed to the whole body of a patient undergoing a series of x-ray examinations in a medical facility is _____ mSv.

(a) 1.0   (b) 2.0   (c) 5.0   (d) 10.0   (e) No limit applies

C. Answers

14-1. Answer = (d). See notes (**A5**). This value is not the risk number. Instead, it is an equivalent radiation dose value for nonuniform irradiation of body organs that can be used to assess the risks of fatal and nonfatal cancers, long-term genetic effects, and nonspecific life shortening.

14-2. Answer = (a). See notes (**A1**). Radiation detectors measure the number of x-rays indirectly by detecting the amount of ionization created in air as the x-rays pass through it.

14-3. Answer = (b). See notes (**A2**). The absorbed dose can be calculated by multiplying the measured exposure by the f-factor. The unit of the absorbed dose is the older term rad, which is equivalent to the newer term cGy.

14-4. Answer = (e). See notes (**A4**). This value is not the risk number. Instead, it is an equivalent radiation dose value for nonuniform irradiation of body organs that can be used to assess the risks of only fatal and first-generation genetic effects.

14-5. Answer = (c). See notes (**A3**). The unit of dose equivalent is the older term rem, which is equivalent to 10 mSv in the newer SI units.

14-6. Answer = (e). In certain tissues, fast neutrons are 20 times more damaging to biologic tissue than the same absorbed dose of x-rays.

14-7. Answer = (a). See notes (**A2**).

14-8. Answer = (d). Entrance skin dose (ESD) is about 1 to 2 mGy for extremity radiographs, 5 to 8 mGy for abdominal images, 9 to 12 mGy for 4.2-cm compressed breast images, 0.10 to 0.30 mGy for PA chest radiographs,

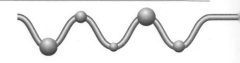

and 3 to 5 mGy for CR skull images. However, mammography doses are usually given as average glandular doses of about 1.5 to 3.0 mGy for 4.2 cm of compressed breast tissue.

14-9. Answer = (d). To convert 3 R to cGy, the 3 R must be multiplied by about 0.94 (f-factor), which yields 2.82 cGy. To convert cGy to mGy, multiply the 2.82 cGy by 10, which yields 28.2 mGy.

14-10. Answer = (b). The MPD for the general public is intended to limit the number of birth defects; the MPD for radiation workers is intended to limit the number of acute somatic effects. Thus, the general public has an effective dose limit that is 50 times lower (at 1 mSv/yr) than that of radiation workers (at 50 mSv/yr).

14-11. Answer = (b). The MPD for radiation workers is 50 mSv/yr. However, this question asks about the limit per month. 50 mSv/yr divided by 12 equals 4.17 mSv/month.

14-12. Answer = (a). 50 mrem per month is equal to 0.50 mSv per month. See notes (**A16**).

14-13. Answer = (d). See notes (**A16**).

14-14. Answer = (c). 10 cGy equals 0.1 Sv. The risks listed are 0.05 per Sv, which is 5% per Sv. This value translates to 0.1 Sv × 5%/Sv, or 0.5% for 10 cGy.

14-15. Answer = (e). For scattered and leakage radiation, the x-rays travel in all directions for all x-ray exposures. The U factor specifies the fraction of workload (W) that sends x-rays in a specified direction toward a given wall. In general, for primary radiation, U = 0.25 for each wall plus the ceiling and floor. This approach adds up to a value greater than 1.0, and it is excessively conservative.

14-16. Answer = (c). See notes (**A19**).

14-17. Answer = (c). The scattered level at 1 meter from the patient can be estimated to be 0.001 times the patient's dose rate (3 cGy/min), or 0.003 cGy/min. At a distance of 0.5 meter, the radiation levels vary as the inverse square of the distance (inverse square law). The closer distance increases the radiation by $[1/(0.5)^2] = [1/0.25] = 4.0$. Being half of 1 meter away increases the radiation levels by a factor of 4.0. Thus, the radiation levels will be 4 × 0.003 cGy/min, or 0.012 cGy/min. Next, the dose rate per minute must be converted to an hourly figure by multiplying by 60: 60 min/hr × 0.012 cGy/min = 0.72 cGy/hr. There are 10 mGy for each 1 cGy. Hence, this value must be multiplied by 10 to yield 7.2 mGy/hr.

14-18. Answer = (d). A 0.50-mm equivalent thickness is the same as two 0.25-mm lead equivalent thicknesses. The transmission of x-rays through a 0.5-mm Pb (lead) thickness is 1 − 0.96 = 0.04. The transmission of 0.25 mm of Pb is called Tr. Tr × Tr = 0.04. Hence, Tr = 0.20. Attenuation for 0.25 mm of Pb is [1.0 − 0.20] × 100% = 80%.

14-19. Answer = (a). If materials with high atomic number (Z), such as metals, are used to shield charged particles, bremsstrahlung x-rays are produced. These x-rays would require significant added shielding because most charged particles are in the MeV energy range and would produce very high energy x-rays. Hence, charged particles should always be shielded with low-Z materials such as plastics.

14-20. Answer = (a). See notes (**A3**).

14-21. Answer = (b). Coul/kg is a unit of measure for exposure; rem/rad is the QF. Risk/rem is related to effective dose and effective dose equivalent. R/mAs at a given kVp and distance is "radiation output."

14-22. Answer = (b). ESD is about 1 to 2 mGy for extremity radiographs, 0.10 to 0.30 mGy for PA chest radiographs, 4 to 7 cGy for head CT, and 9 to 12 mGy for 4.2-cm compressed breast images. However, mammography doses are usually given as average glandular doses of about 1.5 to 3.0 mGy for 4.2-cm compressed breast tissue.

14-23. Answer = (c). See notes (**A13**).

14-24. Answer = (d). Although workers in nuclear power plants do receive considerable doses of radiation, there are very few nuclear power plant workers in the United States. The radiation doses experienced by these workers are averaged in with the doses received by the entire population of the United States—most of whom receive little or no radiation. This lowers the average radiation levels.

14-25. Answer = (e). The fatal cancer risk for effective dose equivalent is about 0.04 per Sv. However, a 4-mSv dose only to the breast must be multiplied by the weighting factor for the breast, which is 0.15. Hence, the effective dose equivalent for a breast exposure is 0.15×4 mSv = 0.60 mSv = 0.0006 Sv. Next, this effective dose equivalent must be multiplied by the risk per Sv, which is $0.0006 \times 0.04 = 0.000024$, or 24×10^{-6}. This risk factor is then multiplied by 1,000,000 patients undergoing mammography. Thus, 24 of the 1 million mammography patients would be at potential risk of contracting fatal cancer from the radiation used in the x-ray examination. The benefit that outweighs this risk is the 1000 to 2000 early breast cancers that would be detected and treated in this population.

14-26. Answer = (d). See notes (**A19**).

14-27. Answer = (c). The equation given in the notes is $0.1 \times (90 \text{ kVp}/100)^2 \times 50 \text{ mAs} \times (100/50 \text{ cm})^2 = 16.2$ mGy. Another approach is to remember the triple 100 rule: 100 kVp at 100 mAs and 100 cm delivers 10 mSv. Ninety kVp is only slightly less than 100 kVp, and 50 mAs is half of 100 mAs. The final number, 50 cm, is half the distance of 100 cm, and, by the inverse square law, the closer distance increases the radiation by a factor of four. Hence, half of the mAs and four times the distance has a net effect of an increase of two more than the triple rule, or 20 mSv. So the correct answer is slightly less than 20 mSv.

14-28. Answer = (d). From the notes, each minute of fluoroscopy delivers a typical skin entrance dose rate of about 3 cGy/min. For 5 minutes, the fluoroscopy dose would be 15 cGy. The notes state that every four digital images deliver about the same radiation dose as a minute of fluoroscopy. Twelve digital images would provide the same radiation dose as 3 minutes of fluoroscopy, or 9 cGy. Thus, the total skin entrance dose would be about $15 + 9 = 24$ cGy. Because 1 cGy is about equal to 10 mSv, the dose from the procedure would be about 240 mSv.

14-29. Answer = (d). The range of charged particles in different materials is inversely related to the densities of the materials. The ratio of tissue density divided by air density is $(1.0 \text{ g/cm}^3)/(0.001293 \text{ g/cm}^3) = 800$. So the range of the particle in air would be 800×1 cm = 800 cm.

14-30. Answer = (e). For patients, there is no MPD. The physician must balance the benefits to the patient, from information provided by the radiologic examination, against the risks of being exposed to radiation. If the benefits outweigh the risks, the examination should be performed despite the radiation dose. Otherwise, perhaps, the examination should be precluded.

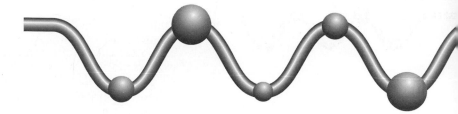

CHAPTER FIFTEEN

Radiation Biology Summary

A. Basic Concepts

1. Radiation biology encompasses both microscopic and macroscopic effects.

   - *Microscopic effects* are at the cellular level.

   - *Macroscopic effects* are observable at the organ level, such as skin erythema and cataracts of the eyes.

2. Ionizing radiation can kill cells in two different ways:

   - *Direct interactions*, in which the radiation breaks the chromosomes in the nucleus and prevents the cell from reproducing.

   - *Indirect interactions*, in which the radiation interacts with the cytoplasm, creating free radicals (OH^-, H_2O_2, H^+, and others). The chemical radicals then interact with the nucleus, damaging the chromosomes and preventing reproduction.

3. *Linear energy transfer (LET)* is a measure of the rate at which ionizing radiation transfers energy to soft tissue. It is measured in units of keV/micron of distance traveled through the tissue.

   - The amount of LET depends on the type and energy of the radiation involved.

   - For charged particles, the greatest charge and slowest velocities produce large LET values.

   - X-rays and gamma rays have very low LET values of about 0.2 to 3.0 keV/μ.

   - Fast neutrons have an LET of about 50 keV/μ.

   - Alpha particles have LET values of about 100 keV/μ.

   - In general, high-LET particles kill every cell along their paths; however, because they lose energy rapidly, they penetrate only small distances.

   - X-rays have low LET values and do not damage cells as much as high-LET radiation—unless there are many x-rays. X-rays affect more cells because they penetrate deeply through the body.

4. Cell sensitivity is described by the law of Bergonié and Tribondeau.

   - Mature cells are more resistant to radiation than are younger cells.

   - Radiosensitivity increases as cell metabolic activity increases.

   - Radiosensitivity increases for cells with a rapid reproduction rate (mitosis).

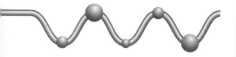

- Differentiated and complex cells are less sensitive (radioresistant) than simple cells.

- For example, lymphocytes and erythrocytes are among the most sensitive, along with skin cells.

- Mature central nervous system (CNS) cells are among the most radioresistant cells.

- The CNS of fetuses and babies is sensitive to radiation effects, which can result in learning disabilities and other neurologic defects.

- Fetuses and babies are more sensitive to radiation effects than adults.

5. Radiosensitivity depends on the stage of the cell cycle.

- Cells are most sensitive to radiation at or near the M (mitosis) stage.

- Late G2 is the next most sensitive portion of the cell cycle.

- The stage most resistant to radiation effects is the S (DNA synthesis) stage.

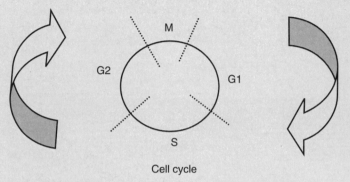

Cell cycle

6. **Cell survival curves** are the key to understanding microscopic effects.

- Graphs plot radiation dose (x-axis) versus $\log_{10}$ (surviving fraction of cells) on the y-axis.

- If a cell cannot continue to reproduce, it is considered nonviable (dead).

- If a cell survival curve has a shoulder at low radiation doses, there are *repair mechanisms* that allow the cells to survive.

- At higher radiation doses, the cell survival curves are always straight lines, meaning that the survival fraction is an exponential function of radiation dose.

- For high-LET radiation, there is no possibility of repair mechanisms to fix the radiation damage; the entire cell survival curve is a straight line.

- D_0 is specified only on the straight line portion of the cell survival curve.

- D_0 is the radiation that reduces the surviving fraction $1/e = 37\%$ of starting point on straight line portion of curve.

- D_{37} is the radiation dose that reduces the surviving fraction from 100% to 37% from the starting point of zero radiation dose—regardless of whether the curve has a shoulder in this region.

- D_q is the "quasi-threshold" of the graph for curves with a shoulder. It is the radiation dose necessary to go from zero radiation to the extrapolated straight line portion of the cell survival curve. A large D_q represents an extended range over which some repairs to cells damaged by radiation can occur.

- n is the extrapolated number. If the straight line portion of the cell survival curve is extended to zero radiation, it intersects the y-axis at some number.

- If n = 1.0, the curve does not have a shoulder, and there is no repair of the radiation damage. If n equals a large number such as 5 or 6, there is a large

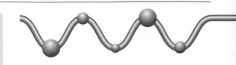

shoulder on the cell survival curve and an extended region over which repair of the cellular radiation damage can occur.

- The equation to relate parameters is as follows:

$$\log_e(n) = D_q/D_0$$

- The equation for the cell survival curve is as follows:

$$S = 1.0 - [1.0 - \exp(-D/D_0)]^n$$

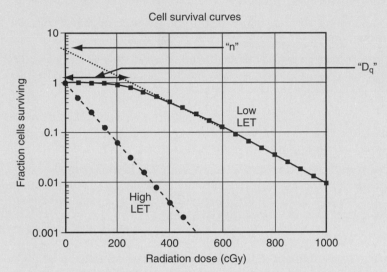

7. To account for the fact that some types of radiation are more damaging than others, the amounts of radiation required to obtain a given cell survival are compared. The ratio of the radiation doses is called the **quality factor** (QF). (The old designation is relative biologic effectiveness [**RBE**].)

- In the cell survival curve shown in the preceding figure, for 0.01 survival, the low-LET radiation requires 1000 cGy and the high-LET radiation requires only 330 cGy.

- The ratio of these two radiation doses is QF = 3.0.

- In other words, for this example, the measured radiation dose for high-LET radiation should be multiplied by 3.0 to yield the same cell damage as the low-LET radiation.

- The "standard" for comparison of biologic radiation effects is x-rays.

8. Similarly, there is a factor to determine the difference in sensitivity to radiation between oxygenated and hypoxic cells. Oxygen has a tendency to bind with the ionization damage caused by radiation, preventing repair. Thus, oxygenated cells are more sensitive to radiation damage. The ratio of the radiation dose required to damage hypoxic cells divided by the radiation dose required to damage the same number of oxygenated cells is called the **oxygen enhancement ratio (OER)**.

9. In **fractionation**, the radiation dose is distributed over time rather than being delivered in one application. With fractionation between radiation doses, the damage is much less than with a single dose of the same amount of radiation.

10. **Macroscopic radiation effects** are divided into two types: stochastic (random chance) and deterministic (or causative).

- With **stochastic effects**, increased radiation enhances the chance that the effect will occur. However, the severity of the effect does not change with more radiation. An example of a stochastic biologic effect due to irradiation is the induction of cancer.

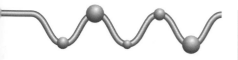

- With *deterministic effects*, more radiation does increase the severity of the effect. An example of a deterministic biologic effect due to irradiation is skin erythema, in which the severity of the skin damage increases with higher radiation doses.

11. Macroscopic biologic effects of irradiation are dependent on many factors, such as the age and sex of the individual; the type, energy, and amount of radiation; the type of tissue involved (part of anatomy); fractionation; and biovariability among individuals.

12. The most radiosensitive organs include the gonads, the skin, blood cells, blood-forming organs (bone marrow), the gastrointestinal tract, and the eyes.

13. The risks of irradiation of body tissue include hematologic effects, cataracts, skin erythema, various types of cancer, genetic effects, birth defects in the fetus, and death (at high, acute radiation dose levels).

14. Some radiation effects have a threshold below which they cannot occur.

15. Many radiation effects are nonlinear with radiation dose. This has sometimes been called the *linear-quadratic dose relationship*.

16. At low radiation doses, a *conservative approach to estimating cancer risk is the linear hypothesis*. The cancer risk increases linearly with the amount of radiation. For example, doubling the radiation dose is assumed to double the risk of cancer induction from the radiation.

17. The *genetic effects* of x-ray exposure to the gonads are as follows:

    - *Genetically significant dose (GSD)* is the average radiation dose to the gonads of all individuals of childbearing age due to radiologic procedures. GSD is about 0.05 to 0.50 mSv (5 to 50 mrem).

    - *Genetic doubling dose (GDD)* is the amount of radiation that would have to be delivered to the gonads of everyone of childbearing age in the United States in order to double the number of birth defects. Without added radiation, the U.S. birth defect rate is about 1% to 2%. To double the rate to 2% to 4%, the radiation dose to the gonads of the entire population would have to be around 0.15 to 0.50 Sv (15 to 50 rem).

GENETIC EFFECT	RADIATION DOSE TO GONADS
1%–2% of chromosomes altered	0.05–0.10 Sv (5–10 rem)
Needed chromosome abnormality for testing	0.25–0.50 Sv (25–50 rem)
Temporary sterility for few months	~1.0 Sv (100 rem)
Temporary sterility for 1–2 years	>2.0 Sv (>200 rem)
Permanent sterility	>5.0 Sv (>500 rem)

18. *In utero exposure of the fetus* is a concern because of the sensitivity of the fetus to radiation.

    - Usually, it is recommend that radiation doses to the fetus be limited to less than 0.05 Sv (5 rem). At fetal doses greater than 0.10 Sv, therapeutic abortion may be recommended.

PERIOD DURING PREGNANCY	TIME LINE	POTENTIAL BIOEFFECT FROM RADIATION	RADIATION AMOUNT AND RISKS
Preimplantation	First 8–10 days	Spontaneous abortion	0.10–2.0 Sv (10–200 rem)
Organogenesis	First 3 months	Microcephaly	15%–40% for 0.10–0.50 Sv (10–50 rem)
	First 3 months	Major deformities	>1.0 Sv (>100 rem)
Second and third trimesters	Fourth through ninth month	Severe mental retardation	10%–40% for Sv (100 rem) [threshold]
	Fourth through ninth month	Diminished IQ, learning disabilities, nervous system disorder	% not well defined for 0.10–1.0 Sv (10–100 rem)
	Fourth through ninth month	Increased cancer incidence, particularly leukemia	0.1%–0.2% for 0.01 Sv (0.1%–0.2% per 1 rem)

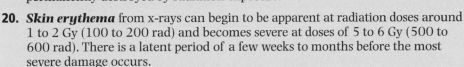

19. **Hematologic effects**, such as reduced red and white cell blood count, begin to appear at 0.25 to 0.50 Sv (25 to 50 rem). There is a delay of a few days to 2 weeks until the peak change is seen. At 7.0 Sv (700 rem), red marrow can be permanently destroyed by radiation exposure.

20. **Skin erythema** from x-rays can begin to be apparent at radiation doses around 1 to 2 Gy (100 to 200 rad) and becomes severe at doses of 5 to 6 Gy (500 to 600 rad). There is a latent period of a few weeks to months before the most severe damage occurs.

21. **Cataract formation** related to x-ray exposure has a threshold of around 2.5 Gy (250 rads). At 12 Gy (1200 rad), there is 100% probability of cataract induction from radiation exposure. The latent period can be 3 to 14 years, with an average latent period of 7 years after irradiation.

22. **Cancer risks** are presumed to be linear without a threshold.

    ● Leukemia usually appears within the first 10 to 15 years after irradiation (seldom at a later date).

    ● Solid tumors rarely appear earlier than 10 years after irradiation and can continue to appear 30 years later.

    ● The estimated risk for all forms of cancer is about 0.05 to 0.06 per Sv (or 0.0005 to 0.0006 per rem).

    ● Cancer incidence without radiation exposure is about 28%.

23. **Epilation** or loss of hair caused by radiation exposure occurs at radiation levels around 5 to 6 Sv (500 to 600 rem).

24. **Death** caused by high levels of acute radiation exposure to the whole body can be expected by several processes, depending on amount of radiation.

    ● $LD_{50/30}$ is the radiation dose that will cause death to 50% of the population within 30 days of receiving whole body, acute radiation exposure. These individuals would be untreated medically.

    ● $LD_{50/30}$ = **4.0 to 4.5 Sv (400 to 450 rem) in humans**.

    ● **Hematopoietic death** refers to death caused by destruction of the blood cells and blood-forming organs of the body. The radiation levels are up to 8 to 10 Sv (800 to 1000 rem). If medically treated with blood transfusions, fluids, and antibiotics, many of these individuals could survive.

    ● **Gastrointestinal death** is due to destruction of the gastrointestinal tract by the radiation, causing ulcers, bleeding, and infections. Death is usually within several weeks. The radiation levels are 8 to 50 Sv (800 to 5000 rem).

    ● **Central nervous system death** is related to damage to the central nervous system, which controls motor functions, breathing, and heart function. This death is usually within 36 hours. The radiation levels required are greater than 50 Sv (>5000 rem).

B. Questions

15-1. Severe skin erythema usually requires an acute skin dose of about _____ Sv.

   (a) 0.25 to 0.50   (b) 1.0   (c) 5 to 6   (d) 7.5 < DE < 12   (e) >12

15-2. For a 100% chance of producing cataracts, the radiation levels need to be ____ Sv.

   (a) 0.25 to 0.50   (b) 1.0   (c) 5 to 6   (d) 7.5 < DE < 12   (e) >12

15-3. The acute whole-body radiation dose necessary to cause a 5% to 6% risk of cancer is _____ Sv.

(a) 0.25 to 0.50   (b) 1.0   (c) 5 to 6   (d) 7.5 < DE < 12   (e) >12

15-4. The acute radiation dose necessary to produce noticeable decreases in the red and white cell blood counts is about _____ Sv.

(a) 0.25 to 0.50   (b) 1.0   (c) 5 to 6   (d) 7.5 < DE < 12   (e) >12

15-5. The lowest amount of acute radiation needed to destroy the bone marrow completely is about _____ Sv.

(a) 0.25 to 0.50   (b) 1.0   (c) 5 to 6   (d) 7.5 < DE < 12
(e) >12

15-6. Leukemia is an example of a(n) _____ effect.

(a) Deterministic   (b) Threshold   (c) Stochastic   (d) Extrapolated
(e) Anachronistic

15-7. Skin erythema is an example of a(n) _____ effect.

(a) Deterministic   (b) Threshold   (c) Stochastic   (d) Extrapolated
(e) Anachronistic

15-8. The portion of the cell reproductive cycle most sensitive to damage from ionizing radiation is the _____ stage.

(a) Mitosis   (b) G1   (c) Synthesis   (d) G2   (e) XY-L2

15-9. The shoulder on the cell survival curve is due to _____.

(a) Latent fading   (b) Synergy   (c) Repair mechanisms   (d) Dilution
(e) Randomization

15-10. The shoulder on the cell survival curve is called the _____.

(a) D_0 (b) n   (c) D_{37} (d) D_q (e) S_X

15-11. The shoulder on the cell survival curve disappears for _____.

(a) Hypoxic cells   (b) Old cells   (c) High-LET radiation
(d) Low-LET radiation   (e) X-rays

15-12. _____ are considered to be the highest LET ionizing radiation from the choices listed.

(a) X-rays   (b) Protons   (c) Beta particles   (d) Gamma rays
(e) Alpha particles

15-13. Fast neutrons have a QF (RBE) of about _____.

(a) 1.0   (b) 10.0   (c) 20.0   (d) 50.0   (e) 100.0

15-14. A factor that corrects for the increased cell-killing power of ionizing radiation related to high oxygen content in the cells is _____.

(a) RBE   (b) OER   (c) D_0 (d) D_{37} (e) f-factor

15-15. The amount of radiation that decreases the cell survival by 63% along the linear portion of the cell survival curve is _____.

(a) RBE   (b) OER   (c) D_0 (d) D_{37} (e) f-factor

15-16. Mechanisms by which ionizing radiation damages human cells include direct damage to the nucleus and _____.

(a) Heating   (b) Cytoplasm leakage   (c) Production of chemical radicals
(d) Electrical current imbalance   (e) Cavitation effects

15-17. The minimum amount of radiation needed to cause central nervous system death by a single whole-body dose is _____ Sv.

(a) 2.0 to 4.0   (b) 8.0 to 12.0   (c) 25 to 35   (d) 50 to 60
(e) 100 to 150

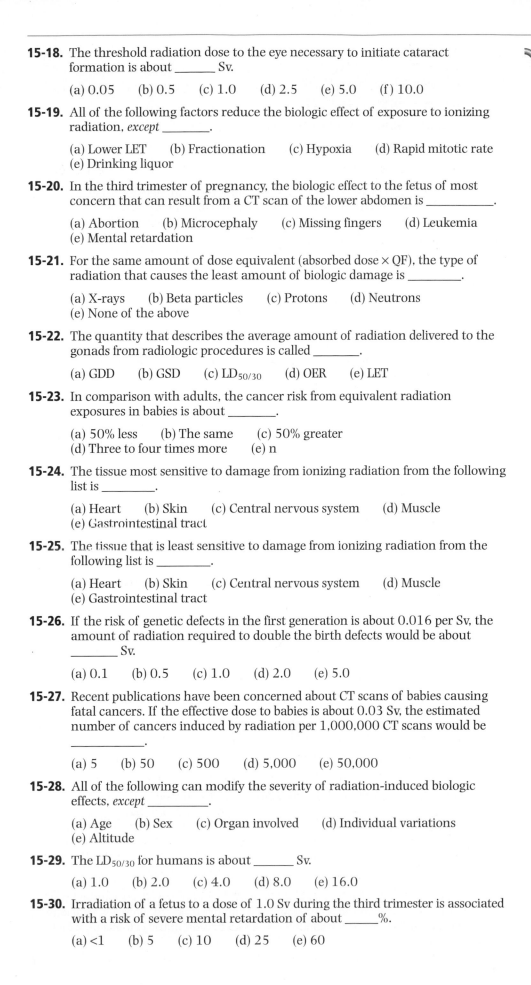

15-18. The threshold radiation dose to the eye necessary to initiate cataract formation is about _____ Sv.

(a) 0.05   (b) 0.5   (c) 1.0   (d) 2.5   (e) 5.0   (f) 10.0

15-19. All of the following factors reduce the biologic effect of exposure to ionizing radiation, *except* _____.

(a) Lower LET   (b) Fractionation   (c) Hypoxia   (d) Rapid mitotic rate
(e) Drinking liquor

15-20. In the third trimester of pregnancy, the biologic effect to the fetus of most concern that can result from a CT scan of the lower abdomen is _____.

(a) Abortion   (b) Microcephaly   (c) Missing fingers   (d) Leukemia
(e) Mental retardation

15-21. For the same amount of dose equivalent (absorbed dose × QF), the type of radiation that causes the least amount of biologic damage is _____.

(a) X-rays   (b) Beta particles   (c) Protons   (d) Neutrons
(e) None of the above

15-22. The quantity that describes the average amount of radiation delivered to the gonads from radiologic procedures is called _____.

(a) GDD   (b) GSD   (c) $LD_{50/30}$ (d) OER   (e) LET

15-23. In comparison with adults, the cancer risk from equivalent radiation exposures in babies is about _____.

(a) 50% less   (b) The same   (c) 50% greater
(d) Three to four times more   (e) n

15-24. The tissue most sensitive to damage from ionizing radiation from the following list is _____.

(a) Heart   (b) Skin   (c) Central nervous system   (d) Muscle
(e) Gastrointestinal tract

15-25. The tissue that is least sensitive to damage from ionizing radiation from the following list is _____.

(a) Heart   (b) Skin   (c) Central nervous system   (d) Muscle
(e) Gastrointestinal tract

15-26. If the risk of genetic defects in the first generation is about 0.016 per Sv, the amount of radiation required to double the birth defects would be about _____ Sv.

(a) 0.1   (b) 0.5   (c) 1.0   (d) 2.0   (e) 5.0

15-27. Recent publications have been concerned about CT scans of babies causing fatal cancers. If the effective dose to babies is about 0.03 Sv, the estimated number of cancers induced by radiation per 1,000,000 CT scans would be _____.

(a) 5   (b) 50   (c) 500   (d) 5,000   (e) 50,000

15-28. All of the following can modify the severity of radiation-induced biologic effects, *except* _____.

(a) Age   (b) Sex   (c) Organ involved   (d) Individual variations
(e) Altitude

15-29. The $LD_{50/30}$ for humans is about _____ Sv.

(a) 1.0   (b) 2.0   (c) 4.0   (d) 8.0   (e) 16.0

15-30. Irradiation of a fetus to a dose of 1.0 Sv during the third trimester is associated with a risk of severe mental retardation of about _____%.

(a) <1   (b) 5   (c) 10   (d) 25   (e) 60

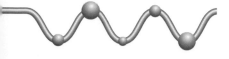

C. Answers

15-1. Answer = (c). See notes (**A20**).

15-2. Answer = (e). See notes (**A21**).

15-3. Answer = (b). See notes (**A22**).

15-4. Answer = (a). See notes (**A19**).

15-5. Answer = (d). See notes (**A19**).

15-6. Answer = (c). For deterministic effects, the severity increases with greater radiation doses. Threshold effects are phenomena that do not occur until some minimum level of radiation exposure has been exceeded. Extrapolation involves continuing a graph along its trend to estimate additional points. An anachronism is something that is unusual and out of place because it is out of its proper chronological order.

15-7. Answer = (a). See answer to Question 15-6.

15-8. Answer = (a). See notes about cell sensitivity (**A6**).

15-9. Answer = (c). In latent image fading, which refers to both film-screen and CR image receptors, the intensity of the image decreases because of delays in processing. Synergy refers to two or more variables that enhance each other in their overall effect. Dilution refers to reducing the concentration of a substance by adding fluid. In randomization, items are selected at random without regard to any criteria.

15-10. Answer = (d). D_q is the quasi-threshold that pertains to the shoulder of the cell survival curve, where repair mechanisms occur. The D_{37} is the first part of the cell survival curve, regardless of whether there is a shoulder or not. It is the radiation dose required to reduce the cell survival from 100% to 37%. The D_0 refers to the linear part of the cell survival curve, not the shoulder. It is the radiation dose required to reduce the cell survival fraction from any starting point to an amount that is 63% less. S_x is the surviving fraction, or the vertical axis, of the cell survival curve.

15-11. Answer = (c). There is a shoulder on the cell survival curve for hypoxic cells, whereas there is no shoulder for oxygen-enhanced cells, where they could repair radiation damage. Old cells have no special effect on the curve. X-rays are low-LET radiation because the ionization is sparse, which allows cells to repair radiation damage. High-LET ionization is concentrated and kills everything in its path.

15-12. Answer = (e). Alpha particles are helium atoms missing the outer shell electrons. Thus, the electrical charge is +2, and the particle is more massive. Even though electrons can be knocked off by x-rays, beta particles (which are electrons), and protons, alpha particles cause more ionization to occur over short distances. Because alpha particles are massive, they travel at slow speeds. The high charge and slow speed of the alpha particles cause high ionization per path length (LET).

15-13. Answer = (c). See notes (**A7**).

15-14. Answer = (b). QF or RBE is the correction for the type of radiation involved. It is used to convert from absorbed dose to dose equivalent. D_0 and D_{37} are radiation doses that describe the cell-killing capacity of different types of radiation and different types of cells. The f-factor also corrects for differences in types of radiation and types of target materials; it converts measurements from exposure to absorbed dose.

15-15. Answer = (c). See definitions in notes under cell survival curve (**A8**).

15-16. Answer = (c). Heating and cavitation are tissue damage effects caused by high-power ultrasound. The radiation is not of sufficient dimensions to cause cytoplasm leakage. The radiation causes ionization in the cytoplasm, which

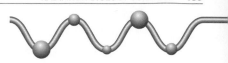

creates free radicals that can chemically damage chromosomes in the cell nucleus. Insufficient electrical charge is created to cause current imbalances.

15-17. Answer = (d). Central nervous system death can occur at 50 Sv (5000 rem) and greater in a single whole-body radiation dose. Some references cite the value for central nervous system death to be as high as 100 Sv (10,000 rem).

15-18. Answer = (d). The threshold or minimum radiation dose to the eyes needed before cataracts form is 2.5 Sv (250 rem). However, there is a long latent period of years, and more than 12 Sv (1200 rem) is required before there is a 100% certainty of causing cataracts.

15-19. Answer = (d). When a cell passes through the mitosis portion of the cell cycle often, it is more vulnerable to damage from ionizing radiation. Lower LET spreads the ionization and allows a chance for repair. Fractionation has a similar effect by spreading the damage over time. Hypoxic cells lack oxygen, which scavenges the electrons knocked loose by the radiation, making the damage permanent. Liquor and other chemicals called *radiation desensitizers* create more free electrons in the tissue, which allow more repair of damaged cells to occur.

15-20. Answer = (d). Spontaneous abortion due to fetal radiation occurs during the preimplantation period; a CT scan is associated with too low a radiation dose for this to occur. Microcephaly and missing fingers occur during the first trimester, and again CT scans deliver too low a radiation dose for this. Radiation can induce mental retardation during the third trimester; however, the radiation dose from a single routine CT scan is too low for this to occur.

15-21. Answer = (e). The dose equivalent has a unit that already corrects for differences among types of radiation. Hence, for a given dose equivalent, all radiation types would be expected to cause similar biologic damage.

15-22. Answer = (b). GDD is a hypothetical dose that would double the number of birth defects if given to the gonads of all persons of childbearing age. The $LD_{50/30}$ is the lethal radiation dose required to cause death to 50% of the population within 30 days—if untreated medically. OER is the oxygen enhancement ratio and has nothing to do with radiology doses delivered to the gonads. Similarly, LET is linear energy transfer, and it is the rate of ionization energy transfer per path length. It is not necessarily related to the radiation dose to the gonads.

15-23. Answer = (d). Fetuses, babies, and young children are more sensitive to ionizing radiation than adults because of the rapid growth of cells in their bodies. From the data given in the notes about the risk of leukemia from fetal radiation exposures, the risks to fetuses (babies) is about three to six times greater than in adults. Babies also live longer, giving the cancer more years to express itself.

15-24. Answer = (b). The cell cycle time for mitosis in the skin is 3 to 5 days; the rapid mitosis rate makes the skin cells sensitive to radiation damage. Heart, muscle, and central nervous system tissue are relatively insensitive to radiation damage. The gastrointestinal tract is a radiation-sensitive tissue, but skin is more sensitive to damage than is the gastrointestinal tract.

15-25. Answer = (c). In adults, the central nervous system is one of the systems least sensitive to radiation damage. In babies and young children, the central nervous system can manifest damage at relatively low radiation doses. See comments in notes.

15-26. Answer = (c). A risk of 0.016 per Sv is equal to 1.6% per Sv. Without radiation, birth defects occur in 1% to 2% of the population. Hence, the radiation required must increase the birth defects by about 1% to 2%. 1 Sv would yield a rate of genetic defects of 1.6%.

15-27. Answer = (d). According to the notes in this chapter, the cancer rate associated with fetal radiation exposure is 0.1% to 0.2% per 0.01 Sv. For a 0.03-Sv whole

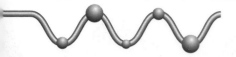

body dose, multiplying the risk by the dose yields (0.15%/0.01 Sv) × 0.03 Sv = 0.45% = 0.0045. Multiplying this number by 1,000,000 babies yields 4500 cancer cases.

15-28. Answer = (e). See note in this chapter (**A11**).

15-29. Answer = (c). See note in this chapter (**A24**).

15-30. Answer = (d). The notes in this chapter suggest a risk of severe mental retardation of about 10% to 40% per Sv. However, there is probably a threshold dose of around 1 Sv.

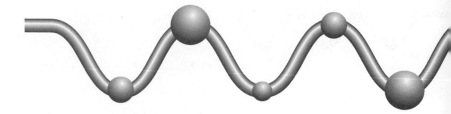

CHAPTER SIXTEEN

Fluoroscopy Systems

A. Basic Concepts

1. Fluoroscopy systems are specialized for the following purposes: positioning for catheter placement, positioning for radiography and digital subtraction angiography (DSA), trauma surveys, and dynamic studies such as swallowing examinations and heart evaluations.

2. Fluoroscopy systems are designed to take many continuous low-mA or pulsed higher mA images over a period of many minutes.

3. A comparison with radiographic imaging is shown in the table.

PARAMETER	FLUOROSCOPY SYSTEM	RADIOGRAPHY
Focal spot size	0.2–0.6 mm	0.6–1.2 mm
kVp used	60–130	50–150
mA used	0.1–5 mA (continuous)	20–1000 mA
	0.5–180 mA (pulsed)	
Exposure times	Multiples of 5 minutes	0.001–4 sec/image
Filter	Min.–0.9 mm Cu added	Min.–2 mm Al added
SID	80–120 cm	100 or 180 cm
Minimum SSD	20–50 cm	68 cm (chest >)
Typ. ESE	3–6 R/min	0.401–0.8 R/image
Image receptor	(II + TV) or FPD	CR, DR, or film

4. The configuration of a fluoroscopic system is shown in the figure.

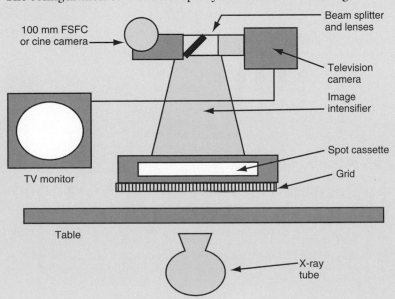

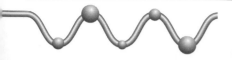

5. Modern fluoroscopy systems use a DR-type receptor called a ***flat panel display (FPD)*** instead of a system with an image intensifier (II), beam splitter, lenses, aperture, and television. As with regular DR systems, the spatial resolution is lower, but the dynamic range is greater than that of the II systems.

6. Components of fluoroscopy systems are listed here along with their function.

   X-ray tube: target where x-rays are produced

   Collimator: device that restricts the size of the x-ray beam

   Filters: substances that remove low-energy x-rays to make the beam more penetrating

   Table: surface on which the patient is placed

   Grid: thin plate containing lead strips that remove many of the scattered x-rays

   Image intensifier: device that captures x-rays passing through the patient and converts the x-ray distribution into a bright light image

   Lens system: device that takes light from the image intensifier and directs and focuses the light image onto the television camera

   Aperture: plate that restricts the light to increase the radiation dose so that quantum mottle is at acceptable levels and distortion at the edge of the lenses is limited

   ADC: component that processes analog-to-digital conversion of the electronic signals

   Television system: system that receives the light image, converts it to an electronic image, and sends it to the television display monitor

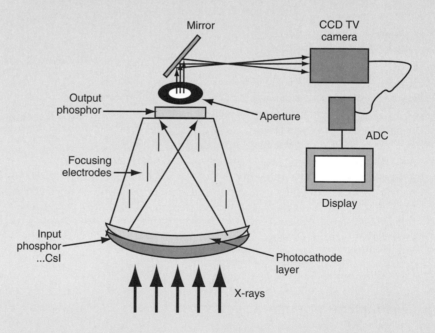

7. The process of image formation in the image intensifier is as follows:

   - X-rays enter thin glass or titanium ***window of image intensifier***.

   - X-rays deposit energy in the ***input phosphor*** of cesium iodide, and a fraction of energy is emitted as light. The amount of light is proportional to amount of input x-rays.

   - Light is then captured in a ***photocathode*** (e.g., antimony sulfide compounds), where light results in electron emission. The number of electrons emitted is in proportion to the amount of light deposited.

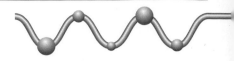

- *High voltage* between the photocathode and the output phosphor accelerates the electrons, and they gain energy. This is called *flux gain* and increases the energy by 50- to 100-fold.

- *Focusing electrodes* focus and invert the position of the electron onto the output phosphor. The inside of the image intensifier is a vacuum, so that accelerated electrons do not bump into air atoms and slow down.

- The *output phosphor* (e.g., $ZnCdSO_2$) is much smaller than the input phosphor (typically 22 to 35 mm). The output converts a portion of the energy deposited in the phosphor to light.

- Some of the increase in light from the output phosphor occurs because the electrons emitted from a large photocathode are confined in the small area of the output phosphor; this is called the *minification gain*. The minification gain is equal to the ratio of the area of the input *field of view (FoV)* divided by the area of the output phosphor. For example,

Input area = $\pi D^2/4 = \pi \times (40 \text{ cm diameter})^2/4 = 1257 \text{ cm}^2$

Output area = $\pi d^2/4 = \pi \times (3.5 \text{ cm diameter})^2/4 = 9.6 \text{ cm}^2$

Minification gain = $1257/9.6 = 130.9$

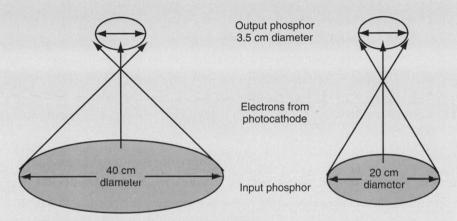

Output phosphor
3.5 cm diameter

Electrons from photocathode

40 cm diameter

20 cm diameter

Input phosphor

- *FoV* is selected by means of the *electron magnification* buttons on the image intensifier. For each "mag mode," the collimators and image intensifier focusing electrodes adjust the image to a smaller portion of the patient's body and spread it over the entire output surface; another way to describe this is *less minification gain. Image intensifiers can have two, three, or four FoVs*. For example, an image intensifier can use a circular area on the input phosphor of 40, 28, 20, or 14 cm in diameter to image the patient.

- *Flux gain* is the energy gained by electrons accelerated by the high voltage applied across the image intensifier.

- *Brightness gain* is the overall gain in light intensity provided by the image intensifier.

    Brightness gain = flux gain × minification gain

8. The energy conversion process in an image intensifier is as follows:

   - X-rays are incident through the input surface into the input phosphor.

   - X-ray energy is converted into light in the input phosphor.

   - Light is converted into electrons in the photocathode.

   - The energy of the electrons is increased by the high voltage (flux gain).

   - The electron energy is converted back to light in the output phosphor.

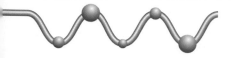

9. ***Automatic brightness control (ABC)*** is an automatic feedback system that senses the light from the output phosphor and adjusts the radiation to maintain a fairly constant light level.

- The ABC can adjust kVp only, mA only, or a combination of mA and kVp (isowatt) or, in pulsed fluoroscopy, a combination of x-ray beam filter, kVp, mA, and pulse width.

- As the FoV is decreased (mag mode), the minification gain decreases in magnitude. Thus, the brightness gain decreases at smaller FoVs.

- The ABC system then increases the radiation to the patient to compensate for the loss in minification gain. Typically, each step in mag mode results in about a 40% to 100% increase in radiation dose to the patient.

- That is, ***the smallest FoVs are associated with the largest fluoroscopic entrance skin exposure (ESE) radiation dose rates and the most electronic magnification of the image***.

10. ***Maximum entrance skin exposure rate (ESER)*** of fluoroscopy systems is set by federal regulations.

- 5.0 R ≥ ESER for manually controlled systems.

- 10.0 R ≥ ESER for ABC systems with one operational level.

- 10.0 R ≥ ESER for the low level of a two-level ABC system; 20.0 R ≥ ESER for the high level of a two-level ABC system.

- The 5-minute timer must sound to remind radiologists of fluoroscopy time.

- Source-to-skin distance (SSD) must be ≥15 inches to reduce radiation dose, except for special surgical units (20 cm).

11. ***F-number (F#)*** is used to describe the light-gathering property of lenses and apertures.

- F# is the ratio of the focal length of the lens divided by the lens diameter.

- The objective lens (at the output phosphor of the image intensifier) is placed one optical focal length away from the output phosphor. The light that exits is in parallel rays.

- The aperture is a plate with a hole in it that blocks some of the parallel light.

- The lens at the television camera refocuses the parallel light onto the camera detector.

- The combined lens system and the aperture have effective F#s.

- Larger F#s gather less light than lower F#s.

- Relative light gathering = [F# 1/F# 2]^2.

- As the F# increases because of a change in the aperture, the radiation dose to the patient increases.

12. ***Pulsed fluoroscopy*** is a system used to reduce the radiation dose to the patient (see figure on next page).

- Pulsed fluoroscopy reduces motion blur.

- Because there are long periods of no radiation between pulses, the radiation dose to the patient is less.

- Pulsed fluoroscopy at 30 pps is about 20% to 30% less than continuous fluoroscopy; 15 pps is about 40% to 60% less; and 7.5 pps is about 75% less.

13. Modern ***fluoroscopic television systems*** use ***charge-coupled device (CCD)*** cameras. Older television systems used tubes such as vidicons and plumbicons.

- The image consists of ***raster lines***, and each line is composed of ***dots***.

- Vertical spatial resolution = [number of raster lines × KF]/[2 × FoV(mm)] where KF = Kell factor ~ 0.7.

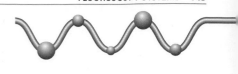

- ***Kell factor*** is the fraction of television lines actually used in image formation. For a 525-line system, only about 360 to 400 lines are actively used in imaging.
- ***To have equal vertical and horizontal resolution, the number of dots per line = number of active raster lines.***
- ***Horizontal spatial resolution*** is proportional to bandwidth (BW)/[(frames/sec) × (number of lines) × FoV (mm)].
- Most televisions display 30 full images each second.
- Interlaced television displays every other line and frame in 1/60 second. Then the alternate lines are scanned in the next 1/60 second.
- Progressive television display scans the raster lines sequentially.
- Bandpass (or bandwidth) = (30 frame/sec) × (number of raster lines) × (number of dots/line)
- For example, BW = 30 × 400 × 400 = 5,000,000/sec = 5 MHz

14. ***Image degradation*** in fluoroscopy "image intensifier + television systems" is related to the following:
    - ***Pincushion distortion***: straight lines curved in large FoV
    - ***Vignetting***: image brighter in center than at edge
    - ***Retrograde light flow***: light from output phosphor illuminates photocathode
    - ***Burn spots***: excessive radiation continually on one spot destroys phosphor
    - ***Lag***: persistence of fluoroscopic image because of slow phosphorescent decay
    - ***Unsharpness***: focal spot blur and lens/electrodes not focused
    - ***Flare (glare)***: high brightness at edge of anatomy or in lung field

15. ***Spatial resolution*** is influenced by the following:
    - Image intensifier resolution is better than television system resolution, which limits the system.
    - Spatial resolution is better in smaller FoVs because of the limitations of television.
    - Horizontal resolution is better for high bandwidth.
    - The number of raster lines affects the vertical resolution. The number of dots per line affects the horizontal resolution.
    - Typical spatial resolutions of the image intensifier + television system for fluoroscopy are shown in the table (for assumed equal numbers of dots and lines and FPD with 200-micron pixels).

FoV (cm)[in]	SPATIAL RESOLUTION (LP/mm) AT 45 DEGREES		
	525-LINE TV	1023-LINE TV	FLAT PANEL
(40) [15.7]	0.7	1.1–1.4	2.5
(28) [11.0]	1.0	1.5–2.0	2.5
(22.9) [9.0]	1.2	1.8–2.4	2.5
(20) [7.9]	1.4	2.1–2.8	2.5
(14) [5.5]	2.0	3.0–4.0	2.5
(11.4) [4.5]	2.5	3.8–5.0	2.5

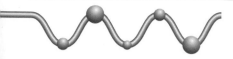

- Because the size of a flat panel detector is fixed at around 200 microns, flat panel spatial resolution does not change much with FoV selection.

16. The entrance skin exposure rate (ESER) for the patient is influenced by the following:

- Smaller FoVs deliver a higher ESER.

- Larger F#s deliver a greater ESER.

- More raster lines use a greater ESER to reduce the quantum mottle.

- Lower pulsed fluoroscopy rates deliver less radiation, and higher pulse rates deliver more radiation.

- Higher brightness gains for the image intensifier deliver less radiation.

- ABC systems, which use more x-ray beam filtration and higher kVp values, deliver much lower ESE radiation levels in fluoroscopy.

- Newer image intensifiers have better conversion gain and deliver a smaller ESER.

- Lowering the image intensifier so that it is closer to the patient delivers less radiation.

- ***Last frame hold (freeze frame)*** can limit fluoroscopy time and reduce radiation dose.

- Limiting the fluoroscopy time reduces the radiation dose.

- Larger patients force the ABC system to deliver a large radiation dose.

- In the lateral projection, scattered radiation to the staff is greatest on the side closest to the x-ray tubes and less on the side closest to the image intensifier.

17. Special features of ***flat panel display fluoroscopy*** systems include the following:

- Spatial resolution does not change with FoV.

- There are no areas of saturation ("blooming") related to the larger dynamic range and window/level adjustments.

- Some image persistence (lag) is visible.

- No pincushion or spatial distortion exists.

- FoV does not provide "mag," but the image is interpolated and expanded to fill the display.

- Radiation dose does not have to increase with FoV, but it usually does increase to limit perception of image noise.

B.   Questions

16-1. If a smaller FoV is selected for a fluoroscopy image intensifier system, the spatial resolution will _____ and the patient's radiation dose will _____.

(a) Increase, increase   (b) Increase, decrease   (c) Decrease, increase
(d) Decrease, decrease   (e) Remain the same, increase

16-2. If a smaller FoV is selected for a fluoroscopy flat panel system, the spatial resolution will _____ and the patient's radiation dose will _____.

(a) Increase, increase   (b) Increase, decrease   (c) Decrease, increase
(d) Decrease, decrease   (e) Remain the same, increase

16-3. Deficiencies of a fluoroscopy image intensifier include all of the following, *except* _____.

(a) Vignetting   (b) Pincushion distortion   (c) Lag
(d) Electronic defocusing   (e) Specular reflection

16-4. All of the following factors affect the radiation dose to the patient during fluoroscopy, *except* _____.

(a) Aperture size   (b) Light flux gain   (c) Conversion gain
(d) Pulse rate   (e) SSD

16-5. A fluoroscopic image intensifier increases brightness gain by _____ and _____.

(a) Aperture reduction, grids   (b) Variable iris, retrograde light flow
(c) Magnification gain, decreased FoV   (d) Minification gain, flux gain
(e) Fractals, filtration

16-6. The spatial resolution of a fluoroscopy television depends on all of the following, *except* _____.

(a) Number of raster lines   (b) Bandpass   (c) FoV   (d) F#
(e) Number of video frames/sec

16-7. The _____ has the lowest spatial resolution of the items listed.

(a) Image intensifier   (b) 525-line television system   (c) Cassette spot film
(d) 100-mm fluoroscopic spot film camera (FSFC)   (e) Objective lens

16-8. All of the following represent different types of television cameras used in fluoroscopy units, *except* _____.

(a) Orthicons   (b) CCDs   (c) Vidicons   (d) Plumbicons
(e) Heptacons

16-9. The maximum ESER permitted by regulations for a standard one-level ABC fluoroscopy system is _____ per minute.

(a) 2.0 R (1.74 cGy)   (b) 5 R (4.35 cGy)   (c) 10 R (8.7 cGy)
(d) 20 R (17.4 cGy)   (e) 30 R (26.1 cGy)

16-10. The maximum ESER permitted by regulations for a two-level system operated in the high-level mode of ABC fluoroscopy is _____ per minute.

(a) 2.0 R (1.74 cGy)   (b) 5 R (4.35 cGy)   (c) 10 R (8.7 cGy)
(d) 20 R (17.4 cGy)   (e) 30 R (26.1 cGy)

16-11. The lowest radiation dose to the patient per single image of the abdomen for an average-sized patient is provided by _____.

(a) Fluoroscopy   (b) DSA   (c) Film-screen cassette
(d) CT scan   (e) CR

16-12. Raising an image intensifier so that it is farther away from the patient during fluoroscopy results in _____.

(a) Higher radiation doses   (b) Less focal spot blur
(c) Less minification gain   (d) Less magnification of the anatomy
(e) All of the above

16-13. Typical 525-line fluoroscopy television systems with equal horizontal and vertical spatial resolution have a bandpass (bandwidth) of about _____ MHz, and 1023-line systems have a bandpass of _____ MHz.

(a) 1, 4   (b) 4, 8   (c) 5, 20   (d) 10, 20   (e) 10, 40

16-14. For ABC fluoroscopy, as the patient's thickness increases, the radiation dose to the patient will _____ and the image contrast will _____.

(a) Increase, increase   (b) Increase, decrease   (c) Decrease, increase
(d) Decrease, decrease   (e) Increase, remain the same

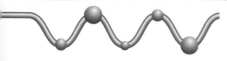

16-15. Pulsed fluoroscopy is important because it _____.

(a) Reduces radiation dose to the patient   (b) Improves image contrast
(c) Improves spatial resolution   (d) Uses lower mA
(e) Has wider dynamic range

16-16. A typical gastrointestinal fluoroscopic examination with barium delivers a total radiation dose of about _____ cGy at the skin entrance point.

(a) 1.5   (b) 5.0   (c) 10.0   (d) 25.0   (e) 50.0

16-17. If the aperture of a fluoroscopy system with an F# of 1.6 is replaced with one with an F# of 3.2, the radiation doses to the patient will _____.

(a) Decrease by 1/4   (b) Decrease by 1/2   (c) Increase by 2 times
(d) Increase by 4 times   (e) Remain the same

16-18. The automatic brightness control of modern fluoroscopy systems regulates all of the following, *except* _____.

(a) kVp   (b) mA   (c) Filtration   (d) FoV   (e) Pulse width

16-19. Switching from continuous fluoroscopy to pulsed fluoroscopy at 15 frames per second affects the radiation dose to the patient as follows:_____

(a) Increases it by 50%   (b) Increases it by 25%   (c) Has no effect
(d) Decreases it by 25%   e) Decreases it by 50%

16-20. In comparison with a conventional fluoroscopy system, a digital (filmless) cardiac cine system has the following characteristic: _____.

(a) Higher power rating   (b) Larger FoVs   (c) Lower lag
(d) Greater dynamic range   (e) Larger focal spot size

16-21. Decreasing the F# of an aperture of a fluoroscopy system results in _____.

(a) Better spatial resolution   (b) More quantum mottle
(c) Less image aberration   (d) Increased magnification
(e) Higher radiation doses to the patient

16-22. In digital subtraction angiography, the contrast-filled vessels are only 1% higher in contrast than the mask. If the mask subtracts 99% of the background from the images, the vessel contrast increases to ____%, and the quantum mottle increases by _____ times more.

(a) 10, 2   (b) 20, 4   (c) 30, 5   (d) 40, 6   (e) 50, 7

16-23. In comparison with image intensifier fluoroscopy, flat panel fluoroscopy systems have all of the following characteristics, *except* _____.

(a) Less spatial resolution   (b) Less blooming
(c) Less pincushion distortion   (d) No lag   (e) Larger dynamic range

16-24. In comparison with an ABC system with fixed kVp and variable mA, when imaging a large patient with an ABC system with fixed mA and variable kVp, the image has _____ contrast, and the radiation dose to the patient is _____.

(a) Increased, increased   (b) Increased, decreased
(c) Decreased. increased   (d) Decreased, decreased
(e) The same, decreased

16-25. The bandpass of a fluoroscopic system affects _____.

(a) Vertical spatial resolution   (b) Horizontal spatial resolution
(c) Both vertical and horizontal spatial resolution
(d) Neither horizontal nor vertical resolution   (e) Artifacts

16-26. In comparison with a 40-cm FoV, a 20-cm FoV has a brightness gain that is_____ that of the large FoV.

(a) One fourth   (b) One half   (c) The same as   (d) 2 times   (e) 4 times

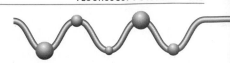

C. Answers

16-1. Answer = (a). Both vertical and horizontal resolution is dependent on [1/FoV (mm)]. Hence, smaller FoVs have better spatial resolution (except for flat panel systems). The minification gain is directly related to the ratio of [input diameter/output diameter]^2. As the FoV of the input diameter becomes smaller, the minification gain decreases, and the brightness gain decreases. As the ABC system senses the reduction in light exiting the image intensifier, the diminished light output is compensated for by more radiation, which brings the light levels back to normal.

16-2. Answer = (e). For flat panel fluoroscopy systems, the spatial resolution does not change with FoV. The spatial resolution is dependent on the pixel size, which is fixed. The radiation dose does not need to increase with flat panel systems; however, the radiation dose is increased to minimize the perception of quantum mottle as the image is expanded and interpolated in size.

16-3. Answer = (e). Specular reflection is an image problem in ultrasonography. Vignetting means that the image brightness fades from the center toward the edges. Pincushion distortion causes the bending of straight structures at the edges. Lag is persistence of the previous image because of slow phosphorescent decay with time. Electronic defocusing is setting the focus point for the electrodes at improper voltages, which results in image blur and loss of spatial resolution.

16-4. Answer = (b). Aperture size controls the image intensifier light to the ABC systems, which regulates the radiation. Light flux gain is a fictitious phrase. Flux gain is a real term, and it refers to the gain in light energy related to the voltage across the image intensifier. Conversion gain is a measure of the light output from the image intensifier for a certain amount of incident radiation; the radiation dose to the patient is related to efficiency of the image intensifier. The radiation dose to the patient is directly related to the selected fluoroscopy pulse rate. The SSD is the source-to-skin distance; the radiation dose increases when the patient is closer to the x-ray tube.

16-5. Answer = (d). The flux gain is the gain in kinetic energy of the electrons accelerated by the voltage across the image intensifier. The minification gain is the concentration of all the electrons released over a large input surface into a very small output phosphor of the image intensifier. Grids and variable iris are not a physical part of the image intensifier. Fractals are a mathematical tool for modeling the branching seen in physical structures, such as the lung.

16-6. Answer = (d). Both vertical and horizontal resolution is inversely proportional to the FoV. Vertical resolution is directly related to number of raster lines. Horizontal resolution is related to bandpass divided by video frame rate, number of lines, and FoV. See notes in this chapter.

16-7. Answer = (b). Any type of lens has a superb spatial resolution. The best resolution at the output phosphor of an image intensifier is about 5 to 6 LP/mm. The spatial resolution of a 525-line television depends on the FoV; the best resolution for a 4.5-inch (11.4-cm) FoV is about 2.2 to 2.5 LP/mm. Cassette spot films have the same resolution as regular film-screen combinations, about 4 to 8 LP/mm. A 100-mm fluoroscopic spot film camera has almost the same (slightly less) resolution as the image intensifier because it images the output phosphor through a lens and beam splitter.

16-8. Answer = (e). Orthicons were the first, very large television camera tubes; these tubes have not been used for years. CCDs are charge-coupled devices, which accumulate charges generated by light exposure in solid-state bins. Vidicons are tubes with antimony sulfate surfaces; these tubes have reduced sensitivity, reduced contrast, increased lag, and less image noise. Plumbicon tubes have lead oxide surfaces; these tubes have improved contrast, reduced lag, and increased image noise in comparison with vidicons. Heptacons is a fictitious word.

16-9. Answer = (c). See note in this chapter (**A10**).

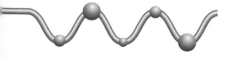

16-10. Answer = (d). See note in this chapter (**A10**).

16-11. Answer = (a). The radiation exposure rate to patients undergoing fluoroscopy is about 3 to 6 cGy per minute, and the image rate is 30 images per second. Thus, radiation exposure to the patient per image is equal to (50 mGy/min)/ (1800 images/min), or about 0.03 mGy/image. DSA delivers about 10 mGy/ image. The radiation levels with a film-screen system are about half the value of the levels with CR. Therefore, film-screen radiation levels would be about 4.0 mGy/image, and CR would deliver about 8.0 mGy per image. CT scans of the body deliver an entrance exposure of about 20 to 40 mGy per image.

16-12. Answer = (a). As the image intensifier moves farther away from the x-ray tube, the radiation output must be increased to maintain a constant level of radiation at the input surface. The focal spot blur increases because the magnification increases. The minification gain does not change with a distance (source-to-image) change.

16-13. Answer = (c). For equal resolution, the number of raster lines must equal the number of dots per line. To double the number of lines from 525 to 1023, the number of dots must also be increased. The amount of data increases by $2 \times 2 = 4$ times. See note in this chapter (**A13**).

16-14. Answer = (b). In imaging thick patients, the transmitted radiation is decreased, and the number of scattered x-rays is increased. The ABC system boosts the amount of radiation by increasing kVp, mA, and pulse width to compensate for attenuation of the x-rays. The increased kVp and scattered x-rays reduce the image contrast.

16-15. Answer = (a). Pulsed fluoroscopy does not affect contrast, spatial resolution, or dynamic range at all. The mA values are higher in pulsed fluoroscopy, but the radiation pulse is "on" only 3 to 10 msec every 33 msec (for 30 pps) or 66 msec (15 pps). The fact that the radiation is turned off for appreciable periods reduces the radiation dose to the patient.

16-16. Answer = (d). For gastrointestinal examinations, the typical fluoroscopy time is about 5 minutes, and there are about 10 to 12 spot films. Assume that the typical entrance dose for fluoroscopy is about 4 cGy per minute and that 4 or 5 spot films equal 1 minute of fluoroscopy. Total fluoroscopy time would be 5 minutes plus 2 minutes for spot films, or 7 minutes. (4 cGy/min) × 7 minutes = 28 cGy entrance dose.

16-17. Answer = (d). As the F# increases, the radiation dose to the patient increases because less light is gathered. A larger aperture number means a smaller hole in the metal plate. The radiation dose increases as the square of the aperture ratio: $[3.2/1.6]^2 = 4.0$.

16-18. Answer = (d). The ABC controls everything except the FoV, which is selectable. The ABC works with all FoVs selected.

16-19. Answer = (e). As the pulse rate of fluoroscopy decreases, the radiation dose to the patient decreases directly with the relative pulse rate. A 50% decrease in pulse rate from 30 to 15 pps would be expected to reduce the radiation dose by about 50%.

16-20. Answer = (d). Higher power x-ray generators and x-ray tubes are not necessarily placed on digital systems. FoVs of digital cardiac systems are generally smaller than or equal to those of image intensifier systems. Flat panel systems can have noticeable lag. The focal spot sizes of the x-ray tubes of digital systems are the same as those of conventional image intensifier systems.

16-21. Answer = (b). A smaller F# aperture collects more light and allows the edges of the lens to be used. The edges of the lens have the most aberration; hence, aberration increases. The effects of using a larger F# on spatial resolution or magnification are minor. Magnification is controlled by FoV or moving the patient away from the image intensifier. Because the larger aperture (smaller F#) gathers more light, the radiation doses to the patient decrease,

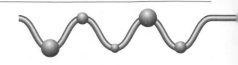

and fewer x-rays are used to create the images. When fewer x-rays are used to form the images, the quantum mottle increases.

16-22. Answer = (e). After subtracting 99% of the background, 1% of the background and 1% of the contrast remain. The ratio of contrast to total radiation is 50%. The relative noise percentage is equal to $100\%/[\text{number of x-rays}]^{0.5}$. The total number of x-rays used in image formation is 2%, or a factor of 50 times fewer x-rays. Noise increases by the square root of 50, or about 7 times more quantum mottle.

16-23. Answer = (d). Because of the fixed pixel size and the arrangement of pixels in a matrix, the spatial resolution does not change with FoV, and there is little or no distortion. The larger dynamic range (12 bits) prevents saturation of the detectors and blooming. However, FPD detectors do contain a CsI scintillator, which has some afterglow that causes lag; the readout/nulling of the pixels and frame averaging to reduce image noise also contribute to the lag.

16-24. Answer = (d). If only the mA is adjusted, the kVp is fixed. Subject contrast is affected by kVp and filtration of the x-ray beam. Therefore, with fixed kVp, contrast remains similar. With variable kVp, the kVp increases with larger patient size, and the contrast degrades. However, because higher kVp x-rays are more penetrating, fewer x-rays can be used, which lowers the radiation dose to the patient.

16-25. Answer = (b). See note in this chapter (**A15**).

16-26. Answer = (a). A smaller FoV is associated with less minification gain. The gain is proportional to the ratio of the diameters squared, or $[20/40]^2 = 1/4$. The flux gain does not change; thus, the overall effect is to have only 25% of the original brightness gain.

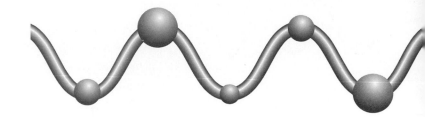

CHAPTER SEVENTEEN

Mammography

A. Basic Concepts

1. Mammography can be done either with special film-screen systems or with digital radiography (DR).

- **Film-screen systems** have a single screen and a single emulsion with high resolution.

- **DR** can be either **direct,** with amorphous selenium detectors, or **indirect,** with CsI coated over a photodiode array.

- Spatial resolution for film-screen mammography is 15 to 20 LP/mm.

- DR systems have different detector element sizes, from 25 to 100 microns, which yield spatial resolution from 5 to 10 LP/mm.

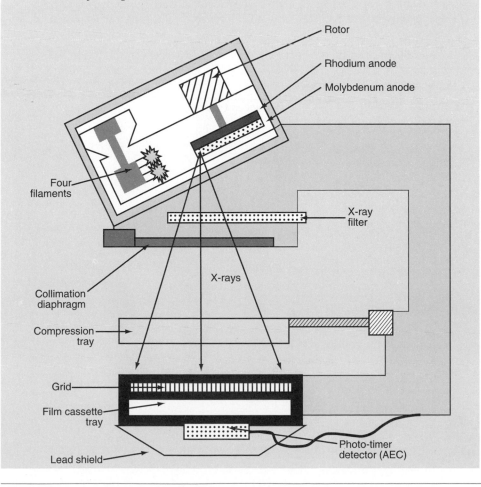

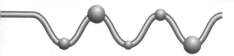

2. The accompanying table compares mammography with regular radiography for film-screen systems.

FACTOR	FILM-SCREEN MAMMOGRAPHY	FILM-SCREEN RADIOGRAPHY
kVp	25–32	60–150
mA	25–175	200–800
Exposure time (sec)	0.5–3.0	0.01–0.25
Focal spot size (mm)	0.1 (small) and 0.3 (large)	0.6 (small) and 1.2 (large)
SID (cm) (distance to film)	65	100 (routine) and 180 (chest)
Grid ratio	5:1	10:1 up to 17:1
Relative film speed	25–50	400 or greater
Screen type	Thin/single	Thick/double
Spatial resolution	15–20 LP/mm	4–8 LP/mm
Anode material	Molybdenum (Mo) or rhodium (Rh)	Tungsten (W)
X-ray filter	0.03 mm Mo or 0.05 mm Rh	1–2 mm Al or 0.1–0.3 mm Cu
HVL (mm Al eq.)	0.3–0.5	3.0–8.0
Compression (lb)	25–40	None
Skin entrance radiation exposure (mR)	200–6000/image (2 to 8 cm thickness)	20–2000/image (chest to thick abdomen)

3. Because the compressed breast thickness is relatively small, and because the calcium deposits in the breast need to be visualized well for clinical reasons, lower energy x-rays (low kVp, special anode, and special filtration) are employed in mammography to emphasize primarily the photoelectric effect, which increases calcium and tissue contrast.

4. For an average (4.2 cm) breast thickness, the ideal x-ray energy that balances image contrast and radiation dose to the patient is around 20 keV, which is obtained with an Mo anode and Mo filter and 25 to 28 kVp.

5. For a thicker or more dense breast, the ideal x-ray energy is slightly higher and is obtained with either just an Rh filter or an Rh filter and Rh anode at approximately 28 to 32 kVp.

6. A significant portion of the mammography x-ray spectra is found in the characteristic x-ray range, whose energy depends on the anode material (see figures below and on next page).

CHARACTERISTIC X-RAY	MOLYBDENUM ANODE	RHODIUM ANODE
K-alpha	17.4 keV	20.2 keV
K-beta	19.6 keV	22.8 keV

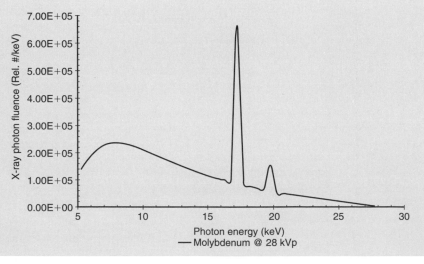

Unfiltered molybdenum mammography x-ray spectra

Molybdenum @ 28 kVp

Unfiltered rhodium mammography x-ray spectra

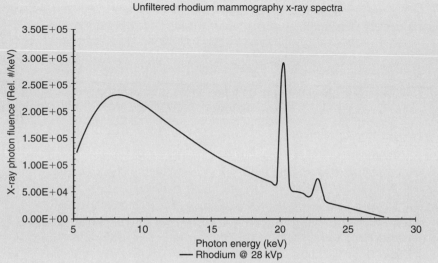

Filtered x-ray spectra: Mo anode and Mo filter

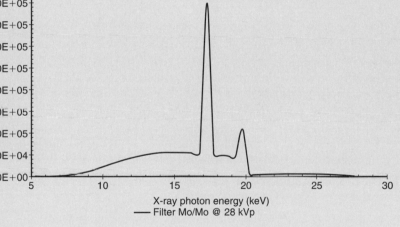

Filtered x-ray spectrum: Rh anode and Rh filter

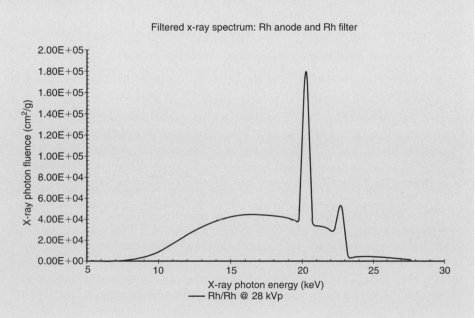

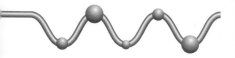

7. The x-ray filters remove the very low energy x-rays, which do not penetrate tissue very well, and they also attenuate many of the bremsstrahlung x-rays above the K-edge of the filter that degrade contrast. The K-edge for Mo is 20 keV and for Rh is 23 keV. The x-rays that have energies just below the K-edge pass through the filters with little attenuation (see figures on p. 155).

8. Hence, an Mo anode with an Mo filter allows the characteristic x-rays to pass through the filter, but it attenuates many of the bremsstrahlung x-rays at low energies (which contribute to dose) and at energies above the K-edge (which degrade contrast).

9. An Rh anode with an Rh filter also permits the characteristic x-rays to escape and attenuates much of the lower and higher energy bremsstrahlung x-rays.

10. ***An Rh filter can be used with an Mo anode*** to allow some of the higher energy bremsstrahlung x-rays to be emitted, but ***an Mo filter is never used with an Rh anode*** because it would attenuate most of the Rh characteristic x-rays.

11. Higher kVp values reduce the radiation dose to the patient, but these kVp values degrade image contrast. Unfortunately, ***higher kVps are necessary for thick and dense breast tissue.***

COMPRESSED BREAST THICKNESS (CM)*	SUGGESTED KVP FOR MO ANODE AND MO FILTER
2.0–3.0	24–26
3.0–4.0	25–27
4.0–5.0	26–28
5.0–6.0	27–29
6.0–7.0	28–31
7.0–8.0	29–32

*For a variety of adipose content.

12. Small ***focal spot sizes*** are used to reduce geometric blur (focal spot blur). A 0.3-mm focal spot is used for contact images where the breast is placed near the cassette. A 0.1-mm focal spot is used for magnification work.

13. The ***compression tray*** is used to apply pressure to the breast tissue. The benefits of compression include the following:

- Breast thickness is less, which allows a lower radiation dose.
- The overlaying tissue is spread out.
- Scattered radiation is reduced, which improves image contrast.
- The breast is immobilized to reduce motion blur.
- Microcalcifications are closer to the image receptor, resulting in less blur.
- The dynamic range of the receptor is improved by reducing variations in breast thickness.

14. ***Exposure time*** should be maintained below 2.0 seconds to minimize motion blur.

15. New mammography units have complex ***automatic exposure controls (AECs, or phototimers)*** that monitor compressed breast thickness and radiation transmitted through the breast in a short (50-msec) test x-ray exposure. The new AECs (called automatic optimization of parameters [AoP] or other names) automatically select anode type, filter type, kVp, and mAs from ***look-up tables (LUTs)*** to maintain film density or image noise for digital units.

16. ***Average glandular dose*** (Dg) is an average of the radiation dose throughout most of the breast tissue, excluding the 3 to 5 mm at the skin surface.

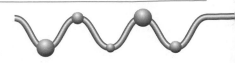

The radiation dose is highest at the point at which the x-rays enter the skin (entrance skin exposure [ESE]), and the radiation dose falls off exponentially as the x-rays pass through the breast.

- Regulations (***Mammography Quality Standards Act [MQSA],*** which went into effect in 1994) specify the permissible Dg.

- Dg ≤ 3.0 mGy (300 mrad) for a film-screen with grid and for a 4.2-cm compressed breast thickness.

- Typical Dg is measured with the American College of Radiology (ACR) quality control (QC) phantom.

- Average Dg is usually 1.50 to 2.0 mGy (150 to 200 mrad).

- Dg increases with thicker breasts.

- ESE values are usually five to seven times the Dg value.

- Dg increases if darker density films are preferred.

17. Half-value layer (HVL) is the amount of tissue thickness needed to decrease the number of transmitted x-rays by half. Each 1 cm of compressed breast tissue is approximately an HVL for mammography.

    - If kVp is kept constant, a 1-cm increase in thickness requires double the mAs, and the ESE dose is doubled. Dg increases but is a little less than doubled.

    - If kVp and x-ray filters change for a 1-cm increase in breast thickness, the mAs and ESE dose will still increase 40% to 70%.

18. Before the use of intensifying screens, plain ***industrial film*** was used for mammography. The ESE for industrial film was about 120 mSv (12 rad).

    - The purpose of the screens was to reduce radiation dose to the patient.

    - However, industrial film had better spatial resolution with less contrast.

    - Calcium specks in the breast can be smaller than 0.05 mm in diameter.

19. ***MQSA provisions*** are extensive:

    - All mammography units must be accredited by ACR or an alternative.

    - All facilities must be certified by the Food and Drug Administration (FDA).

    - Radiologists must have the following qualifications: be licensed to practice medicine, be American Board of Radiology (ABR) certified in radiology, have an initial 60 continuing medical education (CME) credits in mammography with 15 CME credits in the past 3 years, have read 240 mammograms in the previous 6 months, and, after an initial period, must read 960 mammograms every 24 months.

    - Radiologists, technologists, and physicists must earn ***at least 5 CME credits each year*** or 15 CME credits over 3 years.

    - Eight additional CME credits each are needed for digital mammography and stereotactic mammography.

    - Film processors must be monitored using QC daily.

    - Radiologic technologists must do periodic QC and maintain records as follows: daily—sensitometry, viewing conditions, and darkroom cleanliness; weekly—phantom evaluation; quarterly—fixer retention and repeat rate; semiannually—darkroom light leakage, film-screen contact, and compression.

    - Physics QC testing (HVL, kV, collimation, AEC evaluation, focal spot size, and dose) must be done at least annually.

    - There is a requirement for outcome studies to be performed.

    - There is a requirement for quarterly repeat rate analysis.

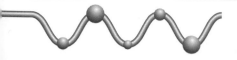

20. Some MQSA equipment performance criteria are as follows:

- X-ray and light field alignment error must be ≤2% of source-to-image distance (SID).

- X-ray field cannot exceed image receptor ≤2% of SID.

- Compression tray edge can exceed image receptor ≤1% of SID.

- Breast thickness inaccuracy (or error of displayed value) must be <±0.5 cm.

- Spatial resolution on a 4.5-cm phantom must be ≥13 LP/mm with bars parallel to anode-cathode axis and >11 LP/mm with bars perpendicular.

- AEC must maintain consistent film density (digital must maintain signal-to-noise ratio [SNR]) within ±0.15 optical density (OD) over used thickness of patient and modes.

- Variation of film-screen density for all cassettes must be ≤0.30 OD.

- ***No appreciable artifacts*** should be seen with uniform phantoms.

- ***ACR phantom image*** must meet criteria; there can be no change in detectability of fibrils, speck group, or masses of more than ±0.5, and the mAs change from previous measurements must be within ±15%.

- ***Measured kVp*** must be accurate to within ±5% and must vary less than 2%.

- Criteria for measured HVL are as follows:

  Measured HVL ≥ [kVp/100] + 0.03 mm Al

  Measured HVL ≤ [kVp/100] + C

  where C = 0.12 for Mo/Mo, 0.19 for Mo/Rh, and 0.22 for Rh/Rh.

- ***Viewbox illumination*** must be ≥3000 nit and background light ≤50 lux.

21. ***ACR phantom image quality test*** must be passed to be accredited.

- Phantom has three sections: fibrils, calcium speck groups, and simulated masses.

- Passing score is visibility of 4 fibrils, 3 calcium speck groups, and 3 masses.

- Density of film is >1.40 OD.

22. Digital mammography units have advantages over film-screen mammography.

- Low-contrast visibility is better because of window and level adjustments.

- Dynamic range of digital units is five orders of magnitude (100,000) compared with film-screen systems, which have only 10 to 100.

- Digital systems do density equalization to see breast periphery and chest wall with same density as average breast thickness.

- Images can be processed for edge enhancement, unsharp masks, and so forth.

- Image can be analyzed with ***computer-aided diagnosis (CAD).***

- Digital images can be transmitted for second opinions and surgery.

- Digital storage (CD) is more compact and can be easily carried by patient.

- Radiation doses are similar to film-screen radiation doses.

- Digital mammography has essentially no repeats.

- Usually, higher kVp values are employed because image receptors are more efficient.

- For digital systems, higher kVp values mean shorter exposure times with little loss in contrast related to window width and level, which allows better display.

- Film processor and chemical are eliminated.

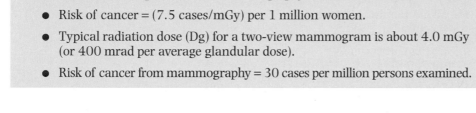

23. Digital systems do have some disadvantages.

- Digital systems have lower spatial resolution than film-screen mammography, with a typical spatial resolution of about 5 to 10 LP/mm.
- Digital units are expensive, about four times the cost of a film-screen system.
- Digital detectors are very sensitive to temperature and mechanical damage.
- Digital systems have image persistence at high radiation doses.
- Software can correct for detector voids and mask clinical problems.

24. Cancer statistics of which to be aware include the following:

- Roughly 10% of women are at risk for breast cancer during their lifetime.
- A large percentage of breast biopsy results are normal.
- The radiation exposure from a mammography examination can induce cancer.
- Risk of cancer = (7.5 cases/mGy) per 1 million women.
- Typical radiation dose (Dg) for a two-view mammogram is about 4.0 mGy (or 400 mrad per average glandular dose).
- Risk of cancer from mammography = 30 cases per million persons examined.

B. Questions

17-1. An anode/filter combination that is not used in mammography is _____.

(a) Mo/Mo   (b) Mo/Rh   (c) Rh/Mo   (d) Rh/Rh
(e) None of the above

17-2. The ACR/FDA requirements limit the average glandular dose (Dg) for a 4.2-cm compressed breast imaged by film-screen mammography with grid to a value less than or equal to _____ mGy/image.

(a) 1.0   (b) 2.0   (c) 3.0   (d) 4.0   (e) 5.0

17-3. The ACR/FDA requirements limit the average glandular dose (Dg) for a 4.2-cm compressed breast imaged by digital mammography to a value less than or equal to _____ mGy/image.

(a) 1.0   (b) 2.0   (c) 3.0   (d) 4.0   (e) 5.0

17-4. To improve the spatial resolution in mammography, all of the following factors are used, *except* _____.

(a) Compression   (b) Special film   (c) Special intensifying screens
(d) Smaller x-ray tube focal spot sizes   (e) Special filters

17-5. The typical spatial resolution is about _____ LP/mm for film-screen mammography systems and about _____ LP/mm for DR mammography systems.

(a) 10 to 12, 3 to 5   (b) 15 to 20, 5 to 10   (c) 5 to 8, 25 to 30
(d) 10 to 15, 10 to 15   (e) 15 to 20, 20 to 25

17-6. If a 4-cm-thick compressed breast requires an exposure of 27 kVp and 80 mAs, a 6-cm compressed breast of the same composition would require approximately _____ mAs at 27 kVp.

(a) 120   (b) 160   (c) 240   (d) 320   (e) 500

17-7. The MQSA program requires a radiologist to complete _____ continuing medical education credits (CMEs) initially and to complete _____ CMEs for every 3-year period thereafter.

(a) 10, 10   (b) 20, 5   (c) 40, 10   (d) 60, 15   (e) 80, 20

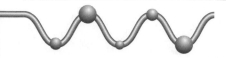

17-8. In comparison with routine radiography, film-screen image receptors for mammography have all the following characteristics, *except* _____.

(a) Single-emulsion film   (b) Higher relative speeds   (c) Low-Z cassettes
(d) High-contrast film   (e) Thin intensifying screens

17-9. The K-characteristic x-rays for a molybdenum anode x-ray tube have an energy of _____ keV.

(a) 17 to 20   (b) 20 to 23   (c) 33 to 36   (d) 55 to 59   (e) 67 to 70

17-10. In comparison with routine radiography, which employs tungsten anodes and aluminum filters, molybdenum anodes and filters are used along with low kVp values for mammography imaging to _____.

(a) Reduce radiation dose   (b) Improve contrast   (c) Improve resolution
(d) Increase latitude   (e) Improve tissue penetration

17-11. MQSA requires that the _____ measurement be performed at regularly specified intervals.

(a) Film processor QC   (b) Repeat rate   (c) Compression pressure
(d) Phantom film   (e) All of the above

17-12. The optimal density of mammography films is about _____ OD.

(a) 0.6 to 0.9   (b) 0.9 to 1.2   (c) 1.4 to 1.8   (d) 2.0 to 2.5
(e) 2.8 to 3.2

17-13. For nonmagnified mammography, the typical x-ray tube focal spot size is about _____ mm; and for magnified mammography, the focal spot size is about _____ mm.

(a) 0.3, 0.1   (b) 0.6, 1.2   (c) 0.3, 0.6   (d) 1.2, 0.6   (e) 2.0, 1.0

17-14. To be accredited, a mammography unit must produce an ACR phantom image that can visualize at least _____ fibers, _____calcium speck groups, and _____ masses.

(a) 2, 3, 2   (b) 3, 2, 3   (c) 3, 4, 4   (d) 4, 3, 3   (e) 4, 3, 4

17-15. The benefits of breast compression include all of the following, *except* _____.

(a) Less scatter   (b) Lower radiation doses   (c) Less contrast
(d) Less motion blur   (e) Less structural mottle

17-16. MQSA requires that an ABR-certified physicist perform all of the following measurements at least annually, *except* _____.

(a) mA accuracy   (b) HVL   (c) AEC consistency
(d) Collimation alignment   (e) Processor artifacts

17-17. Rhodium anodes and rhodium filters are used primarily for _____.

(a) Thin breasts   (b) Fatty breasts   (c) Dense breasts
(d) Biopsy imaging of breast tissue   (e) Mediolateral oblique views

17-18. For all mammography modes and various breast thicknesses, the automatic exposure control is required to maintain the film density to within ± _____ OD.

(a) 0.05   (b) 0.10   (c) 0.15   (d) 0.30   (e) 0.45

17-19. In comparison with film-screen mammography, digital mammography systems have _____.

(a) Improved spatial resolution   (b) Lower radiation doses
(c) Lower scatter sensitivity   (d) Larger dynamic range
(e) All of the above

17-20. To increase mammography film density from 1.20 to 1.70 OD, a mammography film with an average contrast gradient of 3.3 requires an exposure increase of about _____%.

(a) 10   (b) 20   (c) 40   (d) 80   (e) 160

17-21. The HVL for an Mo anode with an Rh filter at 30 kVp would be expected to be around _____ mm of Al equivalent.

(a) 0.25   (b) 0.32   (c) 0.44   (d) 0.51   (e) 1.1

17-22. For mammography from age 40 to death (average 45 years), the risk of radiation-induced cancer in a population of 1 million women is about _____ new cases.

(a) 1   (b) 10   (c) 100   (d) 1,000   (e) 10,000

17-23. Assume that mammography is associated with a 90% probability of detecting cancer early and that the cure rate at this stage is 90%. For the situation described in Question 17-22, the estimated benefit-to-risk ratio for mammography in a population of 1 million women would be about _____.

(a) 10:1   (b) 50:1   (c) 100:1   (d) 500:1   (e) 1000:1

17-24. The perceived advantages of digital mammography over film-screen mammography include all of the following, *except* _____.

(a) Faster throughput of patients   (b) Lower repeat rates
(c) Improved visualization at the chest wall and periphery
(d) Improved spatial resolution   (e) More consistent image processing

17-25. The use of industrial film for mammography examinations provided _____.

(a) Lower radiation doses to patients   (b) Better spatial resolution
(c) Improved image contrast   (d) Better archival storage
(e) Less motion blur

17-26. The K-edges of mammography filters are responsible for all of the following features, *except* _____.

(a) Significantly attenuated low-energy x-rays
(b) Significantly attenuated x-rays with energies greater than the K-edge energy
(c) Maximum attenuation at the binding energy of K-shell electrons in filter
(d) Discontinuity in the attenuation curve
(e) Maximum attenuation at a lower energy than the K-characteristic x-rays

17-27. In comparison with a standard breast composed of 50% adipose tissue, increasing the adipose tissue content will _____.

(a) Increase radiation dose   (b) Increase scatter radiation
(c) Improve spatial resolution   (d) Allow greater x-ray penetration
(e) Increase motion blur

17-28. For a 7-cm compressed breast thickness composed of 50% adipose tissue, a reasonable tube potential for an Mo/Mo combination with a film-screen system might be _____ kVp.

(a) 25   (b) 30   (c) 35   (d) 40   (e) 45

17-29. The HVL of mammography x-rays in a compressed breast composed of 50% adipose tissue is about _____ mm of tissue.

(a) 1.0   (b) 5.0   (c) 10.0   (d) 15.0   (e) 20.0

17-30. If images from a film-screen mammography unit suddenly start having low film density, potential sources of the problems could be all of the following, *except* _____.

(a) Diluted film processor chemicals   (b) Suboptimal detector positioning
(c) AEC set to minus adjustment   (d) kVp selected too high
(e) New batch of film

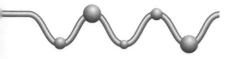

C. Answers

17-1. Answer = (c). X-ray filters attenuate the least at x-ray energies that are just below the K-edge energy, and the most attenuation occurs at energies just above the K-edge energy. For an Mo filter, the K-edge is at 20 keV. For an Mo anode, the K-characteristic x-rays have energies between 17.4 and 19.6 keV; these x-rays easily pass through the Mo filter. Even the Rh filter (which has a K-edge energy of 23 keV) transmits the Mo characteristic x-rays with minimal attenuation. The ideal filter to transmit preferentially the K-characteristic x-rays is composed of the same metal as the anode material. Hence, an Rh filter with an Rh anode easily transmits most of the K-characteristic x-rays of Rh, which are located at energies between 20.2 and 22.8 keV. However, an Mo filter (which has the highest attenuation at energies just above 20 keV) would absorb most of the K-characteristic x-rays of an Rh anode. So, an Mo filter coupled to an Rh anode would remove the Rh characteristic x-rays, which defeats the goal of using characteristic x-rays around 20 keV for mammography.

17-2. Answer = (c). See the note in this chapter (**A16**).

17-3. Answer = (c). The average glandular dose (Dg) for a 4.2-cm compressed breast is limited to 3.0 mGy, regardless of whether film-screen or digital mammography image receptors are employed.

17-4. Answer = (e). Compression reduces breast thickness, which reduces magnification, a component of geometric blur. The other component of geometric blur is focal spot size, which is much smaller in mammography imaging. A single-emulsion film is used to reduce parallax unsharpness and light crossover unsharpness. Film resolution is so good that all double-emulsion films would have practically the same spatial resolution. The intensifying screens used for mammography are very thin to improve spatial resolution. However, the thin screens have low speeds and result in higher radiation doses to patients. The filters used in mammography are directed at improving the contrast of microcalcifications and tissue in the breast; the filters do not affect the spatial resolution.

17-5. Answer = (b). See the note in this chapter (**A1**).

17-6. Answer = (d). If the same kVp and the same breast tissue composition are used, the HVL in mammography is about 1 cm of tissue. A 6-cm breast is 2 cm thicker than a 4-cm breast. The 2-cm thickness difference represents two HVLs, which reduces the transmitted x-rays by $0.5 \times 0.5 = 0.25$. Thus, the incident radiation must be increased by approximately a factor of 4 to keep film density constant. Four times 80 mAs equals 320 mAs.

17-7. Answer = (d). See the note in this chapter (**A19**).

17-8. Answer = (b). Mammography films have single-emulsion coatings. The goal is to reduce parallax blur and crossover blur. The high contrast of the films improves the visualization of microcalcifications and tissue variations. The intensifying screens are thin in order to improve the spatial resolution. The change to single-emulsion film and thin screens reduces the speed of mammography film-screen combinations. The cassettes are made of low-atomic-number plastics to limit the attenuation of low-energy mammography x-rays.

17-9. Answer = (a). See the note in this chapter (**A6**).

17-10. Answer = (b). Low kVp and special filters produce low-energy x-rays that improve subject contrast of microcalcifications. Because contrast and latitude are inversely related, high-contrast film-screen systems have less latitude. However, the low-energy x-rays do not penetrate through tissue well; thus, radiation doses are higher for low-energy x-rays. The energy of the x-rays has no influence on the spatial resolution.

17-11. Answer = (e). See the note in this chapter (**A19**).

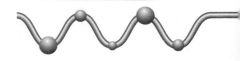

17-12. Answer = (c). The FDA and the ACR require that the minimum film density be equal to or greater than 1.40 OD. High-intensity viewboxes allow higher film densities to be visualized clinically; however, there is a limit to the maximum density. A film density of 2.0 OD allows only 1% of the viewbox light to pass through the film.

17-13. Answer = (a). See the notes in this chapter (**A2** and **A12**).

17-14. Answer = (d). See the note in this chapter (**A21**).

17-15. Answer = (c). Compression improves contrast by reducing the amount of scattered radiation and by allowing lower kVp values to be used because the thickness is less. Structural mottle is the loss of definition of anatomic objects such as microcalcifications because overlying structures cause several images to be superimposed. Compression stretches these structures laterally so that they can be visualized better.

17-16. Answer = (a). Although mAs reproducibility for phototimed exposures of the ACR phantom are measured and evaluated, the mA accuracy is never measured. The fairly complete list of required QC measurements can be found in the note in this chapter (**A20**).

17-17. Answer = (c). An Rh anode with an Rh filter produces higher energy characteristic x-ray energies than an Mo/Mo combination. These higher energy x-rays are useful for penetration of thicker or denser breast tissue.

17-18. Answer = (c). Starting in 2003, the limitations for the variation in film density for different phantom thicknesses and imaging modes became more stringent. The permissible variation changed from ±0.30 OD to ±0.15 OD.

17-19. Answer = (d). Digital mammography systems are associated with less spatial resolution than film-screen systems. Digital systems have a resolution of 5 to 10 LP/mm, versus 15 to 20 LP/mm for film-screen mammography systems. Digital and film-screen mammography systems employ similar radiation doses and have similar sensitivity to scattered radiation. The dynamic range of digital system is 10,000:1 versus 10:1 to 100:1 for film-screen systems.

17-20. Answer = (c). The generalization is that a 10% increase in radiation is needed to result in a 0.10-OD increase. The change in density from 1.20 to 1.70 OD is a change of 0.50 OD. The radiation exposure needed would be expected to be about 50%. The precise calculation is $\Delta D = \gamma \log_{10}(\exp 1/\exp 2)$; $(\exp 1/\exp 2) = 10^X$, where $X = 0.50/3.3$. From this calculation, the necessary increase in exposure would be 42%. The closest choice for both approaches is 40%.

17-21. Answer = (c). From the FDA/ACR specifications for HVL, the minimum HVL = (kVp/100) + 0.03 = 0.33 mm Al. The maximum HVL = (kVp/100) + 0.19 = 0.49 mm Al. The only answer in this range is 0.44 mm Al.

17-22. Answer = (d). The notes of this chapter indicate that the risk of developing cancer from radiation is 30 cases per million persons undergoing one mammographic examination. The risk of cancer is $45 \times 30 = 1350$ cases per million women undergoing 45 years of mammographic examinations. Actually, the risk is a little less because the life expectancy decreases with age and there are fewer years left at old age in which to express cancer.

17-23. Answer = (b). The proportion of women who may develop cancer is 10% of 1 million women, or 100,000. In these women, 90% of the cancers can be detected, and 90% of the detected cancers can be treated, or $0.9 \times 0.9 \times 100,000 = 81,000$. The benefit-to-risk ratio is $81,000/1350 = 60$. The closest answer is 50.

17-24. Answer = (d). See note in this chapter (**A22**).

17-25. Answer = (b). The entrance radiation doses with industrial film were around 120 mGy, which is significantly more than the 10 mGy used in film-screen mammography. The use of an intensifying screen reduces the radiation dose to the patient significantly. However, the spatial resolution of film alone is about 50 to 100 LP/mm, in comparison with mammography film-screen systems, which have a spatial resolution of 15 to 20 LP/mm. The contrast of a film alone exposed directly to x-rays is relatively low; the average contrast gradient of film alone is about 1.5 to 2.0. Archival storage depends only on the film processing; it does not depend on the manner in which the film was exposed. Because film without a screen requires a larger radiation dose, the exposure times are longer, resulting in more motion blur.

17-26. Answer = (e). See answer to Question 17-1 and notes in this chapter. A graph showing the mass attenuation coefficient for molybdenum as a function of x-ray energy is shown here, with the filtered x-ray spectra superimposed.

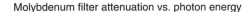

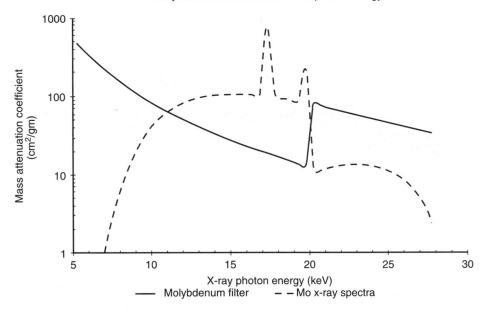

Molybdenum filter attenuation vs. photon energy

17-27. Answer = (d). Adipose tissue has a lower physical density of g/cm³. Hence, adipose tissue attenuates x-rays less than glandular tissue. This feature means lower radiation doses, less scattered radiation, and shorter exposure times, which reduces motion blur. The adipose content has no influence at all on spatial resolution.

17-28. Answer = (b). Thicker and more dense breasts require higher kVp. A compressed tissue that is 7 to 8 cm thick would require near-maximum utilization of 32 kVp. See the note in this chapter (**A11**).

17-29. Answer = (c). The note in this chapter (**A17**) states that the HVL in breast tissue for mammography x-rays is about 1.0 cm, or 10 mm.

17-30. Answer = (d). Dilute developer chemicals react less with exposed silver grains, resulting in lighter film densities. By placing the AEC detector outside the breast or near the periphery, the radiation level is terminated before the central region of the breast is dark enough. A minus setting lowers the radiation level for termination, which produces lighter film densities. AEC systems compensate for kVp variations, and density should not change with different kVp values. The coating of silver grains onto film bases is not consistent. Hence, the density can vary between boxes of film with different film emulsions.

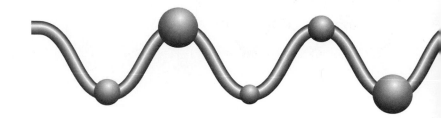

CHAPTER EIGHTEEN

Computed Tomography Scanners

A. Basic Concepts

1. ***The history of computed tomography (CT)*** scanner development is as follows:

   - The first CT scanner was developed by G. Hounsfield at EMI Ltd. around 1969 to1970.

   - The first clinical head CT unit in the United States was EMI Mark I in 1973.

   - The first body CT scanner was developed by R. Ledley at Georgetown University in 1974.

   - Hounsfield received the Nobel Prize in Medicine for his invention of CT in 1979.

2. The following are the five categories of CT scanners:

   - ***First-generation CT:*** translate/rotate motion with a pencil x-ray beam; only two detectors imaging two slices simultaneously; scan time about 5 minutes; matrix 80×80 upgraded to 160×160.

   - ***Second-generation CT:*** translate/rotate motion; 30-degree rotations or greater; fan x-ray beam with many detectors; usually only one slice per image; scan times 20 to 60 seconds, matrix 256×256 up to 512×512.

   - ***Third-generation CT:*** rotate/rotate motion; 360-degree continuous rotation; fan x-ray beam with 1000 or more detectors; 1 to 64 slices per image; scan time 0.5 to 4.0 seconds, matrix 512×512.

   - ***Fourth-generation CT:*** x-ray tubes rotate/detectors are stationary; 360-degree continuous rotation; fan x-ray beam with up to 4800 stationary detectors; one or more slices; scan times of 1.0 to 5.0 seconds, matrix 512×512.

   - ***Fifth-generation CT (electron beam computed tomography [EBCT]):*** no motion; electron beam is scanned across numerous x-ray targets; detectors in a 180-degree arc above the targets; seven simultaneous slices; scan times 50 to 100 milliseconds, matrix 256×256 or 512×512.

   - An ***MDCT*** is a multidetector CT that simultaneously images up to 64 slices in current versions of CT scanners.

   - In a ***helical or spiral CT,*** the x-ray tube rotates continuously, emitting x-rays while the table moves. This produces a volume of images in seconds.

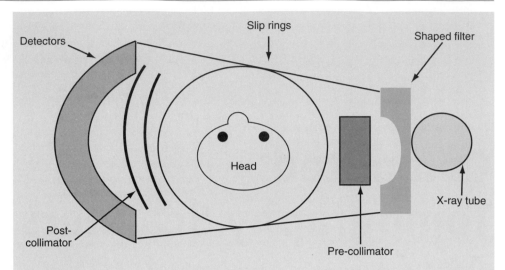

3. **Slip rings** are sliding electrical connections with bearings or brushes that allow the x-ray tube, which is coupled to the detectors, to rotate continuously without the need for cables and wires.

4. **CT radiation detectors** of various types have been used over the years.

   - Early detectors were **scintillation crystals** such as CsI and BGO coupled to **photomultiplier tubes (PMTs)** that detected the light created in the scintillators when x-rays interacted.

   - **Ionization chambers** such as xenon pressure-filled units were used to measure the charges created in the gases by the passage of x-rays.

   - **Scintillators coupled to photodiodes** have been employed.

5. **CT filters** come in two varieties.

   - **Flat filters** uniformly filter the x-ray beam. This results in a larger radiation dose and less CT noise in the periphery of the anatomy than with shaped filters. Flat filters produce a smaller dose and more CT noise in the center of the body than do shaped filters.

   - **Shaped (or Bowtie or parabolic) filters** attenuate the x-ray beam more toward the periphery, where the anatomy is thin, and less in the center, where the anatomy is thick. This type of filtration produces a relatively uniform radiation dose and CT noise.

6. Each CT slice represents a cylindrical section that is divided into volume elements (voxels).

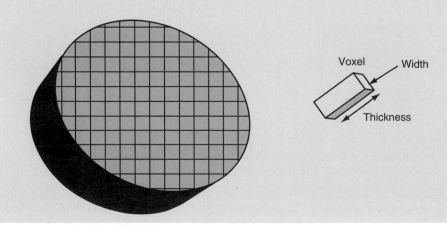

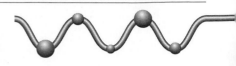

- Each voxel has a thickness that is the same as the CT slice thickness and has the same width on each side as the square surface area.

   Width (W) = [diameter of the field of view (FoV)]/[matrix size]

- For example, width = 25 cm FoV/512 = 0.05 cm = 0.5 mm

7. CT number (CT#) is the average x-ray linear attenuation coefficient for the mixture of materials in each voxel.

   $CT\# = 1000 \times [\mu_X - \mu_{WATER}]/\mu_{WATER}$ in Hounsfield units (HU)

8. The effective linear attenuation coefficients are dependent on many factors.

   - Density (ρ) of the material within a voxel
   - Atomic number (Z) of the material within a voxel
   - Electron density (number of electrons/g) of material within a voxel
   - Effective energy of the x-ray beam (kVp, filtration, and patient's attenuation)

9. There are two materials on which the CT number scale is based.

   - *Air* is always defined as −1000 HU.
   - *Water* is always defined as 0.0 HU.
   - The CT values for air and water do *not* change with kVp or anything else.
   - The CT numbers for other substances such as bone, muscle, and fat change with kVp and filtration.

10. The **CT contrast scale (CS)** is defined by the equation

    $CS = [\mu_X - \mu_{WATER}]/[(CT\#)_X - (CT\#)_{WATER}]$

    - CS is approximately equal to 0.0002 cm^{-1}/HU.
    - It changes with kVp and other factors.

11. The CT# and the effective linear attenuation coefficients are related in a linear fashion.

12. *Pixel is a picture element* on the display matrix.

13. **CT noise** is the variation in CT# of a uniform material caused by quantum mottle and computational errors in the reconstruction of data.

    - It is expressed as one standard deviation variation (σ_{WATER}) of the CT number of uniform water given as a percentage.

      $\% \, \sigma_{WATER} = [\sigma_{WATER} \times CS \times 100\%]/\mu_{WATER}$

    - The CT noise increases when the part of the anatomy being scanned is large or dense and the x-ray attenuation by the body (B) increases.
    - The CT noise increases for small voxel widths (W).
    - The CT noise increases for thin CT slices (H).
    - The CT noise decreases for higher radiation doses (D) to the patient.
    - The relationship between CT noise and these factors is usually expressed as

      $\% \, \sigma_{WATER} = constant \times [B/(W^3 \times H \times D)]^{0.5}$

    - On modern scanners, the scan FoV may be constant for many display FoVs; therefore, the measured voxel width may not vary much.
    - If a small baby were scanned at the same settings as for an adult, the attenuation (B) would be less and the CT noise would decrease.
    - If the scanned slice thickness were reduced from 10 to 1 mm, the radiation would require an increase of 10 times to produce the same CT noise.

- A decrease in the true voxel width from 1.0 to 0.50 mm would require an increase in the radiation dose by a factor of 8 to maintain the same CT noise.

- If the radiation dose to the patient is increased by four times (four times the mAs), the CT noise decreases only by one divided by the square root of four, or by ½.

- CT noise is also affected by the type of reconstruction algorithm selected (e.g., soft tissue, standard, detail, chest, edge, and bone). High edge enhancement can increase noise by two to five times.

- CT noise affects the visibility of low-contrast structures.

14. Spiral (helical) CT scan characteristics include the following:

- Spatial resolution is similar to that of axial scans.

- Slice thickness is typically larger than specified because extrapolation is used to reconstruct data between measured points along the body axis.

- Volume averaging is more pronounced.

15. *MDCT* uses a cone x-ray beam along the axis with a series of parallel detector arrays to scan several slices simultaneously. The detectors can be regrouped after the scan to produce various slice thicknesses and locations.

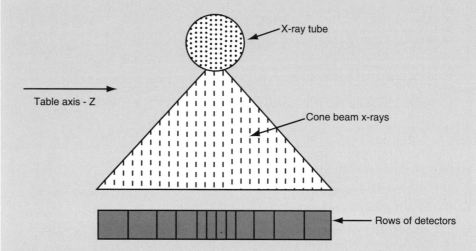

16. *Window and level adjustments* determine which CT numbers appear black, white, or a shade of gray. The CT numbers are not changed; only the gray scale level assigned to a given CT# is changed.

- *Level* is the center CT# at the middle of the gray-scale display.

- *Width* determines the CT# range between black and white. Any CT# greater than one half the width above the CT# level is all white, and any CT# less than one half the width below the level appears all black. CT numbers between these points are different shades of gray.

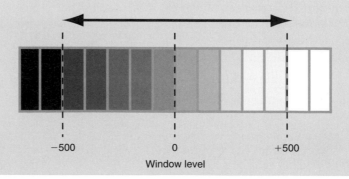

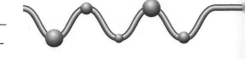

B. CT Image Quality

1. ***Spatial resolution*** of CT scanners is only about 0.5 to 1.2 LP/mm. The spatial resolution of CT scanners is much worse than that of film-screen or CR/DR systems.

2. ***The main advantage of CT scanners is that they can visualize low-contrast structures*** with a contrast in the range of 0.3% to 0.5%. Film-screen system images need at least a contrast level of 7% to 8% to be clearly seen.

3. The ability to see small high-contrast structures (spatial resolution) depends on many factors and is related to the FoV.

   - ***For small FoVs, as in head scans***, the spatial resolution depends on focal spot size (F), magnification geometry (M), detector size (S), and reconstruction algorithm selected.

     $$a_{EFF} = [S^2 + (M - 1)^2 F^2]^{0.5}/M$$

   - ***For large FoVs, as in adult body scans***, the spatial resolution is strictly limited by pixel size (the side of the voxel = W).

4. ***Algorithms*** are a mathematical approach to analyzing the CT measurements to reconstruct the data to obtain the CT numbers of the tissue in the voxels and display the data as anatomic images of the correct dimension.

   - ***Filtered back-projection*** is the method used with most CT scanners.

   - ***Other possible methods*** include iterative schemes, algebraic methods, fast Fourier transforms (FFTs), and others.

   - For each method, there are ***kernels*** that determine the amount of smoothing or edge enhancement that the image reconstruction produces.

   - There are also ***postprocessing schemes*** to remove items such as streaks generated by beam hardening, bone, and metal objects.

5. ***CT artifacts*** represent objects that have been artificially created in the images because of equipment malfunctions, measurement limitations, or the reconstruction process.

   - ***Partial volume effect:*** large voxels sampling a mixture of materials and yielding an average CT number of the mixture.

   - ***Ring artifacts:*** dark or light circular areas in third-generation CT related to either bad or miscalibrated detectors.

   - ***Streak artifacts:*** dark lines related to x-ray tube arcing, table straps, or other items outside the FoV causing attenuation.

   - ***Anode wobble:*** movement of the focal spot because of loose bearings in the x-ray tube anode from use. It causes the image to contain a cross-hatched pattern.

   - ***Beam hardening:*** dark areas between bones or the center of the body related to a large amount of attenuation, which filters the x-ray spectra; this leaves behind higher energy x-rays, which are penetrating and yield a different CT# from the incident lower energy x-rays.

   - ***Motion blur:*** blur areas that can have a partially circular shape because of motion of the body during the acquisition process.

   - ***Star artifacts:*** streaks radiating in a spokelike pattern from a highly attenuating material such as a metal or a pointed bone projection.

   - ***Aliasing:*** pixel so big that it samples two smaller objects as one bigger object.

   - ***Dropout lines or areas:*** usually due to electronics of array processor or computer device that drops data from entire lines or columns.

   - ***Bull's-eye spot:*** a light or dark spot like the center of a target caused by a misalignment of the actual center of rotation with the reconstructed center of data as well as detector miscalibrations.

- *Cone-beam artifact:* wide beam needed for multislice CT causing missing data, which produces swirl-type patterns.
- Care must be taken to avoid diagnosis of an artifact as a clinical abnormality.

C. CT Quality Control Testing

1. *CT# uniformity* is determined by scanning a uniform water or plastic equivalent phantom to look for high- or low-density areas and artifacts.

2. *CT slice thickness accuracy* is measured with either small beads or an aluminum ramp at a small angle to assess the imaged thickness of each setting.

3. *Spatial resolution* is a measurement of the ability to see small objects by using either drilled air holes in plastic or a thin wire from which a point spread function (PSF) is measured; a modulation transfer function (MTF) is calculated from the PSF. The air holes are of different sizes, and there is a CT# difference between the air holes and the surrounding material of more than 1000 HU. The idea is to determine the smallest high-contrast hole that can be seen.

4. *Low-contrast visibility* is measured by use of rods in a background material whose CT# is only a few units different from that of the rods. The rods vary in size, and the goal is to determine the smallest low-contrast rods that can be seen.

5. *CT noise* is measured by determining the standard deviation in the CT# of water or a known uniform material such as water equivalent plastic. It is also important to determine whether water has an average CT value near 0.0 HU.

6. *CT# linearity* is determined by scanning rods composed of different plastics with known linear attenuation coefficients. The measured CT# of each plastic is graphically plotted against its attenuation coefficient. The plot should be a straight line.

7. *Laser slice location* can be determined either by use of film or with known objects positioned at a specified location.

8. *Table incrementation* can be measured either by use of film or with known objects positioned a specified distance apart.

9. *Distance accuracy* is determined by measuring the diameter of a phantom and comparing it with the actual known diameter in two orthogonal directions.

10. *Scan time accuracy* is determined with a radiation detector.

11. *mA linearity* is determined by measuring the amount of radiation for varying mA with fixed kVp and time maintained.

12. *Half-value layer (HVL)* can be measured in a standard format by using the two-dimensional localizer mode in which the x-ray tube does not rotate.

13. *kVp accuracy* requires a special CT kVp meter and is affected by filtration.

14. *CT radiation doses to patients* require a special CT ionization chamber and phantoms.

D. CT Radiation Doses to Patients

1. *Computed tomography dose index (CTDI)* is the radiation dose to the center slice of 15 adjacent, sequential slices without overlap.

- Because CT radiation doses extend outside the CT slice as a result of scattered x-rays in the phantom and some penumbra, the CTDI is about 20% to 40% greater than the dose to a single CT slice without adjacent slices.

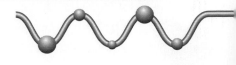

- The radiation dose from a 40-slice CT scan is *not* 40 times the radiation dose of a single CT scan; it is only 20% to 40% greater than that of a single slice.

- If CT slices overlap, by definition, standard CTDI cannot be used.

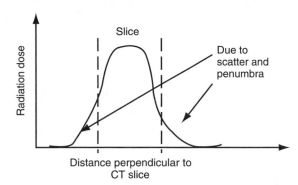

- CTDI is nearly uniform for all locations inside a 16-cm acrylic head phantom.

- CTDI at the center of a 32-cm acrylic body phantom is about 50% of the radiation level near the surface.

- CTDI at the center and the surface decreases nearly exponentially in relation to the radius of the phantom, the kVp, and other factors.

- $CTDI_W$ is a way to average the radiation dose with depth.

  $$CTDI_W = [(1/3) \times CTDI_{Center}] + [(2/3)CTDI_{Surface}]$$

2. **Multiple slice average dose (MSAD) or CTDI $_{VOLUME}$** determines the radiation dose for multiple slices, which may either have gaps between them or be overlapped, or both. It can be calculated from the CTDI.

   - **Pitch** can be used to describe axial slices, helical (spiral) slices, and multidetector CT (MDCT) scans that have either overlap or gaps between the slices.

     Pitch = [table incrementation]/[total width of x-ray beam]

   - If the direct x-ray beam overlaps, the effective pitch is <1.0.

   - If the direct x-ray beam has gaps, the effective pitch is >1.0.

   - If the direct x-ray beam is adjacent without overlap or gap, the effective pitch is 1.0.

   - **Packing factor** is an older term and is just 1.0 divided by the effective pitch.

   - The radiation dose for multiple CT slices that have either gap or overlap can be calculated from the measured CTDI as shown:

     $$CTDI_{VOLUME} = CTDI_W/(pitch)$$

3. **Dose-length product (DLP)** is the product of the $CTDI_W$ and the total length of the scan in centimeters.

   - The American College of Radiology (ACR) accreditation program estimates that the length of a typical head scan is 17.5 cm and the length of a typical adult body scan is 25 cm.

   - Many modern CT scanners calculate an estimated $CTDI_W$ and an estimated DLP for each series of images, assuming an average-sized patient and actual scan settings of kVp, mAs, and pitch.

4. To calculate **effective dose (E),** a radiation exposure to only part of the body is extrapolated to an equivalent exposure of the entire body so that the risks of developing all types of cancers and hereditary effects can be readily evaluated from this single number.

   - There are a number of ways to estimate the effective dose from the measurements. One approach multiplies the DLP by a factor.

- The ACR accreditation program uses $0.0023 \times \text{DLP}$ for head scans and $0.015 \times \text{DLP}$ for body scans.

- Although scattered radiation from adjacent tissue is important, E can be approximated by using the CTDI_W for each organ in the scan region and the risk weighting factors for those organs.

- E does not account for neurologic and learning impediments that might be induced by radiation.

5. The CT radiation dose varies directly **with mAs** (product of mA and scan time). If the mAs is doubled, the patient's radiation dose is doubled.

6. The CT radiation dose varies **with the kVp** squared. For each 20-kVp increase, the patient's radiation dose increases by 40% to 70%.

7. The **average value of CTDI$_W$** for 10 different CT units at 120 kVp is shown in the table.

ACRYLIC DIAMETER PHANTOM (cm)	CTDI$_W$ (cGy/100 mAs)	1 STANDARD DEVIATION (%)
10	2.67	36.7
16	1.91	31.2
24	1.34	22.4
32	0.90	14.1

8. **Typical CT scanner settings** for adult head scans are 120 kVp and 200 to 320 mAs in adjacent axial slice mode and 120 kVp and 150 to 200 mAs in helical (spiral) mode with a pitch >1.2 for body scans.

9. Although the radiation dose values depend on the model of CT scanner, the error is less than ±36% for many different CT units.

10. **Guidelines for clinical CT radiation doses** have been issued by the European Commission (Br J Radiol 2001;74:836–840). Clinical CT radiation doses should be maintained below the values listed.

CT EXAMINATION TYPE	CTDI$_W$ (mGy)	DLP (mGy-cm)	EFFECTIVE DOSE (mSv)*
Brain	60	1050	2.42
Chest	30	650	9.75
Abdomen	35	780	11.7
Pelvis	35	570	8.55

*Based on DLP $\times$ 0.0023 for the brain and DLP $\times$ 0.015 for the other organs listed.

11. Notice that the effective dose is usually between 4% (for the brain) and 33% (for chest and abdomen) of the CTDI$_W$ in adults.

12. **Fetuses, babies, and young children** are much more sensitive (by three to four times) to the risk of induction of cancer than adults for identical radiation doses. Moreover, for the same CT scan settings (kVp, mAs, and pitch), the radiation dose delivered to babies is two to four times more because of their smaller size.

E.   Questions

18-1. The typical radiation dose (CTDI$_W$) for CT scans is about _____ cGy for adult head studies and _____ cGy for adult body studies.

(a) 3 to 6, 1 to 4   (b) 1 to 2, 0.5 to 1.0   (c) 0.5, 0.5
(d) 10 to 15, 5 to 10   (e) 5 to 10, 10 to 15

18-2. The radiation dose from 15 consecutive (no overlap) CT slices is _____ times greater than the radiation dose from a single CT slice.

(a) 15   (b) 7   (c) 3   (d) 1.3   (e) 1.0

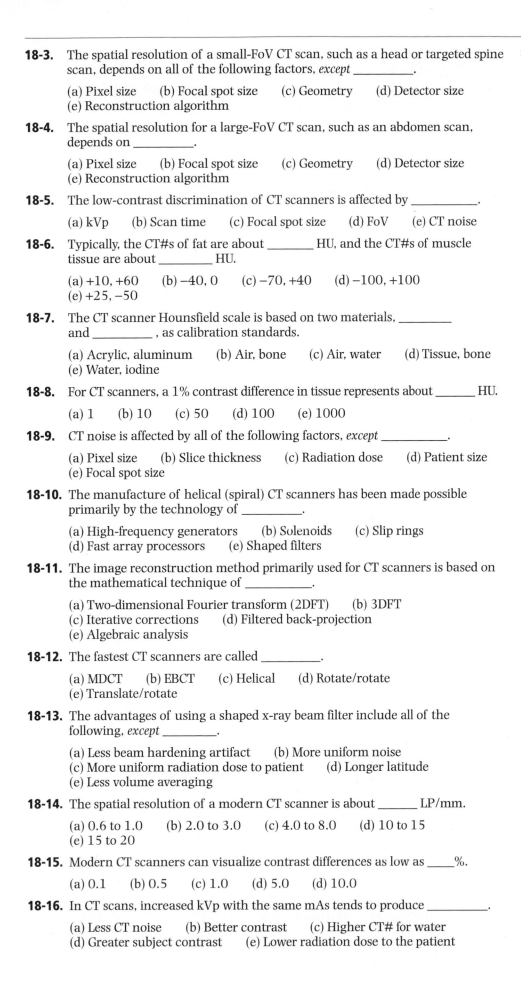

18-3. The spatial resolution of a small-FoV CT scan, such as a head or targeted spine scan, depends on all of the following factors, *except* _____.

(a) Pixel size   (b) Focal spot size   (c) Geometry   (d) Detector size
(e) Reconstruction algorithm

18-4. The spatial resolution for a large-FoV CT scan, such as an abdomen scan, depends on _____.

(a) Pixel size   (b) Focal spot size   (c) Geometry   (d) Detector size
(e) Reconstruction algorithm

18-5. The low-contrast discrimination of CT scanners is affected by _____.

(a) kVp   (b) Scan time   (c) Focal spot size   (d) FoV   (e) CT noise

18-6. Typically, the CT#s of fat are about _____ HU, and the CT#s of muscle tissue are about _____ HU.

(a) +10, +60   (b) −40, 0   (c) −70, +40   (d) −100, +100
(e) +25, −50

18-7. The CT scanner Hounsfield scale is based on two materials, _____ and _____ , as calibration standards.

(a) Acrylic, aluminum   (b) Air, bone   (c) Air, water   (d) Tissue, bone
(e) Water, iodine

18-8. For CT scanners, a 1% contrast difference in tissue represents about _____ HU.

(a) 1   (b) 10   (c) 50   (d) 100   (e) 1000

18-9. CT noise is affected by all of the following factors, *except* _____.

(a) Pixel size   (b) Slice thickness   (c) Radiation dose   (d) Patient size
(e) Focal spot size

18-10. The manufacture of helical (spiral) CT scanners has been made possible primarily by the technology of _____.

(a) High-frequency generators   (b) Solenoids   (c) Slip rings
(d) Fast array processors   (e) Shaped filters

18-11. The image reconstruction method primarily used for CT scanners is based on the mathematical technique of _____.

(a) Two-dimensional Fourier transform (2DFT)   (b) 3DFT
(c) Iterative corrections   (d) Filtered back-projection
(e) Algebraic analysis

18-12. The fastest CT scanners are called _____.

(a) MDCT   (b) EBCT   (c) Helical   (d) Rotate/rotate
(e) Translate/rotate

18-13. The advantages of using a shaped x-ray beam filter include all of the following, *except* _____.

(a) Less beam hardening artifact   (b) More uniform noise
(c) More uniform radiation dose to patient   (d) Longer latitude
(e) Less volume averaging

18-14. The spatial resolution of a modern CT scanner is about _____ LP/mm.

(a) 0.6 to 1.0   (b) 2.0 to 3.0   (c) 4.0 to 8.0   (d) 10 to 15
(e) 15 to 20

18-15. Modern CT scanners can visualize contrast differences as low as ____%.

(a) 0.1   (b) 0.5   (c) 1.0   (d) 5.0   (d) 10.0

18-16. In CT scans, increased kVp with the same mAs tends to produce _____.

(a) Less CT noise   (b) Better contrast   (c) Higher CT# for water
(d) Greater subject contrast   (e) Lower radiation dose to the patient

18-17. In CT scans, increased mAs with the same kVp tends to produce all of the following, *except* _____.

(a) High x-ray tube heat   (b) Less CT noise   (c) Less image unsharpness
(d) Better low-contrast discrimination   (e) Higher radiation dose to the patient

18-18. The main reason that CT scanner rooms need considerable radiation shielding in the walls is _____.

(a) Small room size   (b) High kVp values   (c) Large workload
(d) Motion of x-ray tube   (e) Narrow x-ray beams

18-19. _____ CT artifacts are a result of large voxel sizes.

(a) Volume averaging   (b) Beam hardening   (c) Ring   (d) Streak
(e) Cross-hatched pattern (herringbone)

18-20. _____ artifacts are due to a bad detector in a third-generation CT scanner.

(a) Volume averaging   (b) Beam hardening   (c) Ring   (d) Streak
(e) Cross-hatched pattern (herringbone)

18-21. _____ artifacts produce low CT numbers between two dense structures such as bone or the center of the thorax.

(a) Volume averaging   (b) Beam hardening   (c) Ring   (d) Streak
(e) Cross-hatched pattern (herringbone)

18-22. Helical (spiral) CT images tend to have _____.

(a) Better spatial resolution   (b) Improved low contrast
(c) Lower throughput of patients   (d) Slices thicker than specified
(e) Less CT noise

18-23. To visualize differences in bone structure, a reasonable CT display window level is _____ HU, and a reasonable window width is _____ HU.

(a) 40, 400   (b) −70, 200   (c) 0.0, 4000   (d) 650, 1300
(e) 100, 500

18-24. For helical (spiral) CT scans with 10-mm table incrementation and a cone beam width of 20 mm, the $CTDI_{VOLUME}$ is calculated by multiplying the $CTDI_W$ by a factor of _____.

(a) 0.5   (b) 1.0   (c) 1.4   (d) 2.0   (e) 4.0

18-25. Edge enhancement processing of CT images results in_____.

(a) Better low-contrast discrimination   (b) More CT noise
(c) Lower spatial resolution   (d) Fewer image artifacts
(e) Barrel distortion

18-26. For multiplanar reconstruction (MPR) of CT scans into planes other than axial, the reformatted images have a spatial resolution that is limited primarily by _____

(a) Matrix size   (b) Slice thickness   (c) Detector size   (d) Focal spot size
(e) Array processor

18-27. In comparison with a single axial image, a two-dimensional localizer image (scout view/topogram) delivers a radiation dose to the patient that is_____.

(a) 10% of the axial image   (b) 50% of the axial image
(c) Nearly the same   (d) 1.3 times more than the axial image
(e) 2.0 times more than the axial image

18-28. In helical (spiral) CT scans, the image reconstruction process involves the _____ of the measured data.

(a) Extrapolation   (b) Interpolation   (c) Reclamation   (d) Conjugation
(e) Smoothing

18-29. In helical (spiral) CT, the term "effective pitch" refers to the ratio of _____ divided by _____.

(a) Slice thickness, table motion
(b) Number of slices, length of table travel (cm)
(c) [Tube rotation time × table speed], x-ray beam width
(d) Slice thickness, number of detector channels
(e) Frequency of noise, amplitude of noise

18-30. The radiation dose for a single CT slice (averaged through the patient's abdomen) is about 3.0 cGy. A helical CT study is performed at double the mAs with an effective pitch of 0.5, covering a distance of 20 cm. The $CTDI_{VOLUME}$ (or MSAD) would be expected to be about _____ cGy.

(a) 3.0   (b) 4.0   (c) 8.0   (d) 16.0   (e) 32.0

18-31. The effective dose for the information provided in Question 18-30 would be expected to be about _____ mSv.

(a) 25   (b) 50   (c) 75   (d) 125   (e) 250

18-32. The following represent types of radiation detectors used on CT scanners, *except* _____.

(a) NaI plus PMTs   (b) Xenon ionization   (c) Liquid scintillation plus PMTs
(d) CsI plus photodiodes   (e) Direct charge sensors

18-33. The type of CT scanner that uses the most radiation detectors in its design would be _____ generation CT.

(a) 1st   (b) 2nd   (c) 3rd   (d) 4th   (e) 5th

18-34. As the scan setting of a CT scanner is increased from 120 to 140 kVp, the contrast scale (CS) number is changed by about _____%.

(a) −20%   (b) −5%   (c) 0 (no change)   (d) +15%   (e) +30%

18-35. If the CT slice thickness is decreased from 10 to 2.5 mm and the mAs is decreased from 225 to 100 mAs, the CT noise would be expected to be _____ the previous value.

(a) One half   (b) The same as   (c) 2 times   (d) 3 times   (e) 9 times

18-36. The tails of the radiation dose profiles for a CT scanner are due primarily to _____.

(a) Scattered radiation   (b) Primary radiation   (c) Dose overlap
(d) MTF   (e) Anode wobble

18-37. The effective dose for CT scanners is greatest for _____ examinations.

(a) Routine head   (b) Cervical spinal   (c) High-resolution chest
(d) Abdomen/pelvis   (e) Knee

18-38. All of the following measurements are included in quality control testing of CT scanners, *except* _____.

(a) CT# linearity   (b) AEC tracking   (c) Spatial resolution
(d) CT# uniformity   (e) CTDI

18-39. If the $CTDI_W$ for an adult abdomen CT is about 3.0 cGy, the $CTDI_W$ for a 6-month-old baby using the same CT scanner settings would be expected to be about _____ cGy.

(a) 0.5   (b) 1.5   (c) 3.0   (d) 9.0   (e) 18.0

18-40. The estimated biologic risk of developing cancer for an individual who received radiation as a fetus during an abdominal CT scan is about _____ cases per million examinations of pregnant women.

(a) 25   (b) 120   (c) 600   (d) 3000   (e) 15,000

F. Answers

18-1. Answer = (a). See notes in this chapter. ACR recommends that CTDI$_W$ for head CT be less than 60 mGy or 6.0 cGy (rad) and that the CTDI$_W$ for body CT be less than 35 mGy or 3.5 cGy (rad).

18-2. Answer = (d). The radiation doses from adjacent CT slices without overlap do not add together because different tissue is being exposed. The definition for absorbed dose is the energy deposited per gram of tissue; the total amount of tissue irradiated is not assessed with this measurement. The only additional radiation dose is about a 20% to 40% increase from scattered radiation coming from the adjacent tissue. If it were not for the scattered radiation and some penumbra, the amount of radiation would be the same as with a single-slice absorbed dose. However, the scattered radiation and penumbra radiation increase the single-slice value by a small amount.

18-3. Answer = (a). For small FoV, it is the CT scanner design and reconstruction parameters that matter.

18-4. Answer = (a). The pixel size is the limitation on all FoVs greater than about 25 to 30 cm in diameter.

18-5. Answer = (e). The kVp affects the radiation dose, CT noise, and contrast. The scan time affects motion blur, the total mAs, and the CT noise. The focal spot affects only tube heat capacity and spatial resolution related to focal spot blur (geometric unsharpness). The FoV affects the pixel size, which in turn controls spatial resolution and CT noise. Even though kVp, scan time, and FoV are dependent variables that contribute to CT noise, it is the value of the CT noise that directly affects the visibility of low-contrast structures.

18-6. Answer = (c). Although it only provides an approximation, the CT scanner is basically a density measurement device. The high-energy x-rays from CT interact in tissue primarily by Compton scatter, which is controlled primarily by physical density (g/cm^3). Fat has a density of about 0.92 g/cm^3 and muscle tissue has a density a little more than that of water at 1.04 g/cm^3. The approximation is that CT# is almost equal to 1000 (density difference with water). Water has a density of 1.0 g/cm^3. Thus, the CT# of fat is about $1000 \times (0.92 - 1.0) = -80$ HU. Muscle would have a CT# of about $1000 \times (1.04 - 1.0) = 40$ HU. However, the actual CT# also depends on the kVp, filtration, and reconstruction algorithm.

18-7. Answer = (c). Air must always have a CT# equal to -1000, and water must always have a CT# of 0.0. These two numbers should not change with kVp, filtration, or reconstruction algorithm. However, the CT numbers of other tissues change with selection of different kVp, filtration, patient size, and reconstruction algorithm.

18-8. Answer = (b). See note for this definition (**A13**).

18-9. Answer = (e). Focal spot size is related only to x-ray tube heat capacity and spatial resolution due to focal spot blur. The notes in this chapter provide the relationship between CT noise and pixel width, slice thickness, radiation dose, and attenuation.

18-10. Answer = (c). Although much of the technology listed is necessary for modern CT scanners, slip rings allow the x-ray tube and detectors to rotate continuously, which is needed for helical CT scanning. The slip rings allow the electrical voltage and signal to be transmitted through bearings or brushes that slip along a ring without the need for electrical cables. In the past, the x-ray tube and detectors were connected with cable that would wind up during a single rotation. For the next CT exposure, the x-ray tube would rotate in the opposite direction to unwind the cable.

18-11. Answer = (d). 2DFT and 3DFT are used in image reconstruction in magnetic resonance imaging (MRI). Iterative and algebraic methods are too slow to be employed.

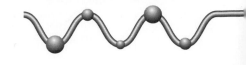

18-12. Answer = (b). See note in this chapter (**A2**). The fastest CT scanners are fifth-generation or EBCT units, which can complete a scan in 50 milliseconds because of a lack of moving parts. Only an electron beam is deflected by electromagnetic fields to produce the x-rays.

18-13. Answer = (e). The shaped filter compensates for the variation in thickness of the body from the central x-ray beam to the edge of the body. Where the body is thin, the filter is thick and vice versa. Hence, beam hardening, radiation dose, and noise are uniform throughout the body. At the edge of the body, the filter is thick to prevent the detectors from being saturated by direct x-ray exposure with no tissue attenuation; this feature improves the system latitude. Volume averaging is not affected by the filter type; it depends only on the voxel size.

18-14. Answer = (a). See note in this chapter (**B3**). The spatial resolution of CT is lower than that of most radiology systems; devices with equal or lower spatial resolution include ultrasound, MRI, and nuclear medicine imagers.

18-15. Answer = (b). Because the CT noise is about 5 to 10 HU, CT scanners are limited by the noise to this small difference in tissue CT numbers. Five HU is equal to 0.5% contrast; this is much better than the 7% to 8% contrast limitation of film-screen systems.

18-16. Answer = (a). Because higher kVp values deliver more x-rays to the detectors (more x-rays as well as more penetrating x-rays), the CT noise is reduced. High kVp values degrade contrast and deliver a larger dose to the patient during CT because the mAs is not necessarily reduced when the kVp is increased. High kVp values have no direct influence on image unsharpness.

18-17. Answer = (c). Greater mAs produces more x-rays, which increases the radiation dose to the patient and decreases CT noise. Because the CT noise decreases, the low-contrast discrimination improves. More mAs means more electrons bombarding the x-ray tube anode, which increases tube heat. If the higher mAs is obtained by using longer scan times, the motion unsharpness increases. If the mAs is obtained strictly by an increase in mA, the focal spot blooming could cause some minor focal spot penumbra (unsharpness).

18-18. Answer = (c). The large number of slices per patient and the large number of patients per week are the main reason for the radiation shielding. Typical workloads for CT scanners are around 5000 to 15,000 mA-minutes per week. This value is much greater than that for radiography, fluoroscopy, angiography, and cardiac catheterization rooms. The motion of the x-ray tube and the narrow x-ray beam do not increase the number of scattered x-rays. Rooms for CT are not necessarily smaller than most x-ray rooms. The higher kVp values do increase the number of scattered x-rays, but it is not the prime consideration.

18-19. Answer = (a). See note in this chapter (**B5**).

18-20. Answer = (c). A bad (or miscalibrated) detector contributes invalid data at all points as the detector rotates around the patient, producing a ring of bad data.

18-21. Answer = (b). As the x-rays are filtered by dense anatomic structures, the energy spectrum changes, leaving higher energy x-rays that have lower linear attenuation coefficients in the remaining tissue. Lower attenuation coefficients result in lower CT numbers.

18-22. Answer = (d). Spatial resolution is affected by focal spot, detector size, scanner geometry, and reconstruction algorithm for small FoVs. For larger FoVs, spatial resolution depends only on pixel size. Pixel size is equal to FoV divided by matrix size. Helical or axial mode has little impact on spatial resolution. Contrast depends on kVp, filtration, window/level, reconstruction algorithm, and patient size. One of the most important advantages of helical scanners is their higher throughput of patients. Because of interpolation between measurements, the helical scanners use slightly thicker CT slices than do axial scans. The CT noise is dependent on the radiation output (kVp and mAs), voxel size, and reconstruction algorithm.

18-23. Answer = (d). To examine differences in bone, all potential values of bone CT numbers should lie within the display window. Various types of bone, including bone marrow with fat, can have CT numbers between −100 and +1200 HU. Ideally, one would set the level in the middle, at 650 HU with a width of 1300 HU.

18-24. Answer = (d). The effective pitch is equal to (table incrementation)/ (x-ray beam collimated width). For the data, the effective pitch is equal to 0.5. The $CTDI_{VOLUME}$ (or MSAD) is calculated by dividing the $CTDI_W$ by the effective pitch. Dividing by 0.5 is like multiplying by a factor of 2.0.

18-25. Answer = (b). Edge enhancement creates more image noise by a factor of 2 or greater, which decreases low-contrast discrimination. Edge enhancement can improve the spatial resolution of high-contrast objects. Edge enhancement artificially increases CT numbers on one side of an edge and decreases them on the other side to improve edge definition. This process can artificially create voids where none existed and can create a ringing effect of the CT number variations. Barrel distortion is found only in nuclear medicine scintillation cameras.

18-26. Answer = (b). In-plane resolution is affected by the other factors, such as focal spot size and detector size. Usually, the slice thickness for most CT scans is equal to or greater than 1.0 mm. For MPR, the slice thickness limitation is much larger than the limitation on in-plane resolution, which is less than 1.0 mm.

18-27. Answer = (a). Localizer scans are done with a thin x-ray beam (~1 mm wide) and low mA without rotation of the x-ray tube. Therefore, any anatomic location is in the x-ray beam for only a very short period of time. The radiation dose to the patient from localizer scans is negligible in comparison with axial or helical CT scans.

18-28. Answer = (b). Interpolation is used to estimate CT numbers located between two measured points. Extrapolation is extension of a trend beyond the point of measured data. Reclamation has to do with restoration of something. Conjugation involves the pairing or coupling of objects. Smoothing is an mathematical averaging process used to reduce image noise.

18-29. Answer = (c). Tube rotation time multiplied by table speed yields table incrementation. See note in this chapter (**D2**) for the definition of effective pitch.

18-30. Answer = (d). CTDI is about 1.2 to 1.4 times the single-slice radiation dose, which in this case is about 4.0 cGy. For an effective pitch of 0.5, the $CTDI_{VOLUME}$ is about two times the $CTDI_W$: $4.0 \times 2.0 = 8.0$ cGy. For double the mAs, radiation dose is doubled: 2×8 cGy = 16 cGy.

18-31. Answer = (b). One approach would be to multiply the $CTDI_{VOLUME}$ by the length scanned to get the DLP. DLP = 20 cm × 16 cGy = 320 cGy-cm. Next, the DLP is multiplied by 0.015 for the abdomen to obtain the effective dose. (See note in this chapter [**D4**].) Effective dose = $0.015 \times 160 = 4.8$ cSv = 48 mSv. The conversion is 1 cSv = 10 mSv. The other approach recognizes that the effective dose for the abdomen is about 33% of the $CTDI_{VOLUME}$. Effective dose = $0.33 \times 16.0 = 5.33$ cSv = 53.3 mSv.

18-32. Answer = (c). See note in this chapter (**A4**).

18-33. Answer = (d). Because (1) fourth-generation CT units need to have detectors in a 360-degree ring around the CT gantry and (2) for high spatial resolution, small detector sizes are needed, this unit has many detectors. In the early days of CT, the detector size was large, so that 600 detectors were adequate to complete the circle. In later versions, 4800 or more smaller detectors were needed. In third-generation CT scanners, the detectors cover only a small arc of about 30 to 60 degrees. The need for a large number of detectors in fourth-generation CT units is one of the reasons that this type of unit has virtually disappeared.

18-34. Answer = (b). The two standards for the contrast scale are air and water. (CS is defined in the notes for this chapter.) Air has a linear attenuation coefficient close to zero. The CT number difference by definition must be 1000 HU. The main variable factor is therefore the linear attenuation coefficient of water, which decreases slowly with increasing kVp. The only possible answers that are negative in value are (a) and (b). The change must be small. These factors limit the only choice to (b).

18-35. Answer = (d). The thinner slices increase the noise by the square root of the amount of change. Similarly, lower radiation doses increase the CT noise by the square root of the amount of change. The radiation dose is directly related to the mAs used. The CT noise increases as the square root of (4.0 for the thickness change × 2.25 for the mAs change). The square root of 9.0 is 3.0 times more CT noise.

18-36. Answer = (a). See note in this chapter (**D1**).

18-37. Answer = (d). The most sensitive organs in the body in regard to cancer risk are the gastrointestinal tract and the gonads. These organs are located in the abdomen and pelvis. The head, the cervical spine, and the knee are relatively insensitive to the risk of cancer. Although the lungs are sensitive to induction of cancer from radiation, high-resolution CT examinations are performed at relatively low radiation doses (about 1 to 4 mSv) as screening studies.

18-38. Answer = (b). AEC tracking is performed in radiography and mammography, where phototimer (AEC) units are used. Although some CT scanners do adjust the mA using measurement of relative radiation transmission through the body, this method (called Smartscan [Smartscan Inc., Livonia, MI] and other names) is not like that in AEC systems. The radiation regulation systems are evaluated with the standard method used for AEC systems. See notes in this chapter (section C) for other quality control tests for CT.

18-39. Answer = (d). For the same scan settings as used for adults, the CTDI for small babies is about three to five times greater in the center of the body and about two to three times greater at the surface because of their small size.

18-40. Answer = (d). The biologic risk for cancer in adults is about 0.05 per Sv, or 0.00005 per mSv. In a fetus or small baby, the cancer risk is about three to four times greater because of the growing tissues and the longer life span during which cancer can be expressed. The risk for the fetus would be about 0.00015 per mSv. If the $CTDI_W$ is 3.0 cGy for a body scan, the surface CTDI would be about 3.6 cGy, and the center CTDI would be about 1.8 cGy. The radiation dose to the fetus would be the center CTDI, or about 1.8 cGy (18.0 mSv). To find the cancer risk, multiply the following: 18.0 mSv × 0.00015/Sv × 1,000,000 persons = 2700 potential cancer cases. The important message is to minimize CT radiation to fetuses and babies unless the examination is deemed clinically urgent.

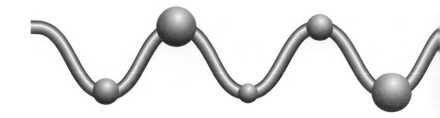

CHAPTER NINETEEN

Ultrasound

A. Basic Concepts

1. Ultrasound is sound waves with frequencies greater than 20,000 Hz, which is beyond the range of human hearing.

2. In practice, clinical ultrasound is operated between 1 and 20 MHz.

3. The origin of ultrasound was during World War II, with "sound navigation and ranging" (SONAR).

4. Two factors affect the **speed of sound** in a given material.

   - **Compressibility:** When a material is very compressible, the speed of sound is much slower.

   - **Density:** As the density of a material increases, the speed of sound decreases if the compressibility coefficient remains the same.

   - V = speed of sound in a material

   - $V_{GAS} < V_{LIQUID} < V_{SOLID}$

   - For example, speed in air = 330 m/sec, speed in water = 1480 m/sec, and speed in bone = 4080 m/sec

   - The speed for different body tissues varies slightly around an average speed of 1540 m/sec.

   - Speed is *not* dependent on the frequency of the sound wave.

5. Sound is a **longitudinal wave**. It moves in the same direction in which it interacts with matter. It is a mechanical wave that causes **compression** and **rarefaction** of the tissue.

6. A transducer is composed of a piezoelectric crystal. When an electrical voltage is applied to the crystal, it expands. When the voltage is removed, it contracts. Thus, a voltage pulse causes the crystal to vibrate.

   - The purpose of the damping material is to stop the vibration as quickly as possible.

   - The thickness of the crystal determines the frequency at which it vibrates.

     λ = wavelength = 2T = 2 × thickness of crystal

     ν = frequency = (4000 m/sec)/λ

   - The piezoelectric crystal is a ceramic material such as lead zirconate titanate (PZT).

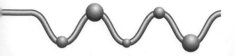

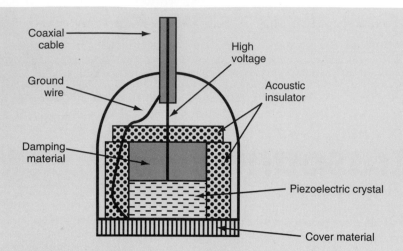

- A piezoelectric crystal can use electrical pulses to create vibrations, or mechanical pressure on the crystal can create electrical signals.

- The transducer is used both to send vibrations into tissue and to receive the echoes of the reflected ultrasound waves and convert them to an electrical signal.

7. **High-Q transducers** produce sound waves with narrow frequency spreads; however, these crystals take a longer time to stop vibrating after an excitation. This long "ring-down" time results in loss of axial resolution and loss of capability to image near the surface.

8. **Low-Q transducers** produce sound waves with wider frequency variations; however, these crystals stop vibration after excitation more rapidly. The short ring-down times result in better axial resolution and better imaging near the surface.

9. The **basic principle of ultrasound imaging** is to send a sound wave into a material and listen for an echo when the wave encounters a dissimilar material. The speed of ultrasound in most tissue is around 1540 meters per second. The time between transmission of the sound and the return of the echo (Δt) is related to the depth of the dissimilar surface (X).

$$X = depth = (1540 \text{ m/sec})(\Delta t)/2$$

- Typically, ultrasound transducers transmit 1% of the time and listen for echoes 99% of the time.

10. The **acoustic impedance (Z)** is the characteristic property of the material. Z is the product of density (ρ) and speed of sound in the material (V).

MATERIAL	SPEED (m/sec)	DENSITY (g/cm³)	Z (RAYLS × 10^{+6})
Air	330	0.001293	0.000427
Water	1480	1.0	1.48
Fat	1460	0.93	1.34
Muscle	1600	1.04	1.66
Bone	4080	1.9	7.75

$Z = \rho \times V$ in Rayls

1 Rayl = (kg/m^2-sec) = (0.1 g/cm^2-sec) or

1 g/cm^2-sec = 10 Rayls

11. The greatest reflection occurs at the interfaces of different materials, where the difference in acoustic impedance (Z) is greatest.

% Reflection = $100\%(Z_1 - Z_2)^2/(Z_1 + Z_2)^2$

% Transmission = $100\%(4Z_1Z_2)/(Z_1 + Z_2)^2$

- If the differences in acoustic impedance are large, most of the power of the wave is reflected.

- If the differences in acoustic impedance are small (the impedance values are nearly the same), most of the power of the wave is transmitted.

- In all cases, some of the power is transmitted through the interface and some of the power is reflected.

12. **Decibel (dB)** is the unit in which the strength of the reflected echo is measured.

$$dB = -10 \times \log_{10}[P_{IN}/P_{ECHO}]$$

where P = power in milliwatts/cm^2.

P_{ECHO}	P_{IN}/P_{ECHO}	DECIBELS (dB)
100%	1.0	0
50%	2.0	−3
25%	4.0	−6
12.5%	8.0	−9
10%	10	−10
1%	100	−20
0.1%	1000	−30
0.01%	10,000	−40

- For each factor of 2 reduction in the power of the echo, add −3 dB.

- For each factor of 10 reduction in the power of the echo, add −10 dB.

13. **Power is removed** from the sound transmission by scatter, attenuation, reflection, and shear losses.

$$Attenuation = \alpha \times \nu \times L$$

where α = attenuation coefficient in dB/(MHz-cm), ν = frequency of ultrasound in MHz, and L = total distance traveled = 2 × depth in cm.

MATERIAL	ATTENUATION COEFFICIENT (dB/MHz-cm) AT 1 MHz
Blood	0.18
Fat	0.6
Muscle	1.0–3.3
Liver	0.9
Kidney	1.0

- It is usually assumed that $\alpha \cong 1.0$(dB/MHz-cm) for most tissues.

- Higher frequency ultrasound waves lose power more rapidly than lower frequency waves.

- Because of the rapid power loss at high frequencies, high-frequency transducers cannot penetrate deeply into the body.

- Low-frequency transducers are needed to image deep in the body.

- Because most ultrasound systems cannot image when the power loss is more than −70 to −80 dB, the depth of penetration can be calculated.

FREQUENCY (MHz)	EST. MAXIMUM DEPTH (cm)
1	35
3	12
5	7
10	3.5

Maximum depth = 70 dB/[2 × α × ν]

- Shear is loss of power laterally because of the viscous nature of tissue through which the ultrasound wave travels.
- Scatter sends power out in all directions so that it does not bounce back to the transducer.

14. **Reflection** occurs when an ultrasound signal bounces off a surface with different acoustic impedance values on opposite sides.

- **Specular reflection** involves bouncing the signal from a smooth interface.
- For specular reflection, the angle of incidence equals the angle of reflection.

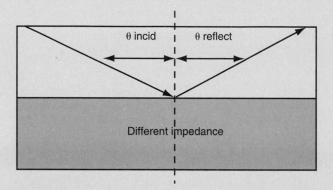

- If the incident ultrasound wave is not perpendicular to the interface, the echo reflects away from the transducer. The surface cannot be imaged.
- **Diffuse reflection** is a bounce from a rough surface that reflects part of the sound wave in many different directions.

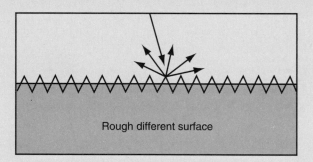

- **Rayleigh scatter** occurs when the scattering objects are much smaller than the ultrasound wavelength. The amount of scatter is proportional to frequency to the fourth power. For very small objects, high-frequency ultrasound has a significant amount of Rayleigh scatter.
- **Refraction** is the change in direction of an ultrasound wave as it is transmitted across an interface with different impedances.

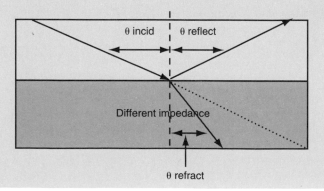

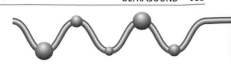

15. ***Snell's law*** for refraction is the following:

$$\frac{\text{Sin}(\theta\,\text{incidence})}{\text{Sin}(\theta\,\text{refraction})} = \frac{\text{speed incidence media}}{\text{speed refraction media}}$$

16. ***Fresnel zone*** is the depth in which the lateral width of the sound wave does not expand. It is the depth to which the sound wave can provide useful images without a significant loss of lateral resolution. For a circular disc element transducer,

Fresnel zone depth $= d^2/(4\lambda)$

where $d =$ transducer diameter in cm and λ is the wavelength in cm.

FREQUENCY	λ (mm)	FRESNEL ZONE FOR d = 1 cm	FRESNEL ZONE FOR d = 2 cm
1 MHz	1.54	1.6 cm	6.5 cm
3 MHz	0.51	4.9 cm	19.6 cm
5 MHz	0.31	8.1 cm	32.2 cm
10 MHz	0.15	16.7 cm	66.7 cm

- In general, transducer diameter is usually equal to >10 wavelengths.
- Higher frequency transducers usually have a longer Fresnel zone.
- However, focused transducers exist that use acoustical lenses and electronic focusing to improve lateral resolution at a specified depth (focal length).
- At the focal depth for a single transducer element, the width (W) of the ultrasound beam is

$W = (1.22\lambda \times F)/d$

where $F =$ focal distance.

- Higher frequency transducers have shorter wavelengths and narrow widths.
- This is important because lower frequencies have better penetration with shorter Fresnel regions.

17. ***Fraunhofer zone*** is the region in which the ultrasound beam continues to expand in width, which degrades the lateral resolution.

18. ***Side lobes*** are regions of ultrasound power that are outside and to the side of the main beam. Echoes from side lobes are thought to be from the main beams and can be misplaced as artifacts in the image.

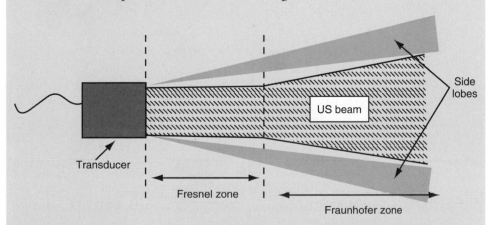

19. ***Doppler effect*** is a shift between the transmitted frequency and the received echo related to motion of the object being imaged.

- If the object is moving toward the ultrasound transducer, the frequency increases.

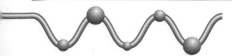

- If the object is moving away from the ultrasound transducer, the frequency decreases.

- This effect is used to measure blood flow. The method is known as "color flow Doppler." Blood flow moving away is displayed as blue and green, and flow toward the transducer is shown as orange and red. The shade and color are related to speed of the blood.

- The measured echo frequency (v_E) depends on the transmitted frequency (v_0); the speed of the sound wave in the medium (V); the speed of the object, such as blood (S); and the angle (θ) between the transducer and the moving object, such as the blood vessel.

$$v_{ECHO} = [2 \times v_0 \times S \times \cos(\theta)]/V$$

- The *key features* are that the Doppler frequency shift increases for faster object speeds and for smaller angles, where the ultrasound beam is aligned nearly parallel to the object's motion.

20. *Frame rate (or refresh rate)* is the number of separate ultrasound images that can be shown per second. A fast frame rate is important to show changing or moving objects.

- The time to image one line of an ultrasound image is equal to twice the maximum depth (D_{MAX}) divided by the speed of sound in the medium.

$$t_R = [2 \times D_{MAX}]/V$$

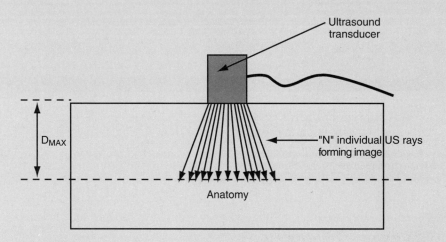

- For example, for a 12-cm maximum depth, the time to scan one ray is [2 × 12]/[1540 m/sec × 100 cm/m] = 0.000156 sec.

- If there are N rays (or lines) per ultrasound image, the time to form one image is $N \times t_R$.

- The maximum number of ultrasound frames per second (frame rate [FR]) is given below.

$$FR = 1.0/[N \times t_R]$$

- For our example with a 12-cm depth and 400 rays, the maximum frame rate is equal to 16 images per second.

- The *key features* are that the FR decreases with longer depths and with more rays in the image.

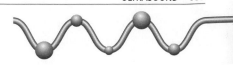

B. Image Quality

1. **Axial spatial resolution** is the ability to see small objects in the direction in which the ultrasound beam is moving through the tissue. The smallest separation of ultrasound echoes is about half of three wavelengths, which is the fastest time in which the transducer crystal can stop vibrating after a pulse.

$$\Delta X = 1.5 \times \lambda = (1.5 \times V)/\nu$$

- Because the speed (V) is about 1540 m/sec in most tissue, the axial resolution improves for higher ultrasound frequencies (ν).

2. **Lateral spatial resolution** is the ability to see small objects perpendicular to the direction of travel of the ultrasound beam. It depends on the width of the ultrasound beam.

- Lateral resolution depends on transducer diameter, frequency, type of acoustic lenses, and electronic focusing.
- Larger diameter transducers and higher frequency transducers have better lateral resolution.

3. **Ultrasound artifacts** fall into several different categories.

- **Reverberation artifacts** are the result of the sound wave bouncing several times inside an object, such as a cyst, producing a ghost image of the original structure spaced at intervals behind the real object.
- **Shadowing** is a dark area behind an object that attenuates most of the incident ultrasound signal.
- **Mirror image artifact** occurs when an echo from an object is reflected from a strongly reflecting structure behind the object, producing a mirror image at a different location.
- **Side lobe artifacts** measure echoes outside the main ultrasound beam and falsely place these objects in the main image.
- **Slice thickness and width artifacts**, like side lobe artifacts, measure echoes of objects outside the main beam and place them in the image.
- **Distortions** are produced because the speed of sound in the body is different from the assumed average speed of 1540 m/sec.

C. Ultrasound Equipment

1. **A-mode** measures the depth of objects along a single ultrasound ray.

2. **T-M mode** (or time motion) plots the change in distance with time and has been used to monitor cardiac valve motion.

3. **Older B-mode mechanical scanners** used linkages to measure locations as the transducer was moved to many positions to form the image.

4. **Rotating sector scanners** have a single-element transducer that either rotates on a wheel or is reflected from an oscillating mirror to produce a triangular image.

5. **Linear array** is a series of individual transducers along a line in which each element images one line or ray to form a rectangular image.

6. **Annular array** is a series of concentric circular transducers that can shape the beam to different focal depths.

7. **Phased array** is a series of transducer elements in a linear or curved array that fire simultaneously with different phase delays to steer the ultrasound beam in various directions to form a trapezoidal image shape.

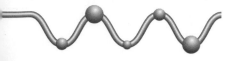

8. A *color Doppler flow scanner* measures blood flow by sensing the Doppler frequency shift.

9. *Specialized transducers* include endorectal and cardiac scanners.

10. To offset *time gain compensation (TGC),* an amplifier is used that can be adjusted to boost the gain of echoes from deep structures more than those from close structures to compensate for the loss in signal by attenuation of signal by tissue.

D. Potential Bioeffects of Ultrasound

1. The *main bioeffects* of ultrasound fall into the following categories, arranged according to the amount of power required (least to most):

    - Central nervous system (CNS) stimulation
    - Tissue heating
    - Cavitation
    - Tissue destruction at very high power

2. *Thermal index (TI)* is the ratio of the power required to cause tissue heating to a temperature increase of around 1° C divided by the actual transmitted power. The 1° increase in temperature is usually taken as the safe limit for diagnostic (nondiathermy) ultrasound. A TI of 1.0 or 2.0 is considered safe.

3. Cavitation is tissue tearing, which occurs at high powers.

4. Destruction, such as emulsification of cells, occurs at high power values.

5. The *mechanical index (MI)* is used to compare the pressure in the ultrasound wave with pressure that could cause mechanical damage. A pressure of less than 0.3 MPa (300,000 newtons/m^2) is generally considered to be safe.

6. CNS stimulation can occur in some fetal scans of pregnant patients.

7. *SPTA* (spatial peak temporal average) is a measure of ultrasound intensity. It is the peak intensity in space averaged over time. Because the transmitting power is turned on only 1% of the time, the SPTA is <1% of the peak intensity.

8. In the United States, it is recommended that the SPTA of a focused diagnostic ultrasound beam should be less than 1.0 watts/cm^2 and that the SPTA of an unfocused beam should be less than 100 mwatts/cm^2. The recommended maximum SPTA depends on the mode being employed.

    - The maximum SPTA for obstetrics and abdominal ultrasound is <100 mwatts/cm^2.

    - Because color Doppler ultrasound employs a high duty cycle and stays in one position for an extended time, its peak intensity and SPTA are nearly the same value.

    - The maximum SPTA for Doppler ultrasonography of peripheral vessels is <700 mwatts/cm^2.

E. Questions

19-1. The speed of sound in body tissue has an average value of about _____ m/sec.

    (a) 100   (b) 330   (c) 960   (d) 1540   (e) 4000

19-2. If an echo arrives 100 microseconds (μsec) after the signal is transmitted, the depth of the structure is about _____ cm below the surface.

    (a) 4   (b) 6   (c) 8   (d) 10   (e) 12

19-3. The speed of sound in any material is dependent on the characteristics of _____ and _____ of the medium. (i) Density (ii) Strain (iii) Bulk modulus (iv) Frequency (v) Polarity

(a) i and ii   (b) ii and iii   (c) iii and v   (d) i and iii   (e) ii and iv

19-4. The frequency of a transducer is primarily determined by the piezoelectric crystal's _____ .

(a) Diameter   (b) Thickness   (c) Density   (d) Conductance
(e) Reynold's number

19-5. The material from which the crystal of an ultrasound transducer is composed is called _____.

(a) Gd_2O_2S (b) NaI   (c) PZT   (d) LiF   (e) $CaHPO_4$

19-6. As an ultrasound wave passes from one material to another, the _____ of the ultrasound wave stays constant and the _____ changes.

(a) Amplitude, frequency   (b) Period, shear   (c) Frequency, wavelength
(d) Wavelength, speed   (e) Impedance, refractive index

19-7. The acoustic impedance of an ultrasound wave is dependent on the _____ and _____ of the material.

(a) Density, velocity   (b) Frequency, elastic modulus   (c) Polarity, pH
(d) Wavelength, diameter   (e) Power, granularity

19-8. If the echo of an ultrasound wave has 0.05% of the initial power, the reduction in intensity is given as _____ dB.

(a) −13   (b) −23   (c) −33   (d) −43   (e) −53

19-9. The percentage of power reflected in the echo of an ultrasound wave primarily depends on _____ differences of the materials at the interface.

(a) Viscosity   (b) Absorption coefficient   (c) Acoustic impedance
(d) Frequency   (e) Refractive index

19-10. The largest reflection of an ultrasound wave would occur at the interface of _____ and _____.

(a) Muscle, bone   (b) Muscle, fat   (c) Muscle, air   (d) Fat, tumor
(e) Aluminum, bone

19-11. The Doppler shift is measured in units of _____.

(a) dB/(MHz-cm)   (b) Rayls   (c) Hz   (d) mwatts/cm^2 (e) Pascals

19-12. Acoustic impedance is measured in units of _____.

(a) dB/(MHz-cm)   (b) Rayls   (c) Hz   (d) mwatts/cm^2 (e) Pascals

19-13. The linear absorption coefficient for ultrasound waves is measured in units of _____.

(a) dB/(MHz-cm)   (b) Rayls   (c) Hz   (d) mwatts/cm^2 (e) Pascals

19-14. The intensity of ultrasound waves is measured in units of _____.

(a) dB/(MHz-cm)   (b) Rayls   (c) Hz   (d) mwatts/cm^2 (e) Pascals

19-15. The pressure of ultrasound waves is measured in units of _____.

(a) dB/(MHz-cm)   (b) Rayls   (c) Hz   (d) mwatts/cm^2 (e) Pascals

19-16. For a 3-MHz ultrasound transducer, the expected axial spatial resolution would be about _____ mm.

(a) 0.4   (b) 0.6   (c) 0.8   (d) 1.0   (e) 1.2

19-17. The maximum depth of penetration of a 3-MHz ultrasound wave would be expected to be about _____ cm, assuming an attenuation coefficient of 1.0 dB/MHz-cm.

(a) 4   (b) 8   (c) 12   (d) 16   (e) 20

19-18. If a 3-MHz sector scanner is used to create an image at a maximum depth of 12 cm with 200 rays of measurement, the maximum expected frame rate is about _____.

(a) 4   (b) 8   (c) 16   (d) 32   (e) 64

19-19. If a 3-MHz ultrasound wave penetrates 5 cm through tissue and then is reflected from a bone surface at that depth, the echo received at the transducer would be expected to be _____ dB.

(a) −10   (b) −20   (c) −30   (d) −40   (e) −50

19-20. The lateral spatial resolution depends on all of the following factors, *except* _____.

(a) Speed   (b) Impedance   (c) Transducer diameter   (d) Apodization
(e) Frequency

19-21. The ultrasound artifact that creates a series of ghost images behind an interface is called _____.

(a) Refraction   (b) Reverberation   (c) Aliasing   (d) Side lobe
(e) Shadowing

19-22. The type of ultrasound scanner that fires an array of transducers one at a(n) time to create a rectangular image is called a _____.

(a) Sector scanner   (b) Linear array   (c) Annular array
(d) Phased array   (e) T-M mode

19-23. Multidirectional scatter of ultrasound waves from a rough surface is called _____ scatter.

(a) Specular   (b) Rayleigh   (c) Elastic   (d) Diffuse   (e) Newtonian

19-24. Quality control testing for ultrasound units should include all of the following, *except* _____.

(a) Distance accuracy   (b) Depth of penetration   (c) Spatial resolution
(d) Uniformity   (e) dB linearity

19-25. The type of transducer needed to damp the "ringing" (continued oscillations) of the transducer element as quickly as possible after each excitation is a(n) _____ crystal.

(a) Fraunhofer   (b) Low Q   (c) Apodization   (d) Annular
(e) Dynamic aperture

19-26. The Fresnel region is longer for transducer crystals that have _____.

(a) Low frequencies   (b) Small diameters   (c) Short wavelengths
(d) Fractionation   (e) Diffraction grating

19-27. To avoid damaging tissue as a result of heating, it is recommended that the SPTA transmit intensity of a focused beam be less than _____ mwatts/cm^2.

(a) 0.5   (b) 10.0   (c) 50.0   (d) 100.0   (e) 1000.0

10-28. The image processing feature that amplifies signal from a deeper depth more than signal from structures closer to the surface is called _____.

(a) ADC   (b) TGC   (c) MCA   (d) RBG   (e) FET

19-29. For color Doppler ultrasound imaging, the measurement of flow velocity requires knowledge of all the following parameters, *except* _____.

(a) Transducer angle   (b) Speed in medium   (c) Focal length
(d) Transmit frequency   (e) Frequency shift

19-30. The reason for using an ultrasound gel between the patient's body and the transducer is to _____.

(a) Dissipate heat   (b) Provide electrical insulation
(c) Provide impedance matching   (d) Reduce friction   (e) Reduce side lobes

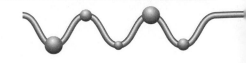

19-31. High-frequency transducers are used primarily to improve _____ .

(a) Spatial resolution   (b) Depth penetration   (c) Scatter rejection
(d) Radiation dose to the patient   (e) Dynamic range

F. Answers

19-1. Answer = (d). Although the speed of sound waves in tissue varies from 1460 m/sec for fat to 1600 m/sec for muscle, the average speed in tissue is 1540 m/sec.

19-2. Answer = (c). The distance is equal to speed times time. However, the depth is traveled twice: once going toward the reflector and once traveling back toward the surface. Thus, depth = $(1.540 \times 10^{+5}$ cm/sec$) \times (100 \times 10^{-6}$ sec$)/2.0 = 7.7$ cm.

19-3. Answer = (d). The speed is dependent on the density and compressibility of the material. Compressibility is inversely related to the bulk modulus. Strain is the change in length divided by the initial length before the application of force. Frequency is determined by the piezoelectric crystal's thickness. Polarity is the electrical charge distribution of the molecular structure of the piezoelectric crystal, which accounts for the property of expanding or contracting linear dimension when a voltage is applied.

19-4. Answer = (b). See note in this chapter (**A6**). Conductance is an electrical property, and Reynold's number refers to flow characteristic of gases and fluids.

19-5. Answer = (c). Gd_2O_2S is the phosphor material of intensifying screens. NaI is a common scintillation material used in nuclear medicine detectors. LiF is the material used in thermoluminescent dosimeters. $CaHPO_4$ is a material used in bone mineral analysis.

19-6. Answer = (c). The frequency is fixed by the transducer design. Both speed and wavelength depend on the properties of the material through which the ultrasound waves travel. Period is equal to one divided by the frequency.

19-7. Answer = (a). The acoustic impedance is the product of density times speed in a material.

19-8. Answer = (c). $0.05\% = 0.0005 = 1/2000$. Each factor of 10 reduction $(1/10)$ in power adds -10 dB. $1/1000 = (1/10) \times (1/10) \times (1/10)$, which adds -30 dB. The extra factor of $\frac{1}{2}$ adds -3 dB, for a total of -33 dB.

19-9. Answer = (c). Viscosity is related to shear loss of power. Absorption coefficient refers to loss in power per linear path length. Frequency differences are related to the Doppler shift and the speed of an object moving toward or away from an ultrasound beam. Refractive index relates to a change in the direction of the ultrasound beam as it crosses boundaries with different sound-wave speeds.

19-10. Answer = (c). The greatest reflection occurs where the acoustic impedance difference is greatest. The acoustic impedances of the various materials in units of Rayls $\times 10^{+6}$ are as follows: air $= 0.33 \times 0.001293 = 0.000427$; fat $= 1.46 \times 0.93 = 1.34$; muscle $= 1.60 \times 1.04 = 1.66$; bone $= 4.08 \times 1.9 = 7.75$; and aluminum $= 6.4 \times 2.7 = 16.2$. The greatest acoustic impedance differences are between air and anything else. For this reason, air interfaces result in almost 100% reflection.

19-11. Answer = (c). Doppler shift is a frequency shift that is measured as a difference in frequencies using units of Hz (or cps).

19-12. Answer = (b). See note in this chapter (**A10**).

19-13. Answer = (a). See note in this chapter (**A13**).

19-14. Answer = (d). See note in this chapter (**D8**).

19-15. Answer = (e). A pascal is equal to 1.0 N/m^2.

19-16. Answer = (c). Resolution = $1.5 \times \lambda = [1.5 \times 1.54 \times 10^{+6}$ mm/sec$]/(3 \times 10^{+6}$ Hz$)$ = 0.77 mm. See note in this chapter (**B1**) for equations.

19-17. Answer = (c). Maximum depth equals -70 dB/$(2 \times (-1)$ dB/MHz-cm $\times 3$ MHz$)$ = 11.67 cm. See note in this chapter (**A13**) for equations.

19-18. Answer = (d). t_R = $(2 \times 12$ cm maximum depth$)/(1.54 \times 10^5$ cm/sec$)$ = 0.000156 sec. Frame rate = $1.0/(200$ rays $\times t_R) = 1.0/(200 \times 0.000156)$ = 32 frames/sec.

19-19. Answer = (c). The attenuation of signal power is about -1 dB per MHz per cm through tissue. At 3 MHz, the power loss is -3 dB/cm. The total distance traveled is 10 cm (5 cm in and 5 cm out). The power loss is -3 dB/cm $\times 10$ cm = -30 dB.

19-20. Answer = (b). The lateral width of the beam is related to $d^2/(4\lambda)$. The wavelength (λ) is equal to the speed of sound divided by the frequency. Apodization is the use of electronic means to reduce the width of the ultrasound beam.

19-21. Answer = (b). See note in this chapter (**B3**).

19-22. Answer = (b). The description is for a linear transducer array of elements.

19-23. Answer = (d). Specular refers to a single beam with an angle of reflection equal to the angle of incidence. Rayleigh scatter involves very small objects that scatter in various directions. Elastic refer to nuclear collisions that conserve energy. Newtonian is a description of basic mechanical interactions.

19-24. Answer = (e). dB linearity is a nonsensical term that has no meaning.

19-25. Answer = (b). Low-Q piezoelectric crystals stop vibrating more rapidly than high-Q crystals. Fraunhofer refers to a zone where the lateral width of the ultrasound beam does not increase. Apodization is electronic focusing for improved lateral resolution. Annular ring is a type of transducer that can be readily focused by electronic means. A dynamic aperture has a sensor that varies the number of elements involved in receiving aperture size as echoes arrive. A small aperture is used for echoes from a shallow region, and the aperture increases as echoes return from deeper structures. This minimizes the variation in beam width with depth.

19-26. Answer = (c). The lateral width of the beam is related to $d^2/(4\lambda)$. Small diameters and long wavelengths are associated with shorter Fresnel regions. Low frequencies are the same as long wavelengths. Fractionation is related to spreading radiation doses over time to reduce bioeffects. Diffraction grating is related to optical effects.

19-27. Answer = (e). See note in this chapter (**D8**).

19-28. Answer = (b). ADC is analog-to-digital converter, which takes a continuously varying signal and converts it into discrete steps. TGC is time gain compensation amplifier, which selectively boosts deep echoes more than shallow echoes. MCA is multichannel analyzer, which is used in nuclear medicine to measure energy spectra. RBG is the use of the three primary colors (red, blue, and green) to yield all combinations of colors. FET is field effect transistor, which is used in control circuits.

19-29. Answer = (c). See note in this chapter (**A19**) about Doppler ultrasound.

19-30. Answer = (c). If there is any air between the transducer surface and the patient's skin, the difference in acoustic impedance is so large that the sound is 100% reflected. The signal never enters the patient's body.

19-31. Answer = (a). High frequency is associated with better spatial resolution because of the shorter wavelength. Higher frequency loses power faster by attenuation and cannot be used for deep structures. High-frequency ultrasound has more scatter. There is no radiation dose to the patient from ultrasound because it does not create ionizations. Dynamic range is related to the weakest echo that can be measured and the number of bits used in the digitization.

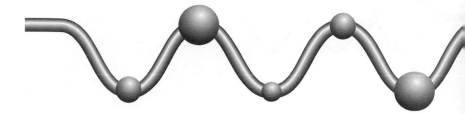

CHAPTER TWENTY

Magnetic Resonance Imaging

A. Basic Concepts

1. All nuclei have neutrons and protons.

- The protons are positively charged.

- Neutrons have a charge distribution but a net charge of zero.

- The net charge of the nucleus is positive.

- The protons and neutrons behave as if they spin on their axes.

- Spinning charges are like an electrical current flowing through a loop of wire.

- Ampère's law states that an electrical charge flowing through a wire loop creates a magnetic field.

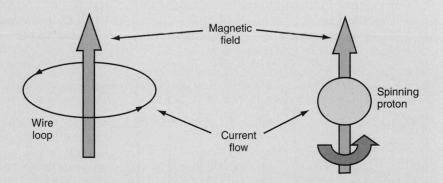

- If a proton in the nucleus pairs with another proton with spin in the opposite direction, the combined magnetic moment of a pair of protons is zero (see figure on next page). This pairing also occurs with neutrons.

- Single neutrons have a smaller magnetic moment than a proton, but paired neutrons have no net magnetic moment.

- Hence, nuclei with an even number of protons and neutrons have no magnetic moment. **_Nuclei with an odd number of protons have the largest magnetic moment._**

- **_Hydrogen is the most important nucleus for magnetic resonance imaging (MRI)._** Hydrogen is found throughout the body in various molecules such as water and has an single (odd) proton that produces a strong magnetic moment.

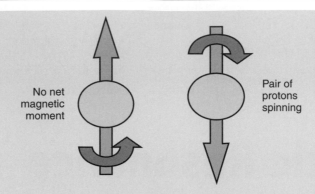

No net magnetic moment

Pair of protons spinning

2. Without the presence of a magnetic field, the magnetic moments of the various nuclei randomly point in all directions. Hence, the **net** magnetic moment of the biologic sample is zero.

3. *If a strong magnetic field is present*, a population of nuclei align so that slightly more than 50% are along the magnetic field (low energy state) and slightly fewer than 50% are antiparallel (high energy state) to the magnetic field.

   ● The nuclei aligned along the magnetic field are at a lower energy.

   ● It requires some input of energy, such as a radiofrequency (RF) wave, to cause the nuclei to flip antiparallel to the applied magnetic field.

   ● The percentage difference between the number of nuclei aligned along the magnetic field and the number opposed to the magnetic field is small (of the order of parts per million) and depends on the temperature of the sample.

   ● The nuclei are not exactly parallel and opposed to the magnetic field. They are at a slight angle to the magnetic field.

   ● If nuclei are slightly misaligned with an external applied magnetic field (B_0), nuclei precess or the nuclear magnetic moment moves in a circular pattern around the applied magnetic field lines.

   ● Because the precession (rotation) about the magnetic field is random, there is no net magnetization perpendicular to the applied main magnetic field, B_0. However, there is a net magnetization along the field from the hydrogen nuclei in the tissue because slightly more nuclei are aligned with the applied magnetic field than are opposed to the field.

   ● The rate of precession is the Larmor frequency.

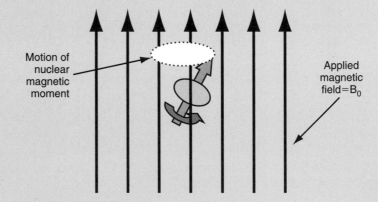

Motion of nuclear magnetic moment

Applied magnetic field = B_0

4. *Larmor's equation* yields the rate of precession or precessional frequency (ω) of the nuclear magnetic moment.

$$\omega = \gamma B_0$$

where γ = gyromagnetic ratio and B_0 = applied external magnetic field.

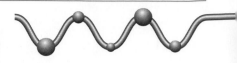

- The gyromagnetic ratio (γ) depends on the element and isotope involved, as shown in the table. It is different for nuclei that have different numbers of protons and neutrons.

ATOM	GYROMAGNETIC RATIO (MHz/tesla)
$_1H^1$	42.58
$_6C_{13}$	10.71
$_9F^{19}$	40.05
$_{11}Na^{23}$	11.26
$_{15}P^{31}$	17.34

5. To provide the energy needed to flip a nucleus from being aligned to the applied magnetic field to being opposed to it, an RF pulse is required whose frequency is the same as the Larmor frequency. RF pulses of other frequencies are not transferred to the nucleus, just as a radio cannot receive music from a given radio station unless the radio is tuned to the proper frequency.

6. The correct Larmor frequency depends on both the strength of the applied magnetic field and the number of neutrons and protons in the nucleus.

7. The strength of an applied magnetic field is measured in tesla (1 T = 10,000 gauss).

   - The Earth's magnetic field is about 0.5 to 1.0 gauss, and the field of a refrigerator magnet is a few hundred gauss.

   - The magnetic field strength of MRI units ranges from 0.3 T for some permanent or smaller units up to 3.0 T for newer clinical units.

   - The most common field strengths of MRI units are 0.5, 1.0, and 1.5 T.

8. All the nuclear magnetic moments in a sample together give rise to a net magnetization along the applied magnetic field. The duration and the amplitude of the RF pulse of the correct Larmor frequency determine how much the **net** nuclear magnetization is tipped relative to the applied magnetic field lines.

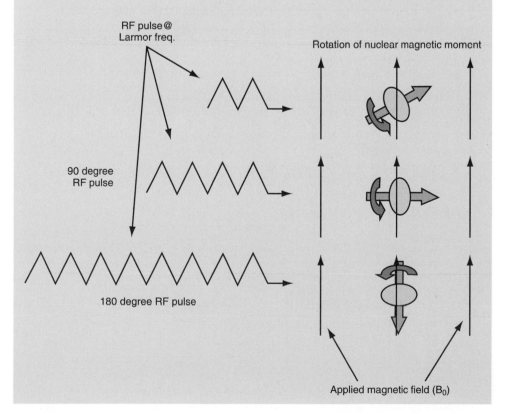

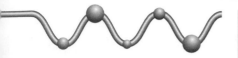

9. After the net magnetization is tipped by the RF pulse, it will recover by realigning itself with the applied magnetic field. The recovery of the magnetization is characterized by a time constant, T1.

   ● ***T1 (or the longitudinal or spin-lattice) relaxation time*** is the time required after a 90-degree tip for 63% of the magnetic moments to realign with the applied magnetic field (B_0).

   ● The time depends on the molecule to which the hydrogen atom is attached.

   ● It is different for various type of tissues and fluids.

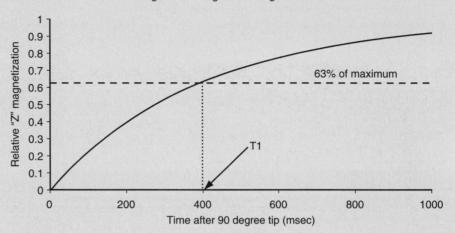

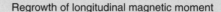

   ● T1 increases with applied magnetic field strength roughly as $(B_0)^{0.3}$.

   ● For an increase in magnetic field from 0.5 to 1.5 T, the T1 relaxation time would increase about 40%.

   ● The T1 of liquids is shorter than the T1 of solids such as bone and plastics.

   $$_{liquid}T1 < {}_{solids}T1$$

   ● Typical T1 times of tissue for a 1.5-T MRI are 300 to 4000 milliseconds.

10. ***Faraday's law*** states that a coil of wire that is located in a changing magnetic field has a current induced in it by the changing magnetic field.

   ● The strength of the current is proportional to the strength of the magnetic field.

   ● The frequency is proportional to the rate of the changing magnetic field.

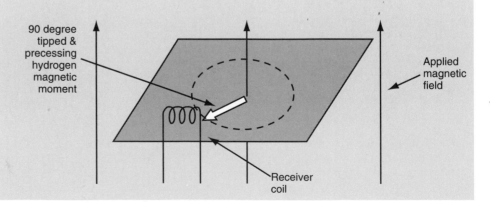

- Hence, a 90-degree RF pulse will tip the net magnetization vector such that there is a component in the transverse plane. The magnetization vector in the transverse plane will rotate, passing a receiver coil that senses the changing magnetic field from the precessing hydrogen nuclei.

- This magnetic moment increases and decreases in strength as it points toward and away from the coil, respectively, creating a sinusoidal current in the wire.

- The strength of the receiver current depends on the strength of the net hydrogen magnetic moment in the 90-degree (X, Y) plane.

- The frequency of the current oscillation in the receiver coils is at the Larmor frequency.

11. **Free induction decay (FID)** represents the rapid loss in signal after a 90-degree tip of the hydrogen magnetic moments with an RF pulse.

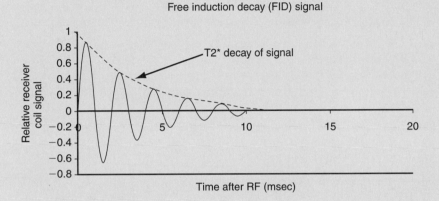

Free induction decay (FID) signal

- **T2* decay rate** of the FID signal is due to two different processes.

  (1) Nonrecoverable dephasing caused by random spin-spin exchanges with adjacent atoms and molecules.

  (2) Recoverable dephasing caused by local nonuniformities in the main magnetic field.

- The **T2 relaxation rate** is the decay rate of just the nonrecoverable portion (spin-spin interactions), which has a different and longer decay rate.

- **Dephasing** means that some of the hydrogen nuclei spin faster and some slower because of local magnet field nonuniformities until the magnetic moments cancel each other. At the point of total dephasing, there is no net magnetic moment in the x-ray plane.

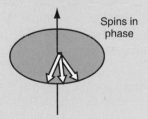

Spins in phase

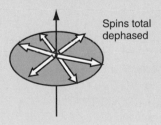

Spins total dephased

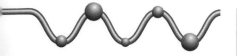

12. The *echo* can be formed by following a 90-degree Larmor RF pulse with a 180-degree RF pulse. (Smaller tip angles than 90 degrees can be used.)

● After the 90-degree RF pulse, the hydrogen atoms dephase rapidly by T2 decay (FID), and the MRI signal disappears.

● However, the magnetic moments of the hydrogen nuclei are still in the X,Y (transverse) plane, but they are randomly oriented.

● *The 180-degree RF pulse changes the direction of precession* of the hydrogen nuclei. The fastest nuclei are in the rear and the slowest in the front.

● Eventually, the *fast spinning nuclei close the gap with the slower spinning nuclei* and the MRI signal reappears, which is called the echo.

● An example is runners going around a track. The faster runners gain the lead, but then the coach blows a whistle to reverse direction (180-degree reversal). The fastest runners are then in the back, but they eventual regroup with the slowest runners, who are now in the front of the pack.

● However, the nonrecoverable signal (T2) will be lost, and the echo will be lower in amplitude because of random spin-spin losses.

● T2 relaxation is a measure of the rate at which the echo amplitude decays.

● T2 is the time for the amplitude of the echo to decay to 37% of the initial FID amplitude.

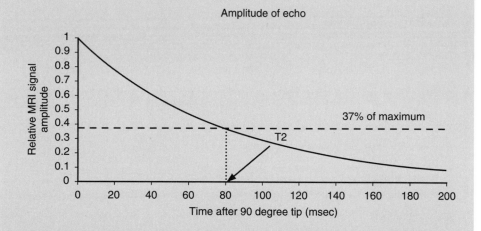

13. T2* << T2 < T1.

14. Typical T2 times for 1.5-T MRI are 50 to 250 milliseconds. In general, T2 relaxation times do not vary much with main magnetic field strength. They are primarily dependent on the molecules to which the hydrogen nuclei are attached and the surrounding molecules.

15. Vector components of the hydrogen magnetic moments are composed of a longitudinal (z-axis) and a transverse (x,y-axis) component.

● Only the transverse (x,y-axis) magnetic moment produces a signal, and only if the magnetic moments are in phase.

● As the longitudinal (z-axis) magnetic vector increases with time constant (T1), the transverse (x,y-axis) decreases.

● The combination of the transverse and longitudinal components is constant.

● After a 90-degree RF pulse, the magnetic moments of the hydrogen nuclei are all in the transverse plane (x,y-axis). With time, the magnetic moments realign so that the net magnetic moment is entirely along the longitudinal plane (z-axis).

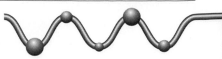

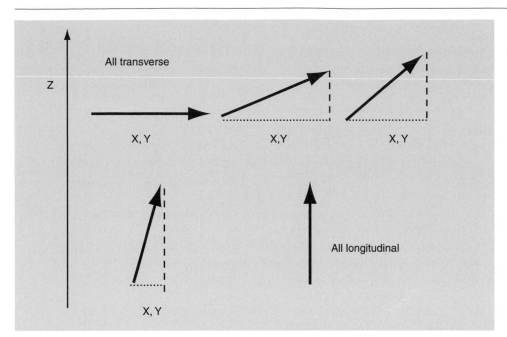

B. MRI Equipment

1. The main magnetic field consists of a series of Helmholtz coils used to produce a strong and nearly uniform magnetic field at the center of the solenoid coils.

- *Superconducting magnets* use liquid helium, which has a temperature near absolute zero (−272° C), to cool the wires so that they have *virtually no resistance*.

- Superconducting magnets are continuously activated once the power is applied.

- *Quenching* can occur if the liquid helium is heated and rapidly "boils off." A big pipe is required to vent the quench gas, which is thousands of times larger in volume than the liquid.

- Typical field strengths are 0.3 to 3.0 T.

2. There are other types of magnets, as follows:

- These magnets are often in the open or vertical configuration.

- *Resistive magnets*, which consume considerable power, require cooling and produce magnetic fields of less than 0.3 T.

- *Permanent magnets*, which are very heavy (>100,000 lb), have very small fringe fields and have main field strengths that are usually less than 0.3 T.

3. *Shim coils* are used to correct for minor nonuniformities in the main magnetic field. Typical uniformity is better than a few parts per million (ppm) over a 30-cm-diameter sphere in the center of the magnet.

4. *Gradient coils* are used to create a small difference in the magnetic field in a linear fashion in the x-, y-, and z-axes.

- Because of the differences in the magnetic fields, only the hydrogen nuclei at the correct magnetic field strength would be affected by the RF field.

- The gradients are used to select the MRI slice and to encode the x and y positions within the slice.

- Higher gradients produce thinner slices, and lower gradient strength produces thicker slices.

- The RF center frequency determines the location of the slice.
- Nonlinearity in the gradients results in spatial distortion (curvature) in images.

5. **RF quadrature coils** are used to send the Larmor excitation pulse and to receive the signal from the tipped hydrogen nuclei.

   - The body coil transmits and receives the RF signals.
   - The head coil is smaller and may transmit and receive the RF signals from head images.
   - Surface coils are placed directly against or around body parts to be imaged (such as the knee, spine, or finger) and usually only receive signals. In these cases, the body coil acts as the transmitter.
   - Head and surface coils produce stronger signals and less noise because they are nearer to the source of the MRI signal.

6. Computer systems are used to control the RF pulses and to receive and organize the MRI signals and process the data from an image.

C. MRI Pulse Sequences

1. A **spin echo (SE) sequence** is a 90-degree RF pulse followed by a 180-degree RF pulse. Then the entire sequence is repeated with a different phase encoding.

   - **Echo time (TE)** is equal to double the time between the 90- and 180-degree RF pulses.
   - TE is selectable by the MRI operator. Longer TE times enhance T2 relaxation time differences in the body tissues.
   - **Repetition time (TR)** is the delay before the 90- and 180-degree RF pulses are repeated.
   - TR is the other parameter that is selected by the MRI operator. Shorter TR times enhance T1 relaxation time differences in the body tissues.

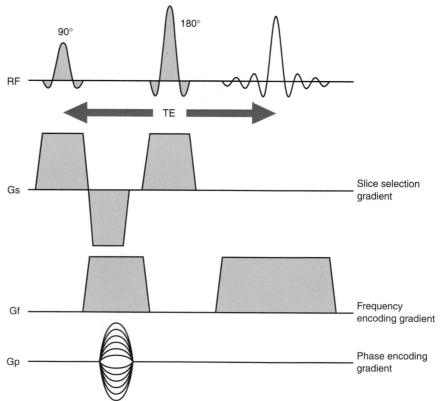

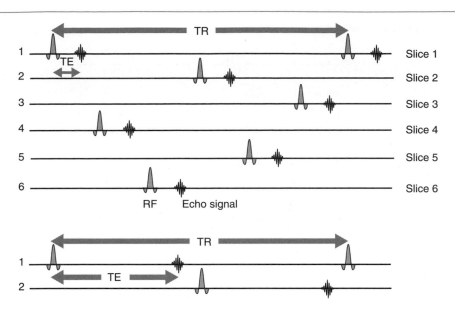

TYPE SE SCAN	TE SELECTION	TR SELECTION
T1 weighted	Short	Short
T2 weighted	Long	Long
Proton density	Short	Long
Not used	Long	Short

2. ***Gradient echo (GRASS = gradient recalled acquisition steady state)*** typically
    uses an RF pulse less than 90 degrees (usually with a 20- to 45-degree tip angle).
    The gradient fields are used to dephase the net magnetization of the hydrogen
    nuclei. The gradients are then reversed to produce an echo without a 180-degree
    RF pulse.

    ● GRE (gradient refocused echo) is usually faster than SE.

    ● The signal is a mixture of T1 and T2 parameter effects.

    ● The signal is usually less, and the image has more image noise and artifacts.

    ● Because the tilt angle for the magnetic moments of the hydrogen atom is less
      than 90 degrees, the hydrogen magnetic moments realign more quickly with the
      applied magnetic field and demonstrate less of a T1 effect, unless the transverse
      magnetization is removed by spoiling (see figures below and at top of next page).

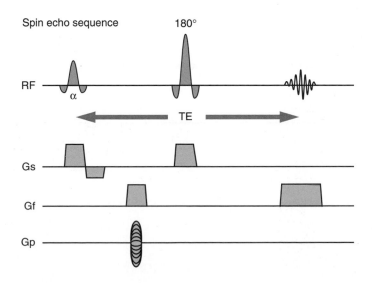

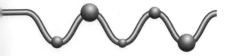

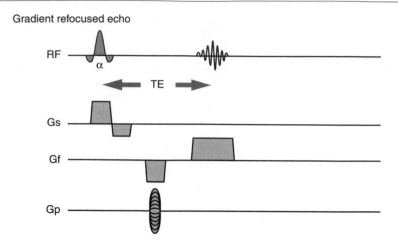

Gradient refocused echo

3. **Inversion recovery** uses a 180-degree RF pulse followed by a 90-degree and 180-degree RF pulse to produce an echo.

- **Inversion time (TI)** is the time between the first 180-degree RF pulse and the following 90-degree RF pulse.

- **STIR** = short T1 inversion recovery

- In STIR imaging, TI can be adjusted so that adipose tissue (fat) has been realigned to the 90-degree position just as the 90-degree RF pulse is applied. This flips the magnetic moment of fat to 180 degrees (90 degrees + 90 degrees) so that the fat in the image has no net signal (see figure below).

- **FLAIR** = fluid-attenuated inversion recovery. As with the technique to nullify fat with STIR, fluid (cerebrospinal fluid) can be nullified by using an appropriate T1 (about 2100 ms).

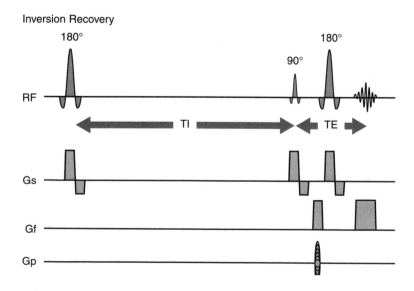

Inversion Recovery

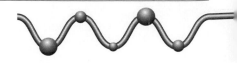

4. **Fast spin echo (FSE)** is a 90-degree pulse followed by a series of 180-degree pulses. Thus, in one sequence, a series of echoes is obtained, one for each phase encode of the image. The image acquisition time is shortened by a factor equal to the number of echoes formed per TR (echo train length or turbo factor).

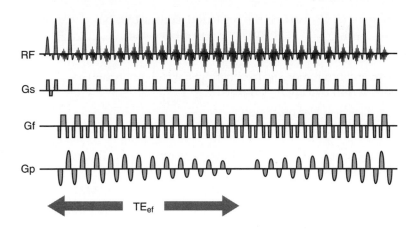

5. **Echo planar imaging (EPI) sequence** employs a continuously oscillating gradient field to gather a significant amount of the total image in a very short period of time.

   ● EPI pulse sequences provide one of the very shortest image times.

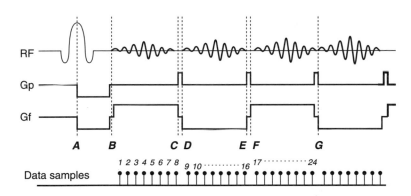

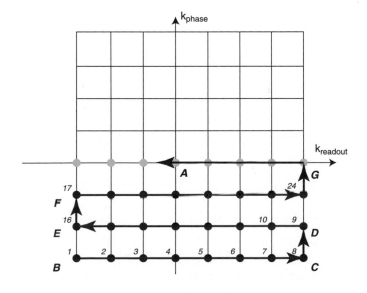

D. MRI Image Quality

1. *Spatial resolution* totally depends on *pixel size*, which is field of view (FoV) divided by the matrix size. A 512×512 matrix has better spatial resolution than a 128×128 matrix.

2. *Signal-to-noise (SNR) ratio* is the key to low-contrast visibility. A strong signal increases the SNR, which improves low-contrast visibility.

   - A larger strength magnet (higher tesla number) produces a better SNR.
   - Large voxels contain more hydrogen atoms, which improves the MRI signal. Therefore, large FoVs improve the SNR.
   - A thicker slice provides more signal.
   - A smaller matrix size provides more signal.
   - Most tissue has a similar (but not the same) number of hydrogen atoms per cubic centimeter.
   - Short TE times and long TR times provide larger amplitude MRI signals.
   - 90-Degree tips for hydrogen nuclei produce a stronger signal than partial angle tips, as used in gradient echo images.
   - Receiver coils close to the body, such as surface coils, have stronger signals.
   - Summation of multiple images (larger NEX [number of excitations]) improves the SNR.
   - Narrow bandwidth improves SNR at the expense of greater chemical shift artifact.

3. *Volume averaging* becomes worse with larger voxels.

4. *Scan times for spin echo* sequences depend on the following factors:

   Scan time = NEX $\times$ (# phase encodings) $\times$ TR

5. The number of spin echo slices that can be simultaneously acquired during a single sequence is given by the following formula:

   # slices per sequence = [TR – load time]/[TE + pulse time]

   where load time is 20 to 100 msec and pulse time is 2 to10 msec.

E. MRI Artifacts

1. *Chemical shift artifact* is due to the Larmor frequency of hydrogen nuclei, which depends on the molecule in which the hydrogen atom is located.

   - The frequency of hydrogen in lipids is about 3 ppm different from that of hydrogen in water, which represents about a 200-Hz difference for 1.5 T.
   - The fats are displaced in the frequency direction, producing a void on one side and a bright area of superimposition on the other side.
   - Chemical shift artifact always occurs in the frequency direction.

2. *Motion ghosts* occur in the phase-encoding direction from fluid flow, respiration, or the patient's movement.

   - There are multiple low-intensity ghosts in the phase-encoding direction due to motion.
   - The direction of ghosting can be changed by reversing phase- and frequency-encoding directions, which may limit ghosting artifacts.
   - Flow effects can produce either dark blood or bright blood, depending on flow and pulse sequence parameters.

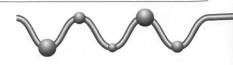

3. ***Aliasing appears as wraparound***, in which a portion of the body is wrapped around onto the other side of the body and overlaps other tissue.

   - This is due to undersampling the data.
   - It can be reduced by using either more pixels or a larger FoV.

4. ***Susceptibility artifact*** is due to differences in the susceptibility coefficients of adjacent structures, such as metal and tissue or air and tissue.

   - Voids appear around metal in the body, and the adjacent area is distorted.

5. ***Volume averaging*** is similar to that seen in computed tomography (CT) when different materials are averaged in large voxels.

6. ***Zipper artifact*** is a light and dark series of short lines (resembling a zipper) along the zero axis due to RF feedback.

7. ***Truncation artifacts*** are alternate light and dark rings at the edges of the body that follow the body contours. They are due to inadequate sampling and have been called ***Gibbs ringing***.

8. ***Cross-talk*** ghosts are faint images of bright structures outside the slice. Because they are close to the edge of the slice, the ghost of the image appears.

9. ***Zebra stripes*** can be due to eddy currents in the MRI or the body.

10. ***Distortion or bending*** of contours can be due to nonlinearity of gradient fields.

F. MRI Safety

1. Static magnetic fields greater than 2 to 10 T can cause the sensation of light flashes in the eyes and can interfere with conduction loops of the central nervous system.

2. Large, rapidly changing magnetic fields (>20 T/sec) can cause currents in the body that affect electrocardiograms and can produce muscular tetanus and respiratory difficulties. The Food and Drug Administration (FDA) limits allowed changes in magnetic fields to <20 T/sec.

3. High-power RF (as in fast spin echo) can cause tissue heating, which should be kept below an increase of 1° C. The FDA specifies the limitation in the specific absorption rate (SAR) from RF of less than 4 watts/kg averaged over the whole body for a 15-minute period and less than 3 watts/kg averaged over the head in a 10-minute period. The peak value in any gram of tissue must be less than 8.0 watts/kg for the head and less than 12 watts/kg for the body in a 15-minute time period.

4. Pacemakers, biostimulators, hearing aids, and similar electronic devices should never be scanned and should be excluded from fringe magnetic fields greater than 5.0 gauss. (Some newer pacemakers have been scanned with no malfunctions.)

5. Credit cards and magnetic storage devices can be erased at fringe magnetic fields greater than 10 gauss.

6. X-ray tubes, computer display screens, and patients' monitors can be affected in 1- to 5-gauss magnetic fields.

7. Ferromagnetic materials (iron, nickel, cobalt, and steel) should be excluded from MRI rooms because they can become flying objects in strong magnetic fields.

8. Patients with shrapnel, metal fragments, metallic prosthetic devices, heart valves, and surgical clips should be screened because the metal could move in a strong magnetic field and cause critical injuries to the patient.

9. The noise of the pulsing MRI gradients can injure hearing, and ear plugs are recommended for patients being scanned. The FDA specifies that the acoustic

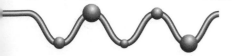

noise levels must be less than 140 dB where patients or staff members are located.

10. Contrast reaction to the gadolinium contrast agent in MRI is a concern.

11. Burns from RF heating of wire leads, jewelry, zippers, dental implants, tattoos, intrauterine devices, and similar devices are a concern.

12. Instruments such as pagers, cell phones, magnetic identification cards, and analog watches can be destroyed if these devices are taken inside MRI rooms.

13. In an emergency (such as a cryogen quench or a heart attack), the patient should be removed from the MRI scanning room.

14. The areas around an MRI room should be zoned, and patients should be surveyed for potential problems.

15. There are no known long-term adverse effects from routine MRI scanning of standard patients.

G. Questions

20-1. Nuclei that have the strongest magnetic moments are those with _____.

(a) High Z   (b) Low N   (c) Odd number [Z and Z + N]
(d) Even number [Z and A]   (e) Only hydrogen

20-2. The Larmor frequency of nuclei depends on _____.

(a) Number of protons and neutrons in the nucleus
(b) Gyromagnetic ratio   (c) Molecule in which nuclei are located
(d) Main magnetic field strength   (e) All of the above

20-3. The shortest relaxation time in MRI is the _____.

(a) T1   (b) T2   (c) T2*   (d) TE   (e) TR

20-4. The spin-lattice relaxation time is also called the _____ relaxation time.

(a) Transverse   (b) T2   (c) T2*   (d) Longitudinal   (e) Gradient

20-5. The coil that provides the best signal-to-noise ratio (SNR) is _____.

(a) Body   (b) Head   (c) Surface   (d) Shim   (e) Gradient

20-6. The relaxation time that controls the free induction decay (FID) signal is the _____ relaxation time.

(a) T1   (b) T2   (c) T2*   (d) TE   (e) TR

20-7. Cryogenic superconductive magnets have their electrical windings cooled by _____.

(a) Liquid oxygen   (b) Liquid fluorine   (c) Liquid hydrogen
(d) Liquid helium   (e) Liquid krypton

20-8. The Larmor frequency of hydrogen nuclei at 1.5 T is about _____ MHz.

(a) 13.7   (b) 23.5   (c) 42.6   (d) 63.9   (e) 89.6

20-9. The brightest signal from a T2-weighted spin-echo MRI image would be from _____.

(a) Pure water   (b) Bone   (c) Fat   (d) Cerebrospinal fluid
(e) Cartilage

20-10. The brightest signal from a T1-weighted spin-echo MRI image of the brain would be from the _____.

(a) Adipose tissue   (b) Gray matter   (c) White matter
(d) Cerebrospinal fluid   (e) Pure water

20-11. A T1-weighted spin-echo image is produced by using a pulse sequence with a _____ TE time and a _____ TR time.

(a) Long, long   (b) Long, short   (c) Short, long   (d) Short, short
(e) Medium, long

20-12. A T2-weighted spin-echo image is produced by using a pulse sequence with a relatively _____ TE time and a relatively _____ TR time.

(a) Long, long   (b) Long, short   (c) Short, long   (d) Short, short
(e) Medium, long

20-13. A proton density–weighted spin-echo image is produced by using a pulse sequence with a _____ TE time and a _____ TR time.

(a) Long, long   (b) Long, short   (c) Short, long   (d) Short, short
(e) Medium, long

20-14. The pulse sequence most often used to nullify the signal from adipose tissue is _____.

(a) Spin echo   (b) Gradient echo   (c) STIR   (d) Echo planar
(e) Fast spin echo

20-15. The fastest MRI pulse sequence is _____.

(a) Spin echo   (b) Gradient echo   (c) STIR   (d) Echo planar
(e) Fast spin echo

20-16. All of the following improve the SNR for a spin echo image, *except* _____.

(a) Thick slice   (b) Large z-gradient   (c) Larger pixel sizes
(d) More NEX   (e) Greater magnet strength

20-17. The "180 degree–90 degree–180 degree" RF pulse sequence is employed in _____.

(a) Spin echo   (b) Partial saturation   (c) Inversion recovery
(d) Magnetization transfer   (e) MRS

20-18. The reconstruction technique used for most MRI images is _____.

(a) Back-projection   (b) 2DFT   (c) Iterative series
(d) Taylor expansion   (e) Matrix inversion

20-19. As the magnetic field strength (B_0) increases, the _____ parameter also increases.

(a) T1   (b) T2   (c) T2*   (d) TI (inversion time)
(e) γ (gyromagnetic ratio)

20-20. The scan time for a spin echo pulse sequence depends on all of the following factors, *except* _____.

(a) NEX   (b) TR   (c) Number of frequency encodings
(d) Number of phase encodings   (e) Use of Fourier symmetry

20-21. The spatial resolution in body MRI images is about _____ LP/mm.

(a) 0.7   (b) 2.2   (c) 4.3   (d) 8.5   (e) 12.1

20-22. The MRI coils that often lead to spatial distortion problems are _____.

(a) Shim   (b) Gradient   (c) Body   (d) Active fringe shield
(e) Eddy shields

20-23. _____ MRI artifacts are repeated low-intensity images in the phase-encoding direction.

(a) Chemical shift   (b) Susceptibility   (c) Motion ghost   (d) Aliasing
(e) Truncation

20-24. _____ MRI artifacts cause images to wrap around to the opposite side and overlap other parts of the anatomy.

(a) Chemical shift   (b) Susceptibility   (c) Motion ghost   (d) Aliasing
(e) Truncation

20-25. _____ MRI artifacts displace fat and tissue to create voids and bright areas of overlap in the frequency-encoding direction of units with large field strength.

(a) Chemical shift   (b) Susceptibility   (c) Motion ghost   (d) Aliasing
(e) Truncation

20-26. _____ MRI artifacts cause voids and distortions near air-tissue interfaces.

(a) Chemical shift   (b) Susceptibility   (c) Motion ghost   (d) Aliasing
(e) Truncation

20-27. Fringe fields from MRI units must be less than _____ gauss in areas where individuals with pacemakers, biostimulators, insulin infusers, and other, similar biologic electronic devices have unrestricted access.

(a) 1.0   (b) 5.0   (c) 10.0   (d) 20.0   (e) 50.0

20-28. Tissue heating from MRI RF signals should be such that the SAR does not deposit more than _____ watts/kg averaged over the body of the patient.

(a) 0.4   (b) 4.0   (c) 8.0   (d) 10.0   (e) 25.0

20-29. Potentially detrimental bioeffects from MRI include all the following, *except* _____.

(a) Acoustic noise   (b) Induced current in central nervous system
(c) Enzyme disassociation   (d) Tattoo heating
(e) Dislodging surgical clips and metal fragments

20-30. The MRI pulse sequence that is most likely to cause the most RF heating in the patient's tissue is _____.

(a) Spin echo   (b) Fast spin echo   (c) Gradient echo
(d) Inversion recovery   (e) Echo planar

H.   Answers

20-1. Answer = (c). Both protons and neutrons have magnetic moments. Both protons and neutrons pair up with particles with the opposite spin so that the net magnetic moment is zero for a pair. Hence, the strongest magnetic moments would be for an odd number of protons and an odd total number of neutrons plus protons. Hydrogen, which has just one proton in the nucleus, is the best example of a strong magnetic moment.

20-2. Answer = (e). The Larmor relationship states that the precessional frequency is a product of the gyromagnetic ratio and the magnetic field strength. However, the gyromagnetic ratio depends on the number of neutrons and protons in the nucleus. From the chemical shift, it is apparent that the precessional frequency for hydrogen depends on the molecules in which the hydrogen atom is located; the frequency is different for hydrogen located in water as compared with hydrogen in lipids. The Larmor frequency is directly related to magnetic field strength.

20-3. Answer = (c). T2* is less than T2, which in turn is less than T1 for most substances. TE and TR are imaging parameters; they do not represent relaxation times, which would be related to the molecule in which the hydrogen is located.

20-4. Answer = (d). See note in this chapter (**A9**). T1 is longitudinal relaxation time, and T2 and T2* are transverse relaxation times.

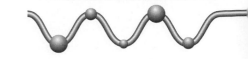

20-5. Answer = (c). Coils that are closest to the hydrogen nuclei being imaged (which are the source of the MRI signal) have the highest signal intensity and SNR.

20-6. Answer = (c). See note and the graph on FID (**A11**).

20-7. Answer = (d). Early cryogenically cooled MRI units used liquid helium in contact with the magnet windings; the liquid helium was surrounded with liquid nitrogen. Modern MRI units only use liquid helium. Liquid nitrogen has a higher temperature and is not conducive to superconduction (zero resistance) in the magnet winding wires. Liquid oxygen is dangerous because it can lead to explosions. Liquid hydrogen could generate extraneous MRI signals and is not used. Fluorine is caustic and usually not in liquid form.

20-8. Answer = (d). See the notes in this chapter, which state that the gyromagnetic ratio for hydrogen is 42.6 MHz/T. Multiplying by 1.5 T equals 63.9 MHz for the Larmor frequency.

20-9. Answer = (a). Pure water has both long T1 and long T2 relaxation times. In a T2-weighted image, water would be one of the last substances to dephase. Therefore, water has the brightest signal, closely followed in brightness by cerebrospinal fluid. Cartilage and bone are solids, which have very little MRI intensity. Adipose (fat) tissue has relatively short T1 and T2 times, resulting in a weak T2-weighted signal.

20-10. Answer = (a). With a very short T1 relaxation time, adipose tissue would have the brightest T1-weighted signal because it realigns rapidly in the z-axis. It would be followed in brightness by white matter and then gray matter. The weakest signal would be from cerebrospinal fluid and water, both of which have very long T1 relaxation times.

20-11. Answer = (d). See table in this chapter (**C1**) for the different combinations of TR and TE.

20-12. Answer = (a). See table in this chapter (**C1**) for the different combinations of TR and TE.

20-13. Answer = (c). See table in this chapter (**C1**) for the different combinations of TR and TE.

20-14. Answer = (c). The IR in the term STIR stands for inversion recovery. The time between the 180-degree and 90-degree pulses (time after inversion, TI) is such that the magnetic moment for fat is zero in the z-direction when the 90-degree pulse is applied. Thus, fat does not produce a signal, and it is nullified from the image.

20-15. Answer = (d). Because of sinusoidally oscillating high-strength gradients, EPI can complete the image in a single shot, which can be on the order of 1 second. However, the images have considerable noise associated with them.

20-16. Answer = (b). Large voxel elements contain more hydrogen atoms, which result in a stronger signal. Therefore, thick slices, smaller matrix, and larger pixel sizes produce a larger voxel. A large z-gradient produces a thin MRI slice, which contains fewer hydrogen atoms. More NEX means that several images are added together, which produces a better SNR. A larger applied main magnetic field produces a stronger signal approximately related to the size of the field, B_0.

20-17. Answer = (c). A spin echo sequence is a 90-degree RF pulse followed by a 180-degree RF pulse. Partial saturation uses a series of 90-degree RF pulses. Magnetization transfer uses a presaturation pulse of a broad, nonresonance frequency to affect the bound versus free proton pools. MRS stands for magnetic resonance spectroscopy. MRS attempts to measure the slightly different resonance frequencies of hydrogen atoms depending on where the nuclei are located in assorted molecules.

20-18. Answer = (b). Because the data in an MRI slice are in the form of phase and frequency encoding, 2DFT is the most direct method of reconstructing MRI images from the measurements. 3DFT can also be used to image volumes,

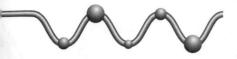

but because of long acquisition times and image problems (aliasing) with the end slices, it is not the most commonly used method.

20-19. Answer = (a). T1 increases the applied main magnetic field. T2 and T2* are relatively insensitive to the strength of the magnetic field. TI is a selectable time between the 180- and 90-degree RF pulses. The gyromagnetic ratio depends on the number of protons and neutrons in the nucleus of the atom, not on the strength of the applied magnetic field.

20-20. Answer = (c). The MRI TR period must be repeated for each phase encoding. However, the frequency encoding is within each TR sequence and does not affect scan time. Each NEX is a repeat of an entire MRI image. Hence, a NEX equal to 2 requires twice the time of a NEX equal to 1. When Fourier symmetry is used, half acquisition can be employed (because of the symmetry of the body) to reduce scan time.

20-21. Answer = (a). Although MRI images typically use a 256×256 matrix, the best resolution would be with a 512×512 matrix. The FoV for body images is around 35 cm. The pixel size for a 512-matrix body image would be about 350 mm/512, or 0.68 mm. The limiting spatial frequency is about $[1.0/(2 \times \text{pixel size})] = 0.7$ LP/mm.

20-22. Answer = (b). The shim coils are used to correct for nonuniformities in the main magnetic field. The body coil is the RF transmit and receive coil for body-sized portions of the anatomy. The active fringe-field shield uses a coil with reverse polarity to attempt to cancel much of the external fringe field of the main magnet. Magnetic shielding or compensation circuits are used to prevent gradient field pulses from inducing currents in the coils or the structure of the MRI unit.

20-23. Answer = (c). Because of motion in the phase-encoding direction (such as breathing), several different images of the chest at different locations are obtained during a typical 6- to 12-minute acquisition. The images appear displaced as low-intensity ghosts.

20-24. Answer = (d). With inadequate sampling, a frequency of 4 Hz can produce results similar to those with a frequency of 2 Hz or 1 Hz. This leads to wraparound of the image from higher frequency to lower frequency.

20-25. Answer = (a). Because fat and tissue have slightly different resonance frequencies, they are slightly displaced in the frequency-encoding direction.

20-26. Answer = (b). Because tissues have a much larger susceptibility to a magnetic field than does air, the applied magnetic lines are drawn toward the tissue, forming signal loss and distortions in the image.

20-27. Answer = (b). See note in this chapter (**F4**).

20-28. Answer = (b). See note in this chapter (**F3**).

20-29. Answer = (c). The strength of the magnetic field, gradients, and RF power are insufficient to break apart chemical substances in the body. The acoustic noise from the gradient coils of some MRI pulse sequences can, however, affect hearing. Small electrical currents can be induced in the patient's body, which could cause arrhythmias and affect the electrocardiogram. RF power can transfer to the metal dyes in tattoos or cosmetics and can cause burns. Magnetic fields can dislodge or rotate ferromagnetic metal shrapnel or surgical clips.

20-30. Answer = (b). Fast spin-echo sequences use multiple 180-degree RF pulses. The SAR values for these sequences are large and cause considerable tissue heating. Echo planar imaging can also be a concern because it uses continuously oscillating gradients and high power to image rapidly; however, the scan times for echo planar imaging are usually short, which limits heating effects.

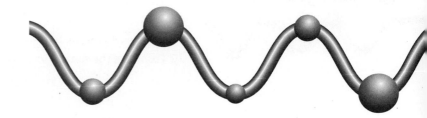

CHAPTER TWENTY-ONE

Nuclear Medicine Physics

A.   Basic Concepts

1. ***The line of stability*** is a graph of the number of neutrons versus the number of protons in the nucleus of stable atoms. For elements with low atomic number (Z), the line of stability is located where there are equal numbers of neutrons and protons. For elements with high Z numbers, the line of stability is located where there are more neutrons than protons. Above or below this line, the nuclei are unstable and decay with radioactive emissions.

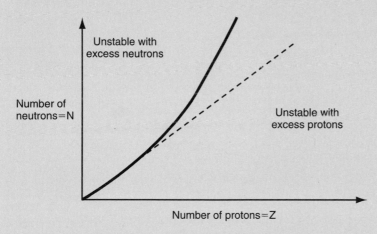

- Atoms with ***excess neutrons*** in the nuclei are created in a ***nuclear reactor***, where there are huge fluxes of neutrons to bombard the stable atoms.

- Atoms with ***excess protons*** in the nuclei are created in ***particle accelerators***, such as linear accelerators and cyclotrons, which bombard stable nuclei with charged particles.

2. Atoms are designated by the following symbols.

- Z = atomic number = number of protons in nucleus

- N = neutron number = number of neutrons in nucleus

- A = mass number = sum of neutrons plus protons in nucleus = $Z + N$

- The symbol for the nucleus is $_Z X^A$; for a carbon atom with six protons + six neutrons, the symbol would be $_6 C^{12}$.

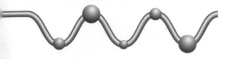

3. The definitions of different types of nuclei can be remembered by looking at the next-to-last letter in the applicable term, which indicates which particle remains the same.

- Isoto*p*e (*p*, proton) has Z same, N different, and A different (e.g., $_6C^{11}$, $_6C^{12}$, $_6C^{13}$).

- Isoto*n*e (*n*, neutron) has Z different, N same, and A different (e.g., $_6C^{12}$, $_7N^{13}$, $_8O^{14}$).

- Isob*a*r (*a*, mass number) has Z different, N different, and A same (e.g., $_6C^{14}$, $_7N^{14}$, $_8O^{14}$).

- Isom*e*r (*e*, everything) has Z same, N same, and A same (e.g., $_{43}Tc^{99m}$, $_{43}Tc^{99}$—everything the same, only the energy in the nucleus different).

4. ***Mass deficit*** is the loss in mass that occurs when neutrons and protons are combined in the nucleus. The lost mass is converted into energy to hold the nucleus together.

- $E = mc^2$ = energy gained from loss of mass. $E = 0.511$ MeV for an electron and $E = 931$ to 932 MeV for a neutron or proton $\cong 1$ amu (atomic mass unit).

- Typically, nuclear binding energy is between 1 and 8 MeV per particle (nucleon), with an average of about 2 to 4 MeV per nucleon.

- Sometimes the binding energy is negative, indicating the possibility of splitting the nucleus (fission).

5. Balancing nuclear equations means that the superscripts and subscripts all add up to the same value on both sides of the nuclear equation.

- For example, $_5B^{11} \rightarrow {_ZX^A} + {_2\alpha^4}$

- Superscripts: $11 = A + 4$ *or* $A = 7$

- Subscripts: $5 = Z + 2$ *or* $Z = 3$

- The decay product is: $_3X^7 = {_3Li^7}$.

6. All radioactive atoms eventually decay. The rate of decay is an exponential process.

- $[N/N_0] = \exp[-\lambda t]$, where exp is the natural number "e" $= 2.7182....$

- $N_0 =$ the initial number of radioactive atoms.

- $\lambda =$ the decay constant for the particular radioactive nucleus $= 0.693/T_{1/2}$.

- $T_{1/2} =$ the half-life or time in which half the radioactive atoms decay.

- $A =$ activity $= \lambda \times N =$ fractional decays per unit time.

- For each multiple of elapsed time (t) equal to $T_{1/2}$, the activity decreases by $^1/_2$.

- Activity can be measured in new SI units of ***becquerels (Bq) = 1 decay per second (dps)***.

- An older unit of activity is ***1.0 curie (Ci) = 3.7 $\times$ 10^{+10} dps***.

- ***Example:*** If the $T_{1/2}$ of Tc-99m is exactly 6 hours and 120 mCi are delivered at 6:00 AM, how much activity will remain at midnight of the same day?

- ***Solution*** to example is as follows:

  t = 18 hours; $t/T_{1/2} = 18.0$ hours/6 hours $= 3.0$ half-lives

  $[N/N_0] = (1/2) \times (1/2) \times (1/2) = (1/8)$

  $A = (1/8) \times 120$ mCi $= 15$ mCi

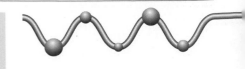

7. ***There are five basic nuclear decay processes*** that occur for most radioactive isotopes in nuclear medicine: positron emission (β+), electron capture (EC), beta decay (β−), isomeric transitions (ITs), and alpha emission (α).

- ***Beta minus (β−) decay occurs for radioactive atoms with excess neutrons.*** In the nucleus, a neutron (n) decays into a proton (P) + electron (β) + antineutrino ($\bar{v}$).

$$_0n^1 \rightarrow {}_{+1}P^1 + {}_{-1}\beta^0 + {}_0\bar{v}^0$$

(a) A ***beta particle*** is an electron that originates in the nucleus. If the electron originates in orbital shells of an atom, it is simply an electron.

(b) The beta electron and the antineutrino are ejected from the nucleus, and the nucleus recoils. Thus, three objects are sharing the energy, and the average energy of the beta is about 33% of the maximum energy.

(c) The nucleus loses one neutron that decays to produce one proton, moving the new nucleus toward the line of stability.

(d) A neutrino (υ) is a particle with no charge and no rest mass that travels very fast and penetrates through most matter.

(e) Following ejection of the beta, there can be further loss of energy by gamma emission.

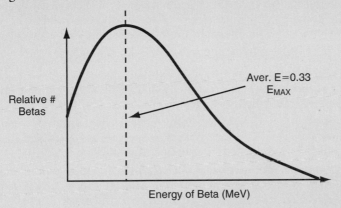

- ***Electron capture (K-capture) occurs for radioactive atoms with excess protons***. A K-shell electron (e) orbiting the atom is captured by the nucleus. The electron combines with a proton in the nucleus to form a neutron.

$$_{-1}e^0 + {}_{+1}P^1 + \text{energy} \rightarrow {}_0n^1 + {}_0v^0$$

(a) The neutrino is ejected from the nucleus.

(b) The number of protons in the nucleus decreases by one and the number of neutrons increases by one, moving the new nucleus toward the line of stability.

(c) After the decay, the K-shell is missing an electron, which results in electron transitions and the emission of characteristic x-rays.

- ***Positron (β+) decay occurs for radioactive atoms with excess protons***. Positron decay begins when 1.02 MeV of nuclear energy is used to create a regular electron and an antiparticle, positive electron (β+). The created electron in the nucleus then combines with a proton to create a neutron. The neutrino and the positron are ejected from the nucleus.

$$1.02 \text{ MeV energy} \rightarrow (\beta+) + (_{-1}e^0) \rightarrow (\beta+) + (_{-1}e^0) + {}_{+1}P^1 + \text{energy}$$
$$\rightarrow {}_0n^1 + (\beta+) + {}_0v^0$$

(a) The neutrino and the positron are ejected from the nucleus, and the nucleus recoils.

(b) The number of protons in the nucleus decreases by one, and the number of neutrons increases by one, moving the new nucleus toward the line of stability.

(c) After the decay, there can be further loss of energy by gamma ray emission.

- *Isomeric transitions* (γ, gamma ray emission) occur for radioactive atoms with excess energy in their nuclei.

  Excess energy in nucleus → γ *or* e + x-ray *or* e + Auger e

  (a) A *gamma ray* is an photon that originates in the nucleus. If the photon originates outside the nucleus, it is called an x-ray.

  (b) *Internal conversion* is a process in which the gamma ray occasionally interacts with an inner shell orbital electron on the way out of the nucleus from which it was emitted. The orbital electron is ejected and is called an *internal conversion electron*. The remaining electrons then make a transition to fill the vacancy in an inner shell and produce a *characteristic x-ray*. Internal conversion electrons can be distinguished from beta particles because betas have a range of energies and conversion electrons are monoenergetic.

  (c) A third alternative is the emission of the *internal conversion electron*, but the characteristic x-ray interacts with an outer shell electron in the same atom, and an *Auger electron* is emitted and the x-ray disappears.

  (d) The alternatives are (1) just a gamma ray, (2) no gamma ray but instead an internal conversion electron + characteristic x-ray, and (3) no gamma ray but instead an internal conversion electron + an Auger electron.

- *Alpha particle emission* typically occurs for radioactive atoms with a high atomic number of $Z > 80$.

  (a) An *alpha particle* is a helium atom missing its orbital electrons. An alpha is two neutrons plus two protons.

  (b) Typically, these radioactive atoms (after decay) continue to emit alpha particles in a series of decays. Each emission reduces the mass number by 4 units and the atomic number (Z) by 2 units.

  (c) The *four well-known series with a chain of alpha particle decays* are thorium (4N), neptunium (4N + 1), uranium (4N + 2), and actinium (4N + 3). The phrase "4N + 1" means that the mass number of each product in the decay can be expressed as 4 times an integer plus one. *The radium-to-radon decay is part of one alpha series decay chain that is "4N + 2."*

8. Energy level diagrams are used to describe three different decay processes.

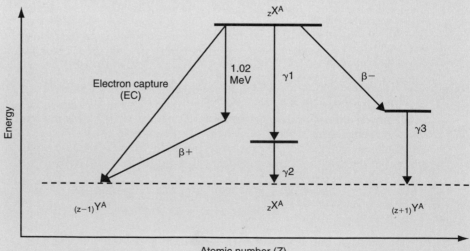

9. Some important radioisotopes that are used in nuclear medicine are listed in the table.

ISOTOPE	PRINCIPAL EMISSION	PERCENT EMISSION	ENERGY (keV)	HALF-LIFE
$_1H^3$	β–	100	18.6	12.5 yr
$_6C^{14}$	β–	100	156.1	5730 yr
$_{15}P^{32}$	β–	100	1708	14.3 days
$_{27}Co^{57}$	γ_2	85.9	122	270 days
$_{31}Ga^{67}$	Many γ's	46	184–394	78.1 hr
$_{36}Kr^{81m}$	γ	100	191	13.0 sec
$_{42}Mo^{99}$	Many β particles	19 →	740–778	66.7 hr
$_{43}Tc^{99m}$	γ_2 and γ_3	88	140.5–142.6	6.05 hr
$_{49}In^{111}$	γ_1 and γ_2	90 and 94	172 and 247	2.81 days
$_{49}In^{113m}$	γ_1	62.1	392	99.4 min
$_{53}I^{123}$	11 γ's	85 (2 γ's)	159 and 529	13.0 hr
$_{53}I^{125}$	γ and X photons	147	27–35	60.2 days
$_{53}I^{131}$	14 γ's	87 →	284–364	8.06 days
$_{54}Xe^{133}$	Many γ's	36 →	81	5.3 days
$_{81}Ti^{201}$	X and γ photons	94 →	69–82	73.0 hr

10. There are other radioactive interactions such as fission, fusion, and (n, γ) interactions. However, most of these processes are not normally included in routine nuclear medicine imaging.

B. Radionuclide Generators

1. A **generator** contains an alumina (or other substrate) **column** unto which is coated a **parent radioactive material**.

   - A **daughter** radioactive material is produced by the decay of the parent material.

   - An **eluant** is a solution that is passed through the generator to dissolve the daughter radioactive material from the column.

   - The parent material is chemically different and is not dissolved by the eluant.

   - A **microscopic filter** is used to stop debris, include flakes of the column with the parent, from passing through to a receptacle.

   - The **elution** contains only the daughter (unless there is **breakthrough**, which is contamination by the parent by flakes from the column). The daughter decays at a rate dictated by its half-life.

   - As more of the parent source decays, more daughter material is created.

   - **There are two competing processes**: The **parent decays** at a rate dictated by its half-life, creating more daughter material, and the new **daughter decays** with a different rate dictated by the daughter's half-life.

   - Equilibrium is reached after a period of time in which the activities of the parent and daughter are nearly equal (see figure shown on next page).

2. **The generator principle** states that at **equilibrium, the activities** of the parent and daughter are almost the same.

$$A_d \cong [\lambda_d/(\lambda_d - \lambda_p)] \times A_p \cong A_p$$

where $\lambda = 0.693/T_{1/2}$.

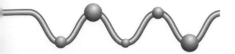

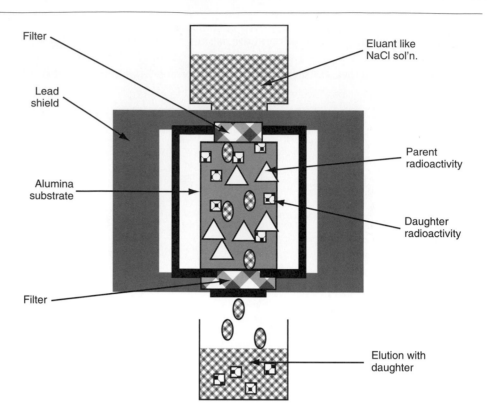

- The ***parent activity*** is decaying at a rate controlled by its half-life.

  $A_p = (1/2)^y$ where $y = (t'/_pT_{1/2})$

  y = (time since calibration/half-life parent).

- ***Buildup of activity*** of the daughter after elution depends on the half-life of both the parent and the daughter.

  $A_d \cong A_p[1.0 - (0.5)^X]$ where $X = (t/_dT_{1/2})$

  X = (time since elution/half-life daughter).

- An example is shown in the table for a Tc-99m generator. The half-life of the parent is about 67 hours, and the half-life of the daughter is about 6 hours.

TIME SINCE ELUTION (HR)	$X = t/T_d$	$[1 - (0.5)^X]$	$Y = t/T_p$	A_p	A_d
0	0	0.0	0	$1.0\,A_0$	0
6	1	0.5	0.090	$0.94\,A_0$	$0.47\,A_0$
12	2	0.75	0.179	$0.88\,A_0$	$0.66\,A_0$
18	3	0.875	0.269	$0.83\,A_0$	$0.73\,A_0$
24	4	0.938	0.358	$0.78\,A_0$	$0.73\,A_0$
36	6	0.984	0.537	$0.69\,A_0$	$0.68\,A_0$
48	8	0.996	0.716	$0.61\,A_0$	$0.61\,A_0$
67	11.2	0.9996	1.0	$0.50\,A_0$	$0.50\,A_0$

3. In ***secular equilibrium***, the half-life of the parent is much, much longer than the daughter's half-life ($T_p \gg T_d$). After elution, it takes about $4T_d$ for the activity of the daughter to approach the activity of the parent. Both materials then

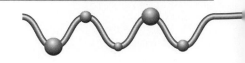

stay at equilibrium without much change in activity for a very long time. See the graph below.

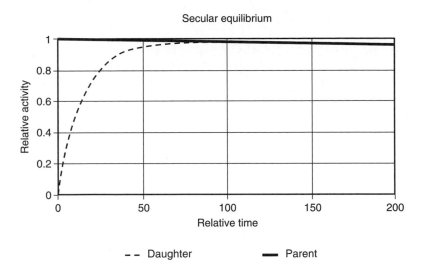

4. In ***transient equilibrium***, the half-life of the parent is appreciably longer than the daughter's half-life by a factor of 10 to 20 times ($T_p > T_d$). After elution, it takes about $4T_d$ for the activity of the daughter to exceed slightly the activity of the parent. Both materials then decay at equilibrium with the decay rate of the parent as long as they are mixed together.

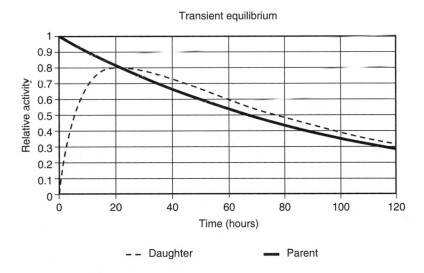

5. For a ***Tc-99m generator, federal regulations*** limit the amount of Mo-99 impurity allowed in the eluant.

- No more than 1.5 µCi of Mo^{99} per 1.0 mCi of Tc^{99m} eluant

- No more than 5.0 µCi of Mo^{99} per patient injection

- The beta particles from Mo^{99} contribute significantly to the radiation dose to the patient.

- ***The Mo breakthrough test*** is done by placing Tc-99m eluant in a leaded container. The lead container attenuates most of the 140-keV gammas from technetium, but the high-energy (740- to 780-keV) gammas of Mo-99 penetrate the lead and are counted.

C. Radiopharmaceutical Dosimetry

1. ***For charged particles and nonpenetrating photons (E < 30 keV),*** the energy is deposited locally. At the location at which the radiopharmaceutical biologic concentrates, the energy is released in emissions deposited at the same organ site.

   $$D_{np} = 3.07 \times F_{organ} \times (A_0/M) \times T_{eff} \times E \text{ in units of cGy}$$

   where F_{organ} = fraction of injected activity concentrating in the organ, A_0 = injected activity in μCi, M = mass of the organ in grams, T_{eff} = effective half-life in hours, and E = average energy of the radiation in MeV.

   - ***Concentration:*** Radiation dose increases with more activity concentration in the organ.

   - ***Activity:*** Radiation dose increases with more injected activity.

   - ***Effective half-life:*** Radiation dose increases with longer effective half-life.

   - ***Energy:*** Radiation dose increases with higher particle energy.

   - ***Organ mass:*** Radiation dose decreases with larger organ mass. If the same radioactivity intended for an adult is injected into a baby, the radiation doses are greater because of the smaller organ sizes.

2. ***The effective half-life (T_{eff})*** is the effective time that the radioisotope stays inside the body. The elimination of radioisotope is by two different methods: excretion with a biologic half-life (T_B) and photon emission decay with a physical half-life (T_P).

   $$T_{eff} = (T_B \times T_P)/(T_B + T_P)$$

   - ***If $T_B \cong T_P$,*** the effective half-life is approximately $0.5 \times T_P$.

   - ***If either the $T_B \gg T_P$ or $T_B \ll T_P$,*** the effective half-life is slightly less than the smaller of the two half-lives.

   - If the two half-lives are just a little different, calculate half of each half-life, and the effective half-life is between those two values.

   - For example, if T_P = 6 hours and T_B = 10 hours, the T_{eff} is nearly midway between 0.5 times each half-life or midway between 3 hours and 5 hours. $T_{eff} \cong 4$ hours. It is precisely equal to 3.75 hours; the approximation is reasonably accurate.

3. ***For gamma ray radiation,*** some of the radiation is deposited locally, and some escapes the body entirely without depositing any energy internally. The activity in some organs irradiates other nearby organs. The calculation for gamma-emitting radiopharmaceuticals is complex; computer Monte Carlo calculations in a simulated human are used to assess the dosimetry.

   $$D_{gamma} = F_{organ} \times (A_0/M_{source}) \times (1.44 T_{eff}) \times S \text{ (organ source} \rightarrow \text{organ target)}$$

   - Many of the effects are the same as for nonpenetrating radiation.

   - The S values are found in tables for different isotopes and different source and target organs.

4. In general, nuclear medicine studies aim to use enough radioactivity to obtain good photon statistics.

   - Critical organ radiation doses for most examinations are nearly 5 cGy.

   - Whole body radiation doses are 0.5% to 5% of the critical organ dose.

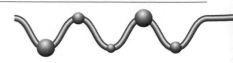

D. Radiation Detectors

1. Efficiencies of detector systems fall into different categories.

   - **Geometric efficiency** is the fraction of all emitted radiation that hits the detector.

   - A **4π detector** has all the radiation impinging on its surface, such as an NaI crystal with a hole drilled into it (a well counter).

   - A **2π detector** has 50% of radiation passing into its surface.

   - **Intrinsic efficiency** is the fraction of the incident radiation that the detectors actually measure.

   - **Overall efficiency** = geometric efficiency × intrinsic efficiency.

2. **Dead time** is the time after a detected event in which the detector cannot register another interaction.

   - With **paralyzable detectors**, additional events occurring during the dead time extend the duration of the dead time. Very high radioactivity can cause the detector system to register zero count rate.

   - With **nonparalyzable detectors**, additional events occurring during the dead time do not extend the dead time, but they are not measured. Very high radioactivity causes the system to reach some maximum count rate that does not increase with more radioactivity.

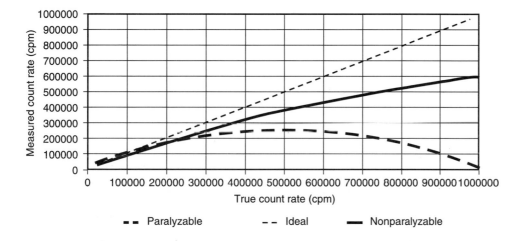

3. Gas detectors have a voltage between a center electrode and an outer shell that collects the charge created by ionizing radiation.

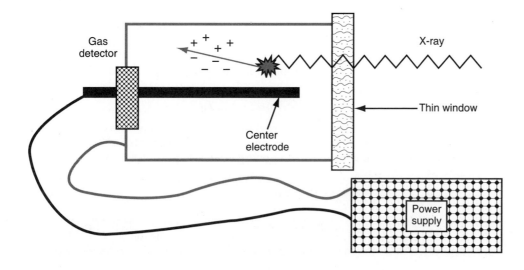

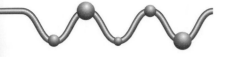

4. Gas detector systems fall into several different categories. There are five voltage regions of gas detectors.

- *Region 1: Recombination region* of the ionization curve; the detector is not useful. Typically at least 200 to 400 volts are needed to prevent recombination.

- *Region 2: Ionization region;* used by the detector to collect all ion pairs created inside the gas detector. In this region, exposure (in mR or R) can be measured.

- *Region 3: Proportional region;* creates additional charge by using higher voltages to create more ion pairs for each initial ionization. The charge is proportional to but greater than the initial ionization. Proportion detectors are use to assess charged particle radiation such as betas and alphas and neutrons.

- *Region 4: Geiger-Mueller (GM) region;* uses a few ionizations in gas to amplify to a large amount of charge. The size of the charge is not related to the initial ionization. The GM region is useful only for detecting and counting a small amount of radioactivity. Radiation doses cannot be determined in this region.

- *Region 5: Avalanche region;* the voltage at which spontaneous discharges can occur without any radioactivity present. The detector can be damaged in this region by continuous discharges initiated by the high voltage, causing a spark.

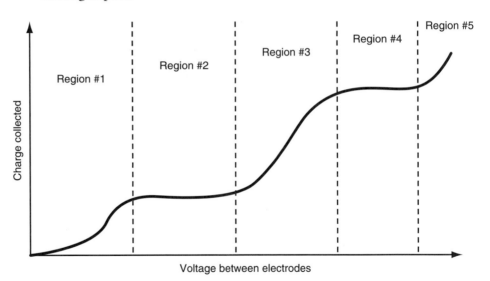

5. *GeLi solid-state detectors* are often used to measure the energy spectra of photons because of their ability to measure small differences in energy of 2 to 3 keV.

- Ionization is created directly in solid-state material and collected.

- These detectors are usually cooled with liquid nitrogen to reduce background signals (see top figure on next page).

6. *Liquid scintillation detectors* are used to measure small amounts of low-energy charged particles in fluids, such as C^{14} in urine or blood, and wipes of radioactive materials that emit low-energy charged particles.

- *Refrigeration* of units is used to reduce photomultiplier tube (PMT) noise.

- *Quenching* by water and other substances can reduce signal.

- *Coincidence detection* uses two PMTs to look for a simultaneous signal to avoid counting noise pulses. In the figure, PHA stands for pulse height analyzer, AMP stands for amplifier circuit (see bottom figure on next page).

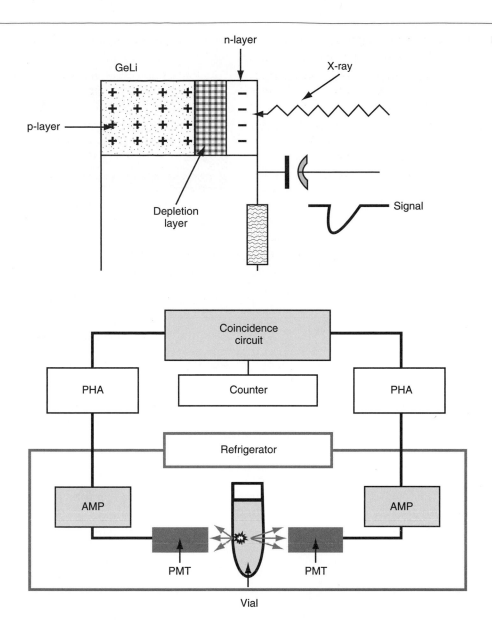

E. NaI Crystal Scintillation Detectors

1. Scintillation crystals such as sodium iodide (NaI) or cesium iodide (CsI) convert some of the energy deposited in the crystal by gamma and x-ray photons into light.

- In photoelectric interactions, all the photon energy is deposited in the crystal.

- For Compton interactions, only a portion of the energy is deposited in the crystal.

- The most energy deposited with Compton scatter is for a 180-degree scatter in the crystal:

$$\Delta E = (2\alpha E_0)/[1 + 2\alpha]$$

where $\alpha = E_0/511$ keV and E_0 = initial energy.

- The least amount of energy deposited is zero in a zero-degree Compton scatter.

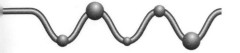

- The light emitted is directly proportional to the energy deposited in the crystal. The percentage varies from about 8% up to 25% to 50%.

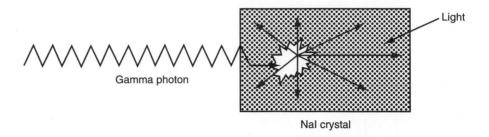

COMPTON SCATTER ANGLE (DEGREES)	ENERGY DEPOSITED IN CRYSTAL FOR Tc-99m 140-keV PHOTONS
0	0
45	10.4 keV
90	30.1 keV
135	44.6 keV
180	49.5 keV

2. PMTs capture the light from the scintillation crystal and convert it into an electrical signal whose amplitude is proportional to the light emitted, which is in turn proportional to the energy deposited in the crystal.

- The photocathode captures the light and converts it into a few electrons.
- There are several hundred volts between dynodes.
- The voltage accelerates the electrons, and, when they collide with the dynodes, the number of electrons is multiplied each time.
- With many dynodes, the number of electrons is multiplied many times to produce a strong signal that is proportional to the amount of energy deposited in the crystal.

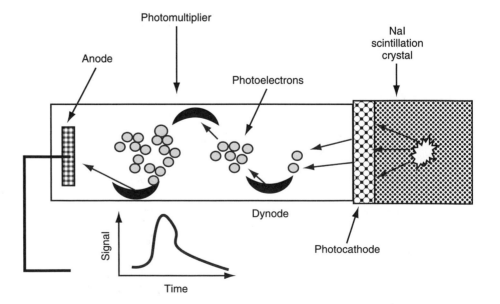

3. A **_pulse height analyzer (PHA)_** counts only signals with an amplitude greater than a lower level threshold (LLT) and less than an upper level threshold (ULT).

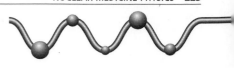

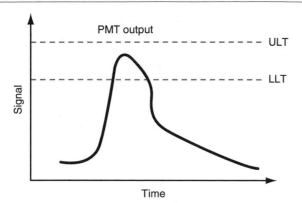

4. A ***multichannel analyzer (MCA)*** is a series of PHAs that are adjacent to one another so that the entire photon spectrum of all gamma photons interacting in the scintillation crystal with different amounts of energy deposited is recorded.

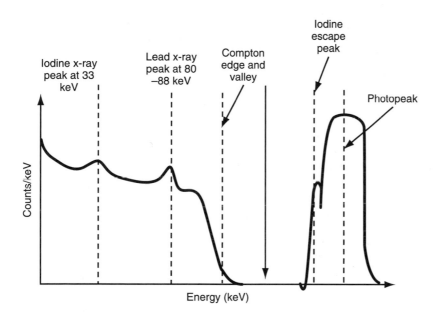

- At the lowest energy, the peak is due to ***dark current*** in the PMT.

- The ***iodine x-ray peak*** occurs at 33 keV. It is a peak related to a photoelectric interaction in the iodine atoms of the crystal followed by escape of ionization and the iodine characteristic x-ray depositing its energy into the scintillator crystal.

- The ***lead x-ray peak*** occurs at 80 to 88 keV. The peak is due to characteristic x-rays coming from the lead that surrounds the detector.

- The ***Compton edge*** is the most energy deposited from a single 180-degree Compton scatter in the scintillation crystal.

- The ***Compton valley*** is the difference between the most energy deposited in a single 180-degree scatter in the crystal and a photoelectric event with all the energy deposited in the crystal.

- ***X-ray escape peak*** refers to the photoelectric deposition of all the energy with the characteristic x-ray of iodine escaping from the crystal. The energy is at 33 keV below the photopeak energy.

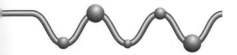

- **FWHM** (full width at half maximum) is the width in energy of the photopeak at half its maximum counts. It is a measure of the energy resolution of the detector.

- A **coincidence peak** occurs when two photons interact simultaneously in the crystal, which causes them to look like a single photon with double the energy.

F. Scintillation Cameras

1. The scintillation camera uses a large-diameter (10- to 14-inch) NaI crystal that is either circular or rectangular to stop the photons and create light in proportion to the energy deposited in the crystal. The light is then detected by a large number of PMTs positioned around the crystal.

   - **Z (or integral) signal** is the sum of the signals from all of the PMTs. This signal is proportional to the **energy deposited** in the crystal by the gamma.

   - **X and Y (or differential)** is related to the **location** of the signal in the crystal.

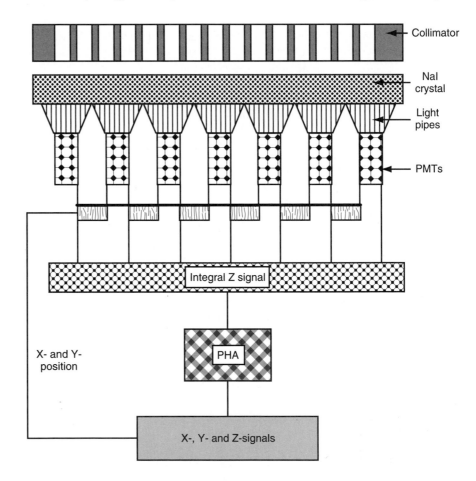

- Light pipes gather light in the crystal and direct it into PMTs.

- NaI crystal thickness ranges from 0.5 to 0.25 inch. Thinner crystals have better spatial resolution, but they are less efficient at detecting gamma photons. Thicker crystals are more efficient at detecting gammas but have degraded spatial resolution.

- The PHA counts only photons that deposit all their energy in the crystal; thereby, scattered photons that have lost energy externally are rejected.

2. ***Collimators*** are used to cause gammas from a particular point in space to interact only with a corresponding point in the crystal. Collimators consist of holes in a thick lead plate that is mounted in front of the scintillation crystal. There are basically four types of scintillation camera collimators.

- ***Parallel hole collimators*** are the most common type. These collimators neither magnify nor minify the image.

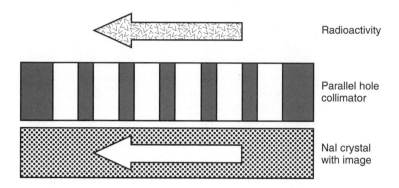

- ***Convergent collimators*** enlarge the image by means of holes that cause the image to converge to a point in front of the collimator.

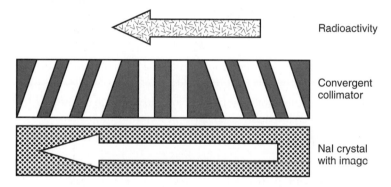

- ***Divergent collimators*** are used to minify the image by means of holes that cause the image to diverge from the view of the NaI crystal to points in front of the collimator.

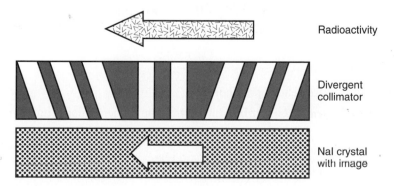

- ***Pinhole collimators*** can either magnify or minify the source object, depending on the distance of the source object from the collimator. If the distance is >L (focal length), the image is minified. If the distance is <L, the image

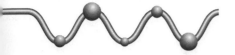

is magnified. The left and right are reversed. This collimator is useful for higher energy gammas when the outer shell of the pinhole can be made thicker. It is also used to enlarge small parts of the anatomy by different amounts.

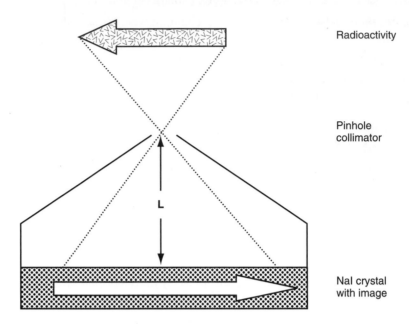

- The efficiency of parallel hole collimators decreases with thicker lead septa (t) between holes. However, thick septa are needed for high-energy photons.

- The efficiency of parallel hole collimators decreases as the length of holes (L) increases. Long holes are needed for better spatial resolution.

- The efficiency of parallel hole collimators increases as the diameter (d) of the holes increases. Wide holes result in worse spatial resolution.

- **_Sensitivity (G, efficiency) for a parallel hole collimator_** with a point source is

  $$G_{pt} = \text{sensitivity} = d^4/[4\pi L^2(d + t)^2]$$

- Sensitivity for a parallel hole collimator with a plane source is

  $$G_{plane} = \text{sensitivity} = Nd^4/[4\pi L^2]$$

  where N = number of holes.

- The **_resolution of a parallel hole collimator_** degrades with distance (X) away from the collimator face. The blur is measured by the **_FWHM_** counts for a point source.

  $$FWHM = [d(X + L)]/L$$

  where d and L were defined previously.

3. **_Problems that degrade the quality_** of scintillation camera images include the following:

   - Motion related to long acquisition times
   - Counting of scattered gamma photons
   - Displacement away from the collimator
   - Septal penetration by high-energy gammas
   - Light and photon scattering in the NaI crystal
   - Collimator limitations

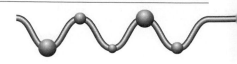

- Tissue attenuation that decreases count rates
- Superimposition of various sources in the body
- Energy uncertainty related to 20% PHA windows
- NaI crystal defects
- Too few counts per image, which results in quantum mottle and limits the ability to see "hot" and "cold" areas in the image

4. ***Uniformity*** is measured in two different ways.

- ***Intrinsic uniformity*** requires removal of the collimator and the placement of a Tc-99m point source far from the crystal. It measures only crystal uniformity.

- ***Extrinsic uniformity*** places a flood source (Tc-99m in water or a Co-57 plastic disk) directly on the collimator. It measures the uniformity of both the crystal and the collimator.

- Uniformity measurements should accumulate at least 1 million counts to limit statistical variation.

- Without correction, uniformity should be better than ±10%. With correction, uniformity can be better than ±5%.

5. Quality control (QC) tests for scintillation cameras include the following:

- Uniformity
- Spatial resolution using bar patterns and a flood source
- Spatial distortion using uniform hole patterns and a flood source
- Centering of PHA around the photopeak
- Dead time measurements of count rate loss

6. SPECT (single photon emission computed tomography) uses one or more scintillation cameras, which rotate around the body and reconstruct the data to form tomographic images.

- Careful balance and mechanical centering of the various detectors are required.

- Transmission measurements with an external source are required to correct for tissue attenuation to quantify amounts of activity.

G.   Positron Emission Tomography (PET) Units

1. PET uses cyclotron-produced short-half-life radioisotopes that emit positrons ($\beta+$). The major positron emitters are listed in the table.

POSITRON EMITTER	HALF-LIFE (MINUTES)	AVERAGE $\beta+$ ENERGY (MeV)
O-16	2	0.72
N-13	10	0.49
C-11	20	0.38
F-18	110	0.28

2. The positrons lose energy by ionization as they travel through tissue. In the process, they slow down. Because the positron is an antiparticle, it eventually combines with an electron (after it slows down), and the two particles are annihilated. As matter is destroyed, two 0.511-MeV photons are produced that travel in nearly 180-degree opposite directions.

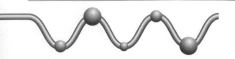
3. PET scanners use banks of detectors to measure two nearly simultaneous events (coincidence circuits) with energies of 0.511 MeV (with PHA) to discern a positron annihilation. The annihilation is on a straight line between the two detectors recording simultaneous 0.511-MeV events.

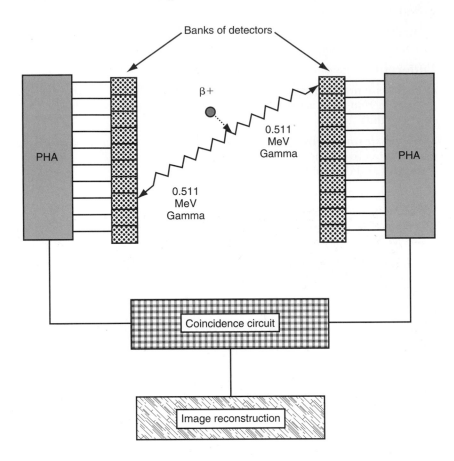

4. To quantify tissue attenuation, corrections must be determined with a separate external ring source.

5. Factors that affect image quality include the following:

    ● The positron travels about 1 to 4 mm before the annihilation occurs, which results in malpositioning of the emission.

    ● The two 0.511-MeV photons are not exactly 180 degrees apart, which causes slight malpositioning of the emissions.

    ● False coincidences occur with one photon from two different decays occurring at the same time.

    ● Detector size and collimator size introduce some uncertainty in positioning.

    ● Uncertainty in PHA windows allows small-angle scattered photons to be accepted.

6. Advantages of PET scanners include the following:

    ● Chemical tracers can be formed with atoms typically found in tissue such as carbon, nitrogen, and oxygen.

    ● High-energy photons are not attenuated much by body anatomy.

    ● Short half-life means activity in patients decays rapidly.

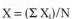

H.   Nuclear Medicine Statistics

1.   **Mean (X)** is the average of a group of measurements (X_i).

$$X = (\Sigma\, X_i)/N$$

where N = number of measurements.

2.   **Standard deviation (σ)** is approximated by the square root of the mean value.

$$1\sigma \cong (X)^{0.5}$$

3.   **Variance** is equal to the standard deviation squared.

$$\text{Variance} = \sigma^2$$

4.   **Confidence interval** is the percentage of the measurements that fall within plus or minus the indicated value above or below the mean value of the measurements.

VALUE AROUND MEAN	CONFIDENCE INTERVAL (%)
±1σ	68.3
±2σ	95.5
±3σ	99.7

5.   The standard deviation for count rates is different.

$$1\sigma_{RATE} = \sqrt{(R/T)}$$

where R = count rate and T = counting time.

6.   **Net counts (or count rate)** are source plus background minus background.

7.   Standard deviation for the sum or difference of two sets of counts is given as

$$1\sigma_{COUNTS} = \sqrt{(N_1)+(N_2)}$$

8.   Standard deviation for the sum of or difference in count rates is given as

$$1\sigma_{RATE} = \sqrt{(R_1/T_1)+(R_2/T_2)}$$

I.   Questions

21-1.   The Tc-99m radioisotope generator is an example of the physics principle of _____.

(a) Cascade process   (b) Retrograde flow   (c) Transient equilibrium
(d) Secular equilibrium   (e) Nuclear propagation

21-2.   Emission from an isomeric decay can include all of the following, *except* _____.

(a) X-ray photons   (b) Gamma ray photons
(c) Internal conversion electrons   (d) Auger electrons   (e) Beta particles

21-3.   The amount of Mo-99 "breakthrough" allowed per mCi of Tc-99m eluant is _____ μCi.

(a) 0.015   (b) 0.15   (c) 1.5   (d) 15.0   (e) 150

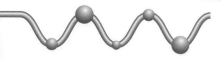

21-4. A 500-mCi Tc-99m radioisotope generator is not used for 137 hours. Then it is eluted. Twelve hours later, the generator is eluted a second time. The two elutions are combined. The total activity in the combined two elutions is about _____ mCi.

(a) 31   (b) 67   (c) 87   (d) 111   (e) 186

21-5. A decay process that occurs in nuclei that have excess protons and is always followed by the emission of characteristic x-rays is called _____.

(a) Beta minus   (b) Beta plus   (c) Isomeric transition
(d) Electron capture   (e) Alpha emission

21-6. A decay process that only reduces the excess energy in the nucleus is called _____.

(a) Beta minus   (b) Beta plus   (c) Isomeric transition
(d) Electron capture   (e) Alpha emission

21-7. A decay process that occurs in nuclei that have excess neutrons is called _____.

(a) Beta minus   (b) Beta plus   (c) Isomeric transition
(d) Electron capture   (e) Alpha emission

21-8. A decay process that occurs primarily in nuclei with Z > 80, such as radium, is called _____.

(a) Beta minus   (b) Beta plus   (c) Isomeric transition
(d) Electron capture   (e) Alpha emission

21-9. Nuclei with an excess number of neutrons are usually created by radiation bombardment in a _____.

(a) Linear accelerator   (b) Van de Graaff generator   (c) Cyclotron
(d) Nuclear reactor   (e) Betatron

21-10. The radiation dose to a critical organ from a beta-emitting radiopharmaceutical increases for greater amounts of the following factors, *except* _____.

(a) Organ mass   (b) Effective half-life   (c) Photon energy
(d) Biodistribution   (e) Injected activity

21-11. The combination of physical half-life (T_P) and biologic half-life that results in the greater critical organ dose is $T_P =$ _____ hours and $T_B =$ _____ hours.

(a) 6, 48   (b) 110, 5   (c) 4, 100   (d) 7, 7   (e) 80, 7

21-12. The number of gamma photons produced per second by a 10-Bq source of Co-60 is _____, and for Tc-99m it is _____.

(a) 5, 5   (b) 10, 5   (c) 20, 9   (d) 10, 20   (e) 10, 10

21-13. Emissions from a positron decay include _____.

(a) Alpha particles   (b) Protons   (c) Neutrinos
(d) Characteristic x-rays   (e) Neutrons

21-14. When $_7N^{13}$ decays by means of positron emission, it produces an atom of _____.

(a) $_8O^{15}$ (b) $_6C^{13}$ (c) $_7N^{12}$ (d) $_9F^{14}$ (e) $_5B^{11}$

21-15. Nuclei that undergo electron capture have _____.

(a) Excess protons   (b) Excess neutrons   (c) Z > 80
(d) Excess electrons   (e) High mass numbers

21-16. For gamma emissions from a radiopharmaceutical, the radiation dose to the spleen from a source in the liver increases with _____.

(a) Higher photon energy   (b) Lower photon energy   (c) Short half-life
(d) Low S value   (e) Low accumulated activity

21-17. The device on a scintillation camera that is used to reject scattered photons is called a _____.

(a) PHA   (b) TOF   (c) PBL   (d) Collimator   (e) Grid

21-18. The energy resolution of a radiation detector is measured by the _____.

(a) MCA   (b) CCD   (c) CNR   (d) FWHM   (e) EMF

21-19. A photon spectrum of a Tc-99m source is recorded with an NaI scintillation detector and a spectrum analyzer. A peak in the spectrum found at 110 keV is called the _____.

(a) Compton edge   (b) Iodine x-ray peak   (c) Coincidence peak
(d) Lead x-ray peak   (e) Iodine escape peak

21-20. An artifact in a scintillation camera image that appears as a "cold spot" could be due to all of the following factors, *except* _____.

(a) Off-center PHA   (b) Nonuniform biodistribution   (c) Defective PMT
(d) Metal in the FoV   (e) NaI crystal defect

21-21. The type of radiation detector that is often used as a survey instrument to locate small amounts of radioactivity contamination without providing measurements related to energy deposited is a(n) _____.

(a) Ionization chamber   (b) GeLi detector   (c) Liquid scintillation detector
(d) GM counter   (e) TLD

21-22. The type of radiation detector that uses coincidence circuits and refrigeration systems to detect low-energy charged particles is a(n) _____.

(a) NaI well counter   (b) Bonner sphere meter
(c) Liquid scintillation detector   (d) Cutie Pie survey meter
(e) MOSFET device

21-23. The typical spatial resolution of scintillation cameras is limited by all of the following factors, *except* _____.

(a) Collimator design   (b) Distance from collimator
(c) Light spread in scintillation crystal   (d) Photon scatter in the patient
(e) Pixel size

21-24. The loss of counts due to high radioisotope activity that affects the ability of the detector system to process data at high speeds is called _____.

(a) Dead time   (b) Vignetting   (c) Pulse pile-up   (d) Quenching
(e) Recombination

21-25. All of the following are positron emitters used with PET scanners, *except* _____.

(a) $_5B^9$ (b) $_6C^{11}$ (c) $_7N^{13}$ (d) $_8O^{15}$ (e) $_9F^{18}$

21-26. Quality control tests for scintillation cameras include all of the following, *except* _____.

(a) Uniformity   (b) Spatial resolution   (c) Coincidence timing
(d) Spatial distortion   (e) PHA centering

21-27. The background count rate is 16 cpm, and the source plus background count rate is 20 cpm. The data must be accumulated for _____ minutes so that the net count rate is different from the background with a confidence level of 95%.

(a) 3   (b) 6   (c) 9   (d) 12   (e) 16

21-28. The type of scintillation camera collimator that can only magnify the portion of the anatomy in the image is a _____ collimator.

(a) Parallel hole (b) Convergent (c) Divergent (d) Pinhole
(e) GAP

21-29. To do quantitative activity measurements, SPECT and PET scanners must correct for _____.

(a) PHA (b) Attenuation (c) Unsharpness (d) Scatter
(e) Conspicuity

21-30. The maximum critical organ dose for most nuclear medicine studies is about _____ cGy, and the whole body dose is usually about _____ cGy.

(a) 5, 0.2 (b) 1, 0.01 (c) 0.2, 2 (d) 0.5, 5 (e) 10, 5

J. Answers

21-1. Answer = (c). Cascade decay is a process in which one photon emission is immediately followed by a second photon emission. Thus, for one decay, two photons are emitted. Retrograde flow is usually applied to anatomic functions when a substance travels in the opposite direction to normal flow. Secular equilibrium occurs in a generator when the parent's half-life is much, much greater (>100) than the daughter's half-life. Thus, for short periods of time, the daughter and the parent stay in equilibrium with approximately equal activity and negligible reduction of activity related to the long half-life of the parent. Nuclear propagation is a term not normally used in nuclear medicine.

21-2. Answer = (e). In an isomeric transition, a gamma photon is released from the nucleus. It may then exit through the orbital electrons surrounding the nucleus. Alternatively, the photon could interact with an inner shell electron and disappear, transferring its energy to the electron that is ejected (internal conversion electron). The vacancy in the inner shell electrons is then filled by rearrangement of the remaining electrons, which produces a characteristic x-ray. Sometimes the characteristic x-ray is not emitted because it interacts with an outer shell electron and ejects it (Auger electron). Beta (either plus or minus) refers to an electron that originates in the nucleus. An electron from an orbital shell is just an electron, *not* a beta.

21-3. Answer = (c). See note in this chapter (**B5**). Mo-99 must be limited because it emits beta particles. Emissions with charged particles result in a considerable radiation dose to the patient.

21-4. Answer = (d). After 137 hours, the Mo-99 has undergone a reduction in activity by two half-lives. Hence, the 500 mCi is reduced to one fourth of its original amount, or 125 mCi. The Tc-99m and Mo-99 activities are at equilibrium, so that 125 mCi is eluted. Now, the Tc-99m decays at a rate determined by its half-life of 6 hours. After 12 hours, the activity of the first elution is reduced by another factor of one fourth to 31 mCi. The activity of the Mo-99 at 149 hours (137 + 12 hours) is 107 mCi. However, after an elution, secular equilibrium is not reached. At 12 hours after elution, the Tc-99m is only $[(1.0 - (0.5)^2] = 0.75$ of the parent activity. Therefore the second elution yields 0.75×107 mCi $= 80.0$. So the total activity is $80 + 31 = 111$ mCi.

21-5. Answer = (d). For nuclei with excess protons, both electron capture and positron emissions can occur. However, only electron capture causes a vacancy in the outer shell electrons, which then rearrange and produce characteristic x-rays.

21-6. Answer = (c). See note in this chapter (**A7**).

21-7. Answer = (a). See note in this chapter (**A7**).

21-8. Answer = (e). See note in this chapter (**A7**).

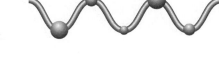

21-9. Answer = (d). To produce nuclei with excess neutrons, the atoms with stable nuclei must be bombarded with neutrons. Of the radiation sources listed, only the nuclear reactor produces significant numbers of neutrons.

21-10. Answer = (a). As the organ mass increases, the radioactivity and radiation dose are distributed over more tissue. Thus, the radiation dose is reduced with more tissue. Similarly, for pediatric patients, the organ sizes are smaller and the radiation doses are greater for injected activity that is the same as that used in adults.

21-11. Answer = (d). The greatest effective half-life results in the greatest critical organ dose. For significantly different physical and biologic half-lives, the effective half-life is slightly less than the smallest value. For nearly equal physical and biological half-lives, the effective half-life is about 0.5 times either half-life. The effective half-lives for the data listed in the answers, in order, are 5.3, 4.8, 3.9, 3.5, and 6.4 hours.

21-12. Answer = (c). Co-60 has a cascade decay in which two photons are emitted per decay. For Tc-99m, 10% of the emitted photons undergo internal conversion. Hence, only 0.9 photons are emitted per decay. 1 Bq is one decay per second.

21-13. Answer = (c). If a real beta is emitted (β– = electron), an antineutrino is also released. If an antiparticle (β+ = positron) is emitted, a real neutrino is emitted.

21-14. Answer = (b). For positron emission, the atomic number decreases by one and the number of neutrons increases by one. The total number of nuclei (neutrons plus protons) remains the same.

21-15. Answer = (a). See notes in this chapter (**A1** and **A7**).

21-16. Answer = (a). Lower energy photons cannot penetrate the tissue of the liver and escape to impinge on the spleen. The radiation dose to the spleen is less for shorter half-lives, a lower S value, and less administered activity. The higher photon energy allows the radiation to penetrate the liver and irradiate the spleen.

21-17. Answer = (a). Scattered photons have less energy, and the pulse height analyzer (PHA) determines the energy deposited in the crystal. TOF is "time of flight," which can be used on PET scanners to partially locate events. PBL is "positive beam limitation," which is the automatic collimation system of x-ray units. Collimators are for the proper placement of photons related to a specific anatomic location, not scatter rejection. Grids are found on x-ray systems, and they are not part of scintillation cameras.

21-18. Answers = (d). FWHM is full width at half maximum, which is the width of the measured energy peak. MCA is a multichannel analyzer, which is a series of PHAs that can measure an entire photon spectrum. CCD is a charge-coupled device, which is a solid-state television camera. CNR is the contrast-to-noise ratio, which is a measure of image quality. EMF is electromagnetic force, which is used to describe radiofrequency interference.

21-19. Answer = (e). The iodine escape peak is created when a 140-keV Tc-99m photon undergoes a photoelectric interaction in the NaI crystal, depositing all its energy. However, an iodine characteristic x-ray is produced by the rearrangement of orbital x-rays to fill the vacancy created by the photoelectric interaction in the crystal. If the x-ray escapes, the deposited energy is 140 keV minus 33 keV (of the iodine characteristic x-ray); the energy deposited is about 110 keV. If only the 33-keV iodine x-ray is deposited in the crystal, it is called the iodine x-ray peak. The Compton edge occurs when a 180-degree scatter photon deposits its energy into the crystal. This energy is equal to $2\alpha E_0/(1 + 2\alpha)$; it is equal to 50 keV for Tc-99m and 478 keV for Cs-137. A coincidence peak occurs when two photons deposit all their energy in the crystal at the same time so that it looks like there is a single photon with double the energy. Characteristic x-rays of lead occur at 80 to 88 keV and are sometimes counted in a peak.

21-20. Answer = (b). A nonuniform biodistribution can cause cold spots. However, these cold spots are real and are not artifacts. A PHA that is off center would not detect real events. A failed PMT would not detect any events, causing a cold spot. Metal-like jewelry would attenuate gamma photons, causing cold spots. A crystal defect such as a crack would also cause cold spots.

21-21. Answer = (d). Ionization chambers measure a charge related to the energy deposited in the detector. Germanium-lithium (GeLi) solid-state detectors are used to obtain good energy discrimination to identify one or more radioisotopes by means of the energy of their gamma emissions. Liquid scintillation detectors are used for low-energy particle detection in fluids such as urine and blood. TLDs are thermoluminescent dosimeters used for personnel dosimetry.

21-22. Answer = (c). Liquid scintillation systems measure low-energy, charged particle emissions, usually in a liquid such as urine or blood. NaI well counters are used to measure samples with gamma ray emissions, as in radioimmune assay (RIA) studies and wipe tests. Bonner spheres are used for neutron detection. Cutie Pie survey meters are used for area surveys and are a type of ionization chamber. MOSFET stands for metal oxide silicon field effect transistors, which are solid-state radiation detectors. They measure directly charges created within the silicon chips.

21-23. Answer = (e). Pixel size in a scintillation camera is the FoV (10 to 12 inch) divided by the matrix (128 to 256), or 1.0 to 2.5 mm. Spatial resolution in scintillation cameras is about 7.5 mm, which is bigger than the pixel size. Light spread in the crystal is measured by numerous PMTs to locate the interaction of the photons in the crystal. Reflections of light in the scintillation crystal cause uncertainty in the event position. Large collimator holes improve sensitivity, but they reduce spatial resolution. Spatial resolution degrades as the source is moved farther from the camera. Photons scattered through small angles would be detected as undeflected photons because of the 20% energy width of the PHA. Thus, these small-angle scattered photons are not positioned properly.

21-24. Answer = (a). Dead time is the period after detection of a radiation event during which a detector cannot sense another event. Vignetting occurs in image intensifiers; the effect is that the center of the image is brighter than the edges. Pulse pile-up occurs at the edge of a scintillation camera because there are no PMTs outside the edge of the crystal to position events properly. Quenching can occur in liquid scintillation detectors or GM counters; it is the loss of counts related to impurities in the detector that absorb the ionizations. Recombination is loss of counts in gas detectors because of low applied voltages that are insufficient to prevent the ion pairs from recombining.

21-25. Answer = (a). See the list of PET radioisotopes in this chapter (**G1**).

21-26. Answer = (c). Scintillation cameras do not use coincidence circuits. Intrinsic uniformity and extrinsic uniformity are major QC tests to prevent false hot and cold spots. Bar patterns are used to assess spatial resolution. Distortion is checked with use of uniform hole patterns. PHA centering is necessary to prevent artificial hot or cold spots.

21-27. Answer = (c). The standard deviation of the result of subtraction of two count rates is equal to $[(R_1/T) + (R_2/T)]^{0.5}$. For 95% confidence regarding the difference between the source plus background minus the background (net count rate), the difference must be at least twice the standard deviation. If both sides of the equation are squared and solved for time (T), $T = [4(R_1 + R_2)]/[R_1 - R_2]^2 = [4(20 + 16)]/[20 - 16]^2 = 4(36)/16 = 9$ minutes.

21-28. Answer = (b). A parallel hole collimator and a general all purpose (GAP) collimator are the same, and both keep the object and image size the same. A divergent collimator minifies the image. A pinhole collimator can either magnify or minify the image depending on the distance from the source object.

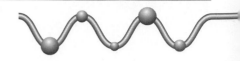

21-29. Answer = (b). Correction for photon attenuation is necessary to obtain the initial number of photons emitted toward the detectors. PHA is used to eliminate the scattered photons from the counts. Unsharpness is blur that affects spatial resolution; it does not affect the count rate. Scatter is eliminated by the PHA. It is part of the attenuation that should not be included in quantification studies. Conspicuity is an term that indicates the relative contrast between the object and the background.

21-30. Answer = (a). Because most nuclear medicine images are limited by the photon statistics (the quantum mottle of too few photons), most studies administer sufficient activity to limit the critical organ dose to less than 5 cGy (rad). Because the radiation levels to the remaining organs are much lower, the average dose (or whole body dose) is usually 5% or less of the critical organ dose.

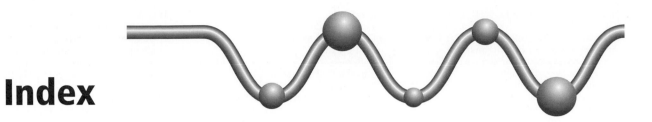

Index

Note: Page numbers followed by the letter f refer to figures and those followed by t refer to tables.